REALIZABILITY:
AN INTRODUCTION TO ITS
CATEGORICAL SIDE

STUDIES IN LOGIC

AND

THE FOUNDATIONS OF MATHEMATICS

VOLUME 152

ELSEVIER

AMSTERDAM • BOSTON • HEIDELBERG • LONDON • NEW YORK • OXFORD
PARIS • SAN DIEGO • SAN FRANCISCO • SINGAPORE • SYDNEY • TOKYO

REALIZABILITY:
AN INTRODUCTION TO ITS
CATEGORICAL SIDE

Jaap VAN OOSTEN
Department of Mathematics
Utrecht University

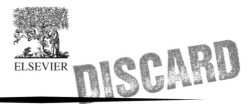

ELSEVIER

AMSTERDAM • BOSTON • HEIDELBERG • LONDON • NEW YORK • OXFORD
PARIS • SAN DIEGO • SAN FRANCISCO • SINGAPORE • SYDNEY • TOKYO

Elsevier
Radarweg 29, PO Box 211, 1000 AE Amsterdam, The Netherlands
The Boulevard, Langford Lane, Kidlington, Oxford OX5 1GB, UK

First edition 2008

Library of Congress Cataloging-in-Publication Data
A catalog record for this book is available from the Library of Congress

British Library Cataloguing in Publication Data
A catalogue record for this book is available from the British Library

ISBN: 978-0-444-51584-1
ISSN: 0049-237X

For information on all Elsevier publications
visit our website at books.elsevier.com

Printed and bound in Hungary

08 09 10 11 12   10 9 8 7 6 5 4 3 2 1

Preface

One good example is worth a host of generalities (Hyland)

"It is too early for a book on realizability", Martin Hyland has said on various occasions. And certainly, the ultimate book about this topic will have to wait until the world of realizability is better understood.

In the meantime, however, one can try to do something about the publicity situation of the field, which leaves something to be desired. Whenever a starting Ph.D. student wishes to work in realizability, he or she has to fumble his/her way forward amidst a mass of scattered papers, unpublished notes, Ph.D. theses which are not all electronically available. It seemed to me that one coherent presentation might help.

The main purpose of this book is to introduce you to the effective topos $\mathcal{E}ff$ and related toposes. The effective topos is a strange thing, and understanding of its logic is rare, even among topos theorists; and although by now there is quite a collection of books on topos theory, none of them treats $\mathcal{E}ff$ in anything like the detail it deserves. True, I am aware that Peter Johnstone is writing the third volume of his monumental *Sketches of an Elephant*, in which there will be a part on this topos; but I am quite sure that the overlap between his and my treatment will be limited.

Instead of aiming for a structural approach, which would first establish as many abstract properties of the object one is studying and then try to view as much as possible as consequences of these, I decided to work *by example* (see the motto of this introduction). I am, as Alex Simpson once remarked, a "details person" and I believe very much in concrete understanding taking place in the mind by working through lots of examples; the concepts, hopefully, come afterwards. Of course, it would be silly to refrain from developing some theory first if this really makes things simpler, and I start by going over the theory of partial combinatory algebras, and then the theory of triposes. When studying the effective topos, it is by interpreting various theories in it, that I hope you get some sort of picture.

Quite a bit of work on realizability takes place entirely in the category of *assemblies*, the separated objects for the double negation local operator; and assemblies are a very nice place to be. But the effective topos is much more, and I have deliberately focused on the *higher order* features of $\mathcal{E}ff$ too, by going over interpretations of higher order arithmetic, set theory and synthetic domain theory, in an attempt to stay clear of Scott's lamented "first order disease" (preface to [18]).

It is my hope that at least the first three chapters of the book are written in a sufficiently leasurely text book style for a graduate student with some requisite preliminary knowledge (which I will detail below) to read it. In the fourth and last chapter, which is a bit of 'capita selecta', the style becomes more succinct and the aim is rather to summarize results and give a guide to the literature.

Preliminaries. The book is aimed at advanced undergraduate students or beginning Ph.D. students, who have at least some knowledge of the following topics:

1. Logic: a course presenting the notions of *language, theory, structures* and Gödel's Completeness Theorem. At least some acquaintance with Peano Arithmetic. However, it would be *very useful* if you have studied Intuitionistic logic too.

2. Category Theory: the first five chapters of MacLane's *Categories for the Working Mathematician*, as well as acquaintance with the notion of a topos, and the general idea of interpreting a theory in a category. As I said, there is by now quite a range of books on topos theory but if you really want to *learn* the subject, in my opinion the best book is still the old [80]. Yes, it is tough going.

3. Recursion Theory: the basics of computable functions, Kleene's *T*-predicate and normal form, the recursion theorem and the notion of Turing reducibility.

Style. There is only one aspect in which I have deliberately deviated from standard scientific usage: and that is, that being not a group of authors or of royal descent, I see no point in writing 'we' when I mean 'I' (which doesn't mean I don't use 'we', like in: '...now we shall see...'), and therefore also none in writing 'the reader' when I mean 'you'. But, I have not been very consistent in this.

Terminology and Notation. I have tried to be as conservative and uncontroversial as possible, but as this has become a somewhat contentious issue in Category Theory, I should maybe clarify my position. Over the last 20 years, a few attempts have been made to improve categorical terminology, with varying degrees of success. Category theory has a lot of redundant terminology (just think of the number of ways you can say that a category 'has finite limits'); despite this, words are often used with multiple meanings; and then, sometimes terminology is not very well chosen.

The most radical attempt to rename everything, was [48]. Unless you have read this book from cover to cover, it is impossible to find anything, because the index will be meaningless to you. In this particular case my advice would be: just *read* it from cover to cover (it is a wonderful book), but forget about the new terminology since it didn't catch on.

The choice of good terminology, it is too often forgotten, requires a bit of literary talent. Such talent is not displayed by calling a terminal object a 'terminator'. Good examples of imaginative terminology are Paul Taylor's 'prone' and 'supine' in the context of fibrations.

In general my position is that there is only one thing worse than bad terminology, and that is *continually changing* terminology. Therefore, even if I agree with some criticisms made, I stick in most cases to the old names. I do avoid 'left exact' because one can just say 'has finite limits'. Using the word 'cartesian' for this (as in [83]) creates confusion and is ineffective if one still has to write on p. 161 (l. -10): 'cartesian (i.e. preserves finite limits)'. For 'exact category' I see no alternative. If this is horrible, is 'effective regular' an improvement?

Acknowledgements. Since this book contains a large part of my work done in the last two decades, I should thank the people who were influential to me during that period.

I feel privileged in having had *Anne Troelstra* as thesis advisor. His work [161] has been immensely useful to me for a long time. This is such a neat arrangement of systems and interpretations (with a lot of original work in between), that in my view he is the Linnaeus of realizability. He might be pleased with this title, having had a passion for botany all his life.

I have learned very much from discussions with great people in the subject; the greatest of all is *Martin Hyland*. But I also mention *Pino Rosolini* and *Dana Scott*, whom I visited and who in different periods of my development, opened my eyes to new visions. I have moreover been extremely fortunate to be working in the group of *Ieke Moerdijk*, who always has ideas and questions which stimulate research.

Since part of what I report in this book has been joint work with others, I thank my coauthors *Lars Birkedal*, *Martin Hofmann*, *Pieter Hofstra*, *Claire Kouwenhoven*, *Alex Simpson* and *Thomas Streicher*. Especially with the last two I have had long discussions at times.

Albert Visser and *Dick de Jongh* have generated questions which find their way into this book. It is clear from the text to what extent I am indebted to *John Longley*, whose work I admire. *Bas Terwijn* helped me with the proof of 3.2.32.

Also inspiring has been reading work of, and discussing with, *Andrej Bauer*, *Benno van den Berg*, *Peter Lietz* and *Matías Menni*.

Introduction

In 1945, Stephen Cole Kleene published a paper ([88]) in which he showed that the partial recursive functions (the theory of which he had been developing himself during the 1930-ies) could be used to give an interpretation of the logic of Brouwer's Intuitionism. By means of this interpretation any classical mathematician, whatever his philosophical views, could study intuitionistic logic.

Every partial recursive function can be assigned a *Gödel number* or *index*, in such a way that, if we denote by φ_e the partial recursive function with index e, and write $\varphi_e(x)\!\downarrow$ for 'x is in the domain of φ_e', we have the following properties:

> The partial function sending the pair (e, f) to $\varphi_e(f)$ is partial recursive as function of e, f;
>
> there are primitive recursive functions S_n^m with the property that for every e and every $m + n$-tuple $x_1, \ldots, x_m, y_1, \ldots, y_n$, we have
>
> $$\varphi_{S_n^m(e, x_1, \ldots, x_m)}(y_1, \ldots, y_n) \simeq \varphi_e(x_1, \ldots, x_n, y_1, \ldots, y_m)$$
>
> where $\simeq$ means: either side is defined iff the other is; and if defined, they are equal.

There is, moreover, a primitive recursive bijection $\langle \cdot, \cdot \rangle : \mathbb{N} \times \mathbb{N} \to \mathbb{N}$. We say that the number $\langle a, b \rangle$ *codes the pair* (a, b). From the code of a pair one can, primitive-recursively, recover both components of the pair.

Kleene's interpretation was given in the form of a relation between numbers and sentences of arithmetic, which he called 'realizes': a number could realize (that is: witness, carry information to the truth of)

a statement. The relation is defined by recursion on the logical structure of the sentence. Two significant clauses (for the full definition, see
section 3.1) read:

> n realizes $(\phi \vee \psi)$ if and only if n codes a pair (a, b) and either
> $a = 0$ and b realizes ϕ, or $a \neq 0$ and b realizes ψ;

> n realizes $(\phi \rightarrow \psi)$ if and only if for every m such that m realizes
> ϕ, $\varphi_n(m)\downarrow$ and $\varphi_n(m)$ realizes ψ.

Kleene proved that the axioms and rules of first-order intuitionistic arithmetic are sound for this interpretation. That is: if ϕ is a consequence of
these axioms and rules, then there is a number n which realizes ϕ.

The converse does *not* hold: there are sentences which have a realizer,
yet are unprovable in intuitionistic arithmetic. This makes Kleene's
interpretation an interesting model.

In subsequent years, many variations of this idea were developed,
and interpretations given. At the same time (the 1950-ies and 1960-
ies) a school of 'recursive constructive mathematics' was working; these
people investigated which theorems of mathematics would remain valid
if 'everything is recursive'. For example, a group would be a subset
G of $\mathbb{N}$ together with partial recursive functions $(\cdot)^{-1} : G \rightarrow G$ and
$\cdot : G \times G \rightarrow G$ satisfying the group axioms, and a group homomorphism
$G \rightarrow H$ would have to be a partial recursive function. Which theorems
of algebra would remain?

Or, more sophisticatedly, a group would be a set G together with,
for every $x \in G$, a set of numbers $E(x)$ thought of as carrying 'recursive
information' about x; a function from such a construct (G, E) to another
(H, E') would be a function $f : G \rightarrow H$ for which there exists a partial
recursive function ϕ such that for every $x \in G$ and every $n \in E(x)$, $\phi(n)\downarrow$
and $\phi(n) \in E'(f(x))$. Such objects (G, E) are now called *assemblies*, f
is a morphism of assemblies and ϕ *tracks* f.

If 'everything is recursive' then certainly all functions from natural
numbers to natural numbers are; what about functions on functions
from $\mathbb{N}$ to $\mathbb{N}$, etcetera? Well, every function $\mathbb{N} \rightarrow \mathbb{N}$ has an index e, so
a function from functions $\mathbb{N} \rightarrow \mathbb{N}$ to $\mathbb{N}$ is a partial recursive function
acting on indices. But it has to be *extensional*: if e and e' are indices

of the same function (and every function has infinitely many indices), they should be sent to the same number. This leads to the construction of the type structure HEO of hereditary effective operations, which I define now.

We have *types*: a type o for natural numbers; if σ and τ are types then we have a type $(\sigma \to \tau)$ of functions from things of type σ to things of type τ. For every type σ we define a set HEO_σ of natural numbers and an equivalence relation $\equiv_\sigma$ on this set, as follows:

$$
\begin{aligned}
\mathrm{HEO}_o &= \mathbb{N} \\
n =_o m \quad &\text{iff} \quad n = m \\
\mathrm{HEO}_{\sigma \to \tau} &= \{e \mid \forall f \in \mathrm{HEO}_\sigma(\varphi_e(f)\!\downarrow \wedge \varphi_e(f) \in \mathrm{HEO}_\tau) \wedge \\
&\qquad \forall f f' \in \mathrm{HEO}_\sigma(f \equiv_\sigma f' \Rightarrow \varphi_e(f) \equiv_\tau \varphi_e(f'))\} \\
e \equiv_{\sigma \to \tau} e' \quad &\text{iff} \quad \forall f \in \mathrm{HEO}_\sigma(\varphi_e(f) \equiv_\tau \varphi_{e'}(f))
\end{aligned}
$$

Then HEO gives some interpretation of the hierarchy of higher-type functions from a recursive point of view.

Now the objects $(\mathrm{HEO}_\sigma, \equiv_\sigma)$ can also be seen as assemblies, in the following way. Given two assemblies (X, E) and (Y, E') we can form an assembly of functions $(X, E) \Rightarrow (Y, E')$: this is an assembly (V, E'') where V is the set of all functions $f : X \to Y$ which are tracked by a partial recursive function, and $E''(f)$ is the set of indices of partial recursive functions which track f. Let us now form a type structure of assemblies: we take for o the assembly $A_o = (\mathbb{N}, n \mapsto \{n\})$ and, supposing that for types σ and τ we have defined assemblies A_σ and A_τ, then at type $\sigma \to \tau$ we take the assembly $A_{\sigma \to \tau} = A_\sigma \Rightarrow A_\tau$. So for each σ we have an assembly $A_\sigma = (X_\sigma, E_\sigma)$. With this notation we can verify that for every σ, there is a bijection between X_σ and the set of equivalence classes of HEO_σ under $\equiv_\sigma$ such that for every $x \in X_\sigma$, the set $E(x)$ is equal to the $\equiv_\sigma$-equivalence class to which x corresponds.

Inspired by this phenomenon, Martin Hyland constructed a topos in which HEO is really the structure of *all* higher type functionals over the natural numbers.

This topos is the *effective topos*.

At the same time, his student Andy Pitts worked out a general theory on how to obtain such toposes: *tripos theory*. It turned out that various modifications of the realizability interpretation that had been studied in the past, also gave rise to toposes, and these came often out of standard topos-theoretic constructions applied to the efective topos.

The enormous advantage of the topos-theoretic approach is, that there is a uniform notion of truth for any higher-order language, and mathematical constructions like function space, power set and so on are already given to you. You don't have to wonder about what real-valued functions are, and in the effective topos *all* functions from the reals to the reals are continuous.

The natural numbers are not the only set which can act as a set of 'realizers'. The properties of indices of partial recursive functions, given at the beginning of this introduction, mean that $\mathbb{N}$ is an example of a so-called 'partial combinatory algebra'. This notion, first formally defined by Feferman but going back to the work of Schönfinkel, embodies exactly what one needs in order to construct a 'realizability topos'.

In this book, I start with a chapter on partial combinatory algebras. Then, tripos theory is developed. In the third, and most voluminous chapter, I present the effective topos in detail. This topos harbors interpretations of a number of theories, and in some cases I have found it necessary to also introduce you briefly into the particular theory at hand. Finally, chapter 4 gives a number of variations, with emphasis on how these can be topos-theoretically constructed.

If you are only interested in the effective topos, you can skip chapter 1, but you'll need at least some parts of chapter 2 (which give the tripos-to-topos construction and the internal logic of the constructed topos out of that of the tripos).

Contents

Chapter 1

Partial Combinatory Algebras

Combinatory algebras are models of so-called 'Combinatory Logic', invented by M. Schönfinkel ([143]) around 1920. Some authors call them therefore 'Schönfinkel algebras'. Curiously, it took over 50 years before the partial notion was defined (by Feferman in [42]). Since then, quite a bit of theory has been developed from many points of view, the most important being λ-calculus, term rewriting and combinatory logic.

In this chapter, I will take a pragmatic attitude and restrict myself to those aspects of the theory that are relevant to realizability.

1.1 Basic definitions

We start with the following definitions.

Definition 1.1.1 A *partial applicative structure* or *pas* is a nonempty set A together with a partial map from $A \times A$ to A.

We denote this map by $(a, b) \mapsto ab$. For reasons which will become clear later, this map is often called *application*; ab, if defined, will be called the result of applying a to b.

Application need not be associative (in fact, will *never* be in the cases of interest to us, see proposition 1.3.1 below); therefore we adopt, for the

1

sake of economizing on brackets, the usual convention of association to the left: we write $(ab)c$ as abc. However whenever ambiguity is possible, we use brackets.

Let A be a pas, and V an infinite set of variables. The set $E(A)$ of *terms over* A is the least set such that the following conditions hold:

  i) $A \subseteq E(A)$;

  ii) $V \subseteq E(A)$;

  iii) if $t \in E(A)$ and $s \in E(A)$ then $(ts) \in E(A)$.

Again, in the manipulation of terms over A we use aasociation to the left as much as is convenient.

A term in which no variables occur is called *closed*. We define the relation $t{\downarrow}a$, "term t denotes element a" between closed terms and elements of A, as the least relation satisfying:

  i) $a{\downarrow}a$ for all $a \in A$;

  ii) $(ts){\downarrow}a$ if and only if there are $b, c \in A$ such that $t{\downarrow}b$, $s{\downarrow}c$, and $bc = a$.

Clearly, if $t{\downarrow}a$ and $t{\downarrow}b$, $a = b$ must hold. We use the abbreviation $t{\downarrow}$, "t denotes", if there is an $a \in A$ such that $t{\downarrow}a$. We shall then not distinguish notationally between t and the element it denotes. For example, $ab{\downarrow}$ if and only if (a, b) is an element of the domain of the application map. Given two closed terms t and s, we write $t = s$ if t and s both denote the same element of A; we write $t \simeq s$ for the statement that if either of t, s denotes, then $t = s$. If we indicate variables, like in $t(x_1, \ldots, x_n)$, we understand by this that all variables occurring in t are among $x_1, \ldots, x_n$. There is of course a straightforward notion of substitution; given $t(x_1, \ldots, x_n)$ and elements $a_1, \ldots, a_n$ of A, $t(a_1, \ldots, a_n)$ has the expected meaning.

We extend the notation $t \simeq s$ to possibly non-closed terms: then it means that for every possible substitution instance (substituting elements of A for variables), $\simeq$ holds between the resulting closed terms.

We can also have a substitution of a term t_2 for a variable x in t_1; this will be written $t_1[t_2/x]$.

Definition 1.1.2 A pas A is *combinatory complete* if for any $n \in \mathbb{N}$ and any term $t(x_1, \ldots, x_{n+1})$ there is an element $a \in A$ such that for all $a_1, \ldots, a_{n+1} \in A$ the following statements hold:

i) $aa_1 \cdots a_n{\downarrow}$;

ii) $aa_1 \cdots a_{n+1} \simeq t(a_1, \ldots, a_{n+1})$.

A pas is called a *partial combinatory algebra* or *pca* if it is combinatory complete. A *total combinatory algebra* or *combinatory algebra* for short, is a pca for which the application map is a total function.

The following theorem is essentially due to Feferman ([42]).

Theorem 1.1.3 (Feferman) *Let A be a pas. Then A is a pca if and only if there are elements $k, s \in A$ satisfying for all $a, b, c \in A$:*

i) $sab{\downarrow}$;

ii) $kab = a$;

iii) $sabc \simeq ac(bc)$.

Proof. Given combinatory completeness, choose for k an element satisfying definition 1.1.2 for the term $t(x_1, x_2) = x_1$. Clearly, (ii) is satisfied. For s, choose an element satisfying 1.1.2 for $t(x_1, x_2, x_3) = x_1x_3(x_2x_3)$. Then (i) follows from the corresponding item (i) in 1.1.2, and (iii) also holds.

Conversely, assume k and s satisfy (i)–(iii) of the statement of the theorem. For further reference, we make a definition.

Definition 1.1.4 Define for every variable x and every $t \in E(A)$ a term $\langle x \rangle t$ by induction on t, as follows:

$\langle x \rangle t = kt$ if t is a constant $b \in A$, or a variable y different from x;

$\langle x \rangle x = skk$ (we also use i for this term);

$\langle x \rangle t_1 t_2 = s(\langle x \rangle t_1)(\langle x \rangle t_2)$

One proves easily by induction on t, that the variables of $\langle x \rangle t$ are exactly those of t minus x, that every substitution instance of $\langle x \rangle t$ denotes, and that if $t = t(x, x_1, \ldots, x_n)$ then for all $a, a_1, \ldots, a_n \in A$ one has

$$(\langle x \rangle t)(a_1, \ldots, a_n)a \simeq t(a, a_1, \ldots, a_n)$$

For the element $a \in A$ corresponding to the term $t(x_1, \ldots, x_{n+1})$ as required by definition 1.1.2, one can then take the element denoted by

$$\langle x_1 \rangle (\langle x_2 \rangle (\cdots (\langle x_{n+1} \rangle t) \cdots))$$

∎

Remark. Item (i) in definition 1.1.2 is hard to motivate and, as we will see shortly (see 1.2.3), in fact redundant. Anticipating the argument, we call a pas A *conditionally combinatory complete* ([75]), or a *conditional partial combinatory algebra* (c-pca) if for any term $t(x_1, \ldots, x_{n+1})$ as in 1.1.2, there is a closed term u such that for all $a_1, \ldots, a_{n+1} \in A$,

$$ua_1 \cdots a_{n+1} \simeq t(a_1, \ldots, a_{n+1})$$

Note the difference: we don't require that $ua_1 \cdots a_n$ denotes.

The analogue of theorem 1.1.3 holds: A is a c-pca if and only if A contains elements k and s such that (ii) and (iii) of 1.1.3 are true (pick terms $[k]$ and $[s]$ as in the proof of 1.1.3, according to the definition of conditional combinatory completeness; then $[k]$ denotes since A is nonempty, and $[s]$ also denotes since for every $a \in A$, $[k]a([k]a) = [s][k][k]a$ denotes). Conversely, one constructs terms $\langle x \rangle t$ just as in the proof of 1.1.3 and one has all required properties except for the statement that every substitution instance of $\langle x \rangle t$ always denotes. In general, if $t = t(x, x_1, \ldots, x_n)$ then $\langle x \rangle t(a_1, \ldots, a_n)$ denotes if for *some* a, $t(a, a_1, \ldots, a_n)\!\downarrow$.

Remark. The terms $\langle x \rangle t$, defined in 1.1.4 are often in the literature written as $\Lambda x.t$ or $\lambda^* x.t$, suggesting a connection to the λ-calculus. Since I do not wish to explore this connection here in any precise way, I do not adopt this notation. It is potentially confusing because these terms do not obey the usual conversion rules of the λ-calculus. For example, it is not generally true that $((\langle x \rangle t_1)t_2 \simeq t_1[t_2/x]$: if t_1 is a variable y different from x then $(\langle x \rangle t_1)t_2 \simeq kyt_2$ and $y[t_2/x] = y$. Now $y \simeq kyt_2$ does *not* always hold, because t_2 need not denote.

Neither does one have that $(\langle x \rangle t_1)[t_2/y] \simeq \langle x \rangle t_1[t_2/y]$: take $t_1 = y$, $t_2 = ss$. The terms $k(ss)$ and $s(ks)(ks)$ may denote different elements of A.

1.1.1 Pairing, Booleans and Definition by Cases

We distinguish a few closed terms we shall use frequently. It is convenient to abbreviate successive uses of definition 1.1.4: instead of $\langle x \rangle(\langle y \rangle(\langle z \rangle t))$ we write $\langle xyz \rangle t$, etc. Let p be $\langle xyz \rangle zxy$ so $pab = \langle z \rangle zab$. As in 1.1.4, i denotes skk so $ia = a$ for all $a \in A$. Let $\bar{k}$ be ki so $\bar{k}ab = b$; p_0 is $\langle v \rangle vk$ and p_1 is $\langle v \rangle v\bar{k}$. With these definitions, we have:

$$p_0(pab) = (pab)k = (\langle z \rangle zab)k = kab = a$$
$$p_1(pab) = (pab)\bar{k} = (\langle z \rangle zab)\bar{k} = \bar{k}ab = b$$

In view of this, we can use pab as an element of A which codes the *pair* (a, b); by p_0 and p_1, a and b can be unequivocally retrieved from pab. The elements p, p_0,p_1 are called *pairing* and *projection* operators.

In any pca, one can use the elements k and $\bar{k}$ as codes for the 'Booleans' *true* and *false*, in the following sense: there is a 'definition by cases' term

$$t = \langle vxy \rangle(\text{if } v \text{ then } x \text{ else } y)$$

such that $tkab = a$, $t\bar{k}ab = b$ (in fact, one can take i for t). This can be extended to closed terms: there is a term $t=$'if v then u else u'' for closed terms u, u', such that $tk \simeq u$, $t\bar{k} \simeq u'$: let

$$t = \langle v \rangle v(\langle y \rangle u)(\langle y \rangle u')k$$

1.2 $\mathcal{P}(A)$-valued predicates, conditional pcas and Longley's Theorem

At this point we introduce one of the main motivating constructions for the study of pcas. Let A be a pas; $\mathcal{P}(A)$ denotes, as usual, the powerset of A. A $\mathcal{P}(A)$-*valued predicate* on a set X is a function $\phi : X \to \mathcal{P}(A)$. If $a \in \phi(x)$ we call a a *realizer for* the statement that $\phi(x)$ holds.

We define a relation on the set of $\mathcal{P}(A)$-valued predicates on X: $\phi \leq \psi$ if there is an $a \in A$ such that for all $x \in X$ and all $b \in \phi(x)$, $ab\downarrow$ and $ab \in \psi(x)$. We say that a realizes $\phi \leq \psi$.

If A is just a pas there is not much one can say about the relation $\leq$ (not even, that it is reflexive). Some sort of justification for the notion of a pca is given by the following proposition.

Proposition 1.2.1 *If A is a pca, the relation $\leq$ between $\mathcal{P}(A)$-valued predicates on a set X is a preorder, and the partial order reflection forms a Heyting algebra.*

Proof. Since i realizes $\phi \leq \phi$ for all ϕ, $\leq$ is reflexive; and if a realizes $\phi \leq \psi$ and b realizes $\psi \leq \chi$, then $\langle x \rangle b(ax)$ realizes $\phi \leq \chi$, so $\leq$ is transitive.

We define some operations on predicates. First, $\top$ is the predicate given by $\top(x) = A$ for all $x \in X$; and $\bot$ is defined by $\bot(x) = \emptyset$ for all $x \in X$. Clearly, $\bot \leq \phi \leq \top$ holds for every ϕ (for the second relation, use i). Furthermore, given ϕ and ψ, define

$$
\begin{aligned}
(\phi \wedge \psi)(x) &= \{pab \mid a \in \phi(x) \text{ and } b \in \psi(x)\} \\
(\phi \vee \psi)(x) &= \{pka \mid a \in \phi(x)\} \cup \{p\bar{k}b \mid b \in \psi(x)\} \\
(\phi \Rightarrow \psi)(x) &= \{a \in A \mid \forall b \in \phi(x)(ab\downarrow \text{ and } ab \in \psi(x))\}
\end{aligned}
$$

For any triple ϕ, ψ, χ we have $\chi \leq \phi \wedge \psi$ if and only if both $\chi \leq \phi$ and $\chi \leq \psi$. One implication follows because p_0 realizes $\phi \wedge \psi \leq \phi$ and p_1 realizes $\phi \wedge \psi \leq \psi$; conversely if a realizes $\chi \leq \phi$ and b realizes $\chi \leq \psi$, then $\langle x \rangle p(ax)(bx)$ realizes $\chi \leq \phi \wedge \psi$.

Analogously we have $\phi \vee \psi \leq \chi$ if and only if both $\phi \leq \chi$ and $\psi \leq \chi$; for $\langle x \rangle pkx$ realizes $\phi \leq \phi \vee \psi$ and $\langle x \rangle p\bar{k}x$ realizes $\psi \leq \phi \vee \psi$, and if a realizes $\phi \leq \chi$ and b realizes $\psi \leq \chi$, then $\phi \vee \psi \leq \chi$ is realized by

$$[a, b] = \langle x \rangle p_0 x(\langle y \rangle a(p_1 x))(\langle y \rangle b(p_1 x))k$$

since

$$
\begin{aligned}
[a, b](pkc) &= k(\langle y \rangle ac)(\langle y \rangle bc)k = (\langle y \rangle ac)k = ac \\
[a, b](p\bar{k}c) &= \bar{k}(\langle y \rangle ac)(\langle y \rangle bc)k = (\langle y \rangle bc)k = bc
\end{aligned}
$$

So the preorder $\mathcal{P}(A)^X$ has finite joins and meets. Moreover, for any ϕ, ψ and χ, $\phi \wedge \psi \leq \chi$ holds exactly when $\phi \leq \psi \Rightarrow \chi$: if a realizes $\phi \wedge \psi \leq \chi$ then $\langle xy \rangle a(pxy)$ realizes $\phi \leq \psi \Rightarrow \chi$, and if a realizes $\phi \leq \psi \Rightarrow \chi$ then $\langle x \rangle a(p_0 x)(p_1 x)$ realizes $\phi \wedge \psi \leq \chi$, as can be easily checked. ∎

Some sort of justification for requirement (i) in definition 1.1.2 (equivalently, that sab always denotes) is given by the following observation.

Proposition 1.2.2 *Suppose A is a pas such that the relation $\leq$ on $\mathcal{P}(A)^X$ as defined above, is always a preorder. If the operation $\Rightarrow$, defined by*

$$(\phi \Rightarrow \psi)(x) = \{a \in A \mid \forall b \in \phi(x) ab \in \psi(x)\}$$

is a Heyting implication on every $\mathcal{P}(A)^X$, then there are elements k and s in A such that (i) and (ii) of theorem 1.1.3 hold, and moreover, for all $a, b, c \in A$, if $ac(bc)\downarrow$ then $sabc = ac(bc)$.

Proof. For the existence of k, let $X = \mathcal{P}(A) \times \mathcal{P}(A)$ and ϕ and ψ respectively the first and second projection. Since $\Rightarrow$ is a Heyting implication, $\phi \Rightarrow (\psi \Rightarrow \phi)$ must be the top element of $\mathcal{P}(A)^X$; that means that

$$\bigcap_{U,V \subseteq A} U \to (V \to U)$$

is inhabited, where $U \to V = \{a \mid \forall b \in U ab \in V\}$. Any element in this set satisfies (ii) of 1.1.3, as is seen by specializing to $U = \{a\}, V = \{b\}$.

Similarly, if $X = \mathcal{P}(A) \times \mathcal{P}(A) \times \mathcal{P}(A)$ and ϕ, ψ and χ are the first, second and third projections, then because

$$(\phi \Rightarrow (\chi \Rightarrow \psi)) \Rightarrow ((\phi \Rightarrow \chi) \Rightarrow (\phi \Rightarrow \psi))$$

must be the top element of $\mathcal{P}(A)^X$, we must have an element

$$s \in \bigcap_{U,V,W \subseteq A} (U \to (V \to W)) \to ((U \to V) \to (U \to W))$$

For any $a, b \in A$ we have $a \in (\emptyset \to (V \to W))$ and $b \in (\emptyset \to V)$, so $sab\downarrow$; if moreover $ac(bc)\downarrow$ then by taking $U = \{c\}$, $V = \{bc\}$, $W = \{ac(bc)\}$

we see that $a \in U \to (V \to W)$, $b \in U \to V$, $c \in U$. So $sabc \in W$, that is: $sabc = ac(bc)$. ■

Two remarks are in order here. The first is, that from the hypotheses of Proposition 1.2.2 it is not possible to prove that A is a pca, that is: that if $sabc\downarrow$, then $sabc = ac(bc)$. This will become clear when we discuss an important generalization of the notion of pcas, namely order-pcas (see section 1.8).

The second remark is that given the preorder $\leq$ on $\mathcal{P}(A)^X$, it may well be the case that its partial order reflection is a Heyting algebra (and in a natural way), without condition (i) holding. This means that the Heyting implication is then given in a different way from that in 1.2.2. I proceed to show this now; this result is a pretty theorem discovered by John Longley. Its upshot is that also if A is just a conditional pca, the preorders $\mathcal{P}(A)^X$ (note that they are always preorders, if A is a c-pca) have all the properties that they have for pcas.

Theorem 1.2.3 (Longley) *Suppose A is a conditional pca, with application written as $a, b \mapsto ab$. Choose k and s satisfying the c-pca analogue of theorem 1.1.3. Define a new application $*$ on A by*

$$a * b = akb$$

Then the following two statements are true:

i) *$(A, *)$ is a pca;*

ii) *For any set X, the two preorders on $\mathcal{P}(A)^X$ defined with respect to the two application maps, are identical.*

The proof of theorem 1.2.3 goes via the construction of a strong "if..., then..., else..." operator. Recall the Booleans and definition by cases operator from subsection 1.1.1. For the closed term

$$t = \langle v \rangle v(\langle y \rangle u)(\langle y \rangle u')k$$

defined there, reading 'if v then u else u'', we have that $tk \simeq u$ even if u' does not denote.

However this is by virtue of the fact that, in a pca, $\langle y \rangle u$ always denotes. In case A is a c-pca, one has to be a bit more delicate.

Proof. We start with a lemma:

Lemma 1.2.4 *Let A be a conditional pca. For every term t and every element $c \in A$ there is a term $\mathrm{Th}(t, c)$ such that the following two statements are true:*

i) $\mathrm{Th}(t, c)\bar{k} = c$, *in particular* $\mathrm{Th}(t, c)\!\downarrow$;

ii) *if* $t\!\downarrow$, *then* $\mathrm{Th}(t, c)k = t$.

Proof. $\mathrm{Th}(t, c)$ is constructed by recursion on t:
$\mathrm{Th}(x, c) = \langle y \rangle yxc = s(si(kx))(kc)$ if x is a variable or a constant;
$\mathrm{Th}(tt', c) = \langle y \rangle (\mathrm{Th}(t, kc)y)(\mathrm{Th}(t', k)y)$.

The properties (i) and (ii) are proved by induction on t.

For the base case, $t = x$, since we have $si(kx)\bar{k} = \bar{k}(kx\bar{k}) = \bar{k}x$, $kc\bar{k} = c$ and $\bar{k}xc = c$, we see that $s(si(kx))(kc)\bar{k} = c$, which proves (i). Moreover, since $si(kx)k = k(kxk) = kx$, $kck = c$ and $kxc = x$, we have $s(si(kx))(kc)k = x$, proving (ii).

For the induction step, check that

$$\mathrm{Th}(tt', c) = s(s(\langle y \rangle \mathrm{Th}(t, kc))i)(s(\langle y \rangle \mathrm{Th}(t', k))i)$$

By induction hypothesis, $\mathrm{Th}(t, kc)\bar{k} = kc$ and $\mathrm{Th}(t', k)\!\downarrow$ hence a fortiori $\langle y \rangle \mathrm{Th}(t, kc)\!\downarrow$ and $\langle y \rangle \mathrm{Th}(t', k)\!\downarrow$.

Hence $(\langle y \rangle \mathrm{Th}(t, kc))\bar{k}(i\bar{k}) = kc$. It follows that $s(\langle y \rangle \mathrm{Th}(t, kc))i\bar{k} = kc$. Similarly, $s(\langle y \rangle \mathrm{Th}(t', k))i\bar{k} = k$. Since $kck = c$ we have that $\mathrm{Th}(tt', c)\bar{k} = c$, which proves (i).

For (ii), assume $tt'\!\downarrow$. Then $t\!\downarrow$ and $t'\!\downarrow$, so the induction hypothesis gives $(\langle y \rangle \mathrm{Th}(t, kc))k(ik) = t$, hence $s(\langle y \rangle \mathrm{Th}(t, kc))ik = t$. By a similar deduction, $(\langle y \rangle \mathrm{Th}(t', k))k(ik) = t'$. Since $tt'\!\downarrow$,

$$s(s(\langle y \rangle \mathrm{Th}(t, kc))i)(s(\langle y \rangle \mathrm{Th}(t', k))i)k = tt'$$

which is (ii). ∎

Continuing the proof of theorem 1.2.3: for the terms $\mathrm{Th}(t, c)$ it is easy to prove by induction on t that if x is a variable and $a \in A$, then $\mathrm{Th}(t[a/x], c) = (\mathrm{Th}(t, c))[a/x]$.

We are now ready to prove that $(A, *)$ is a pca. Let $k' = k(s(kk)k)$. Since $s(kk)ka = kka(ka) = k(ka)\downarrow$, $k'\downarrow$. Moreover,

$$
\begin{aligned}
k' * a * b &= s(kk)kakb &= \\
k(s(kk)k)kakb &= s(kk)kakb &= \\
kka(ka)kb &= k(ka)kb &= \\
kab &= a
\end{aligned}
$$

Let $s' = \langle txuyvz \rangle \mathrm{Th}(xkzk(ykz), \bar{k})v$. Then

$$
\begin{aligned}
(s' * a * b)\bar{k}c &= s'kakb\bar{k}c \\
&= \mathrm{Th}(akck(bkc), \bar{k})\bar{k} \\
&= \bar{k} \text{ by the Lemma}
\end{aligned}
$$

Hence, $s' * a * b\downarrow$. Moreover,

$$
\begin{aligned}
s' * a * b * c &\simeq s'kakbkc &\simeq \\
\mathrm{Th}(akck(bkc), \bar{k})k &\simeq akck(bkc) &\simeq \\
&& a * c * (b * c)
\end{aligned}
$$

So s' has the right properties.

It remains to prove that the preorders $\mathcal{P}(A)^X$ are equal. Suppose $\phi \leq \psi$ w.r.t. the original application: let $a \in A$ such that for all $x \in X$ and all $b \in \phi(x)$, $ab \in \psi(x)$. Then for all $x \in X$ and all $b \in \phi(x)$, $(ka) * b = kakb = ab \in \psi(x)$, so $\phi \leq \psi$ w.r.t. $*$, realized by ka.

Conversely if a is such that for all x and all $b \in \phi(x)$, $a * b \in \psi(x)$, we distinguish cases: if $\bigcup_{x \in X} \phi(x) = \emptyset$ then trivially $\phi \leq \psi$ w.r.t. the original application; if $\bigcup_{x \in X} \phi(x) \neq \emptyset$ then $\phi \leq \psi$ is realized by $\langle y \rangle aky$ (note that in this case, $\langle y \rangle aky\downarrow$).   ∎

Remark. The case split at the end of this proof may bother constructively-minded readers. A way to avoid it is to define the preorder $\leq$ on $\mathcal{P}(A)^X$ differently, so that $\phi \leq \psi$ may be realized by a closed *term* instead of an element of A. Reasoning classically, one has then the same preorder; and the identity in theorem 1.2.3 is then established constructively.

Example. The main example of a genuine c-pca is the set SN of strongly normalizing λ-terms (w.r.t. β-reduction), with the ordinary application (juxtaposition) map. For k and s, there do not seem to be other choices than the terms $\lambda xy.x$ and $\lambda xyz.xz(yz)$, respectively. SN is a conditional pca, but if $w = \lambda x.xx$ then ww does not normalize; hence $s(\lambda v.w)(\lambda v.w)$, which reduces to $\lambda z.ww$, is not defined in SN.

Another example of a strictly conditional pca is given in [21].

1.3 Further properties; recursion theory; finite types

Before we start on examples of pcas, it is useful to record some further properties. The first proposition is rather a curiosity.

Proposition 1.3.1 *Let A be a nontrivial pca, that is: one with more than 1 element. Then the following statements are true:*

i)   The application map is not associative;

ii) the application map is not commutative;

iii) if k and s satisfy the properties of theorem 1.1.3, then $k \neq s$;

iv) if A is nontotal, there is an element $a \in A$ such that for all $b \in A$, ab is not defined.

Proof. (i) Since $k = kkk = (kk)k$, associativity would imply that $k = k(kk)$; hence $a = kak = k(kk)ak = kkk = k$ for all $a \in A$, contradiction with nontriviality.

ii) Commutativity would imply $i = ki(\bar{k}i) = \bar{k}i(ki) = ki$, hence $b = ib = kib = i$ for all $b \in A$, again contradicting nontriviality.

(iii) $k = s$ implies $i = ii = skki = kkki = ki$; see (ii).

(iv) If $c, d \in A$ are such that cd is not defined, $a = \langle x \rangle cd$ does the job. ∎

1.3.1   Recursion theory in pcas

We now show that in any nontrivial pca A, there is a copy $\{\bar{n} \mid n \in \mathbb{N}\}$ of the natural numbers, such that every partial recursive function is represented by an element of A in a suitably defined way.

Definition 1.3.2 (Curry numerals) The *Curry numerals* in a pca A are defined by:

$$\begin{aligned} \bar{0} &= i \\ \overline{n+1} &= p\bar{k}\bar{n} \end{aligned}$$

where p is the pairing operator.

Note, that the Curry numerals depend on a choice of k and s.

Proposition 1.3.3 *There are elements* $S, P, Z \in A$ *such that for all* $n \in \mathbb{N}$:

$$S\bar{n} = \overline{n+1}; \quad P\bar{0} = \bar{0}; \quad P\overline{n+1} = \bar{n}; \quad Z\bar{0} = k; \quad Z\overline{n+1} = \bar{k}$$

Proof. Recall the pairing and projection operators $p = \langle xyz \rangle zxy$, $p_0 = \langle v \rangle vk$ and $p_1 = \langle v \rangle v\bar{k}$. Define $S = \langle x \rangle p\bar{k}x$, $P = \langle x \rangle p_0 x \bar{0} (p_1 x)$ and $Z = p_0$. The stated properties are left as exercises for the reader. ∎

Recalling the use of k and $\bar{k}$ as Booleans, the element Z acts as a 'zero test' on the numerals.

Proposition 1.3.4 (fixed point operators) *There are elements* $y, z \in A$ *such that for all* $f \in A$:

i) $\quad yf \simeq f(yf)$;

ii) $\quad zf\downarrow$ *and for all* $x \in A$, $zfx \simeq f(zf)x$

Proof. Let $w = \langle xv \rangle v(xxv)$, $u = \langle xyz \rangle y(xxy)z$, $y = ww$, $z = uu$. Then: $yf \simeq wwf \simeq ((\langle y \rangle y(ww)y))f \simeq f(wwf) \simeq f(yf)$, and $zf \simeq uuf \simeq \langle z \rangle f(uuf)z$. So $zf\downarrow$, and $zfx \simeq f(uuf)x \simeq f(zf)x$. ∎

Proposition 1.3.5 (primitive recursion operator) *There is an element* $\mathcal{R} \in A$ *such that for all* $a, f \in A$ *and all* $n \in \mathbb{N}$:

$$\mathcal{R}af\bar{0} \simeq a$$

$$\mathcal{R}af\overline{n+1} \simeq f\bar{n}(\mathcal{R}af\bar{n})$$

Proof. Define R by

$$R = \langle rxfm \rangle Zm(kx)(\langle y \rangle f(Pm)(rxf(Pm)i))$$

and

$$\mathcal{R} = \langle xfm \rangle zRxfmi$$

where Z and P are as in 1.3.3 and z as in 1.3.4. Then
$\mathcal{R}af\bar{0} = zRaf\bar{0}i \simeq R(zR)af\bar{0}i \simeq$
$Z\bar{0}(ka)(\langle y \rangle f(P\bar{0})(raf(P\bar{0})i))i \simeq$
$k(ka)(\langle y \rangle f(P\bar{0})(raf(P\bar{0})i))i \simeq kai = a$; and
$\mathcal{R}af\overline{n+1} \simeq zRaf\overline{n+1}i \simeq R(zR)af\overline{n+1}i$
$\simeq Z\overline{n+1}(ka)(\langle y \rangle f(P\overline{n+1})(zRaf(P\overline{n+1})i))i$
$\simeq \bar{k}(ka)(\cdots)i$
$\simeq (\langle y \rangle f(P\overline{n+1})(zRaf(P\overline{n+1})i))i$
$\simeq f\bar{n}(zRaf\bar{n}i) \simeq f\bar{n}(\mathcal{R}af\bar{n})$,
as desired. ∎

Theorem 1.3.6 (Recursion in pcas) *In a nontrivial pca A, there is for every partial recursive function F of k variables, an element $a_F \in A$ such that for all $n_1, \ldots, n_k \in \mathbb{N}$: $a_F\overline{n_1} \cdots \overline{n_k}$ denotes if and only if $F(n_1, \ldots, n_k)$ is defined, and $a_F\overline{n_1} \cdots \overline{n_k} = \overline{F(n_1, \ldots, n_k)}$ if this is the case.*

Proof. Since F is constructed from the basic functions using primitive recursion and the fixed point operator, such an a_F can be constructed using propositions 1.3.3, 1.3.4 and 1.3.5. ∎

Using primitive recursion in A, we can define a *coding of finite sequences* of elements of A in A. Moreover, for a number of basic operations F on these sequences there are elements a_F in A such that, if u is the code of a sequence σ, then $a_F u$ is the code of $F(\sigma)$.

First define, inductively, maps $J^n : A^n \to A$ for $n > 0$ by putting

$$
\begin{aligned}
J^1(a) &= a \\
J^{n+1}(a_1, \ldots, a_{n+1}) &= pa_1 J^n(a_2, \ldots, a_{n+1})
\end{aligned}
$$

Then if $u_0, \ldots, u_{n-1}$ is a finite sequence of elements of A, we define its code $[u_0, \ldots, u_{n_1}]$ as follows:

$$
\begin{aligned}
[] &= p\overline{0}\overline{0} & (n = 0) \\
[u_0, \ldots, u_{n-1}] &= p\overline{n}j^n(u_0, \ldots, u_{n-1}) & (n > 0)
\end{aligned}
$$

It is now straightforward to work out, using proposition 1.3.5, that there are elements $\mathsf{lh}, b, c, d \in A$ such that

$$
\begin{aligned}
\mathsf{lh}[\,] &= \bar{0} \\
\mathsf{lh}[u_0, \dots, u_{n-1}] &= \bar{n} \\
b[u_0, \dots, u_{n-1}]\bar{i} &= u_i \ (i < n) \\
c[u_0, \dots, u_{n-1}]\bar{i}\bar{j} &= [u_i, \dots, u_{j-1}] \ (i < j < n) \\
d[u_0, \dots, u_{n-1}][v_0, \dots, v_{m-1}] &= [u_0, \dots, u_{n-1}, v_0, \dots, v_{m-1}]
\end{aligned}
$$

and so on.

Finally, we include in this section a few definitions for later use.

Definition 1.3.7 A pca is called

i)   *decidable* if there is an element $d \in A$ such that for all $a, b \in A$, $dab = k$ if $a = b$, and $dab = \bar{k}$ otherwise;

ii) *extensional* if for all $a, b \in A$ it holds that if for all $c \in A$, $ac \simeq bc$, then $a = b$.

Definition 1.3.8 (Finite Types over a pca) The *finite types* are the expressions built up from the constant $*$ and the binary operation $\rightarrow$. Given a pca A, the *intensional finite type structure* over A associates to any type σ a subset I_σ of A as follows:

$$
\begin{aligned}
I_* &= \{ \bar{n} \mid n \in \mathbb{N} \} \\
I_{\sigma \rightarrow \tau} &= I_\sigma \Rightarrow I_\tau \\
&= \{ a \in A \mid \forall b \in I_\sigma (ab{\downarrow} \text{ and } ab \in I_\tau) \}
\end{aligned}
$$

The *extensional finite type structure* over A associates to any type σ a subset E_σ of A as well as an equivalence relation $\approx_\sigma$ on E_σ, as follows:
$E_* = \{ \bar{n} \mid n \in \mathbb{N} \}$; $\approx_*$ is the equality relation;
$E_{\sigma \rightarrow \tau}$ is the set

$$
\{ a \in A \mid \forall b \in E_\sigma (ab{\downarrow} \text{ and } ab \in E_\tau) \text{ and } \forall bb' \in E_\sigma (b \approx_\sigma b' \Rightarrow ab \approx_\tau ab') \}
$$

and $a \approx_{\sigma \rightarrow \tau} a'$ holds if for all $b \in E_\sigma$, $ab \approx_\tau a'b$).

Definition 1.3.9 A pca is *finite type extensional* if $I_\sigma = E_\sigma$ for every type σ (note that this implies that $\approx_\sigma$ is the equality relation for each type σ).

1.4 Examples of pcas

1.4.1 Kleene's first model

The best known pca, also called *Kleene's first model* or $\mathcal{K}_1$, is the set $\mathbb{N}$ with partial recursive application: $a, b \mapsto \varphi_a(b)$.

1.4.2 Relativized recursion

Generalizing $\mathcal{K}_1$, for every partial function F on $\mathbb{N}$ there is the notion of "partial recursive application with oracle F": a program may, at any stage of the computation, ask for values of F at certain arguments (with the stipulation that the program will not terminate if the argument presented to the oracle is not in the domain of F). We shall call this model $\mathcal{K}_1^F$.

1.4.3 Kleene's second model

For our next model, *Kleene's second model* $\mathcal{K}_2$ or the pca for *function realizability*, we consider the set of functions $\mathbb{N}^{\mathbb{N}}$ as an infinite product, with the product topology (where the topology on $\mathbb{N}$ is discrete). This means that a basis for the topology on $\mathbb{N}^{\mathbb{N}}$ is given by sets of the form U_σ where $\sigma = (\sigma_0, \ldots, \sigma_{\text{lh}(\sigma)-1})$ is a finite sequence of natural numbers of length $\text{lh}(\sigma)$, and

$$U_\sigma = \{\alpha \in \mathbb{N}^{\mathbb{N}} \mid \forall n < \text{lh}(\sigma)\, \alpha(n) = \sigma_n\}$$

A partial map $F : \mathbb{N}^{\mathbb{N}} \to \mathbb{N}$ is continuous on its domain if for every $\alpha \in \text{dom}(F)$ there is an n such that for every $\beta \in \text{dom}(F)$:

$$\text{if for all } i < n,\ \alpha(i) = \beta(i),\ \text{then } F(\alpha) = F(\beta)$$

We use a 1-1, surjective coding of finite sequences of natural numbers by natural numbers; let $\bar{\alpha}n = \langle \alpha(0), \ldots, \alpha(n-1) \rangle$ ($\bar{\alpha}(0) = \langle \rangle$). Using this coding, every $\alpha \in \mathbb{N}^{\mathbb{N}}$ determines a partial map F_α from $\mathbb{N}^{\mathbb{N}}$ to $\mathbb{N}$ in the following way:

$F_\alpha(\beta) = k$ if there is an n such that $\alpha(\bar{\beta}n) = k + 1$ and $\forall m < n\, \alpha(\bar{\beta}m) = 0$, and is undefined if such an n does not exist.

It is easy to see that F_α has the following properties:

a) F_α is continuous on its domain;

b) $\mathrm{dom}(F_\alpha)$ is an open subset of $\mathbb{N}^\mathbb{N}$.

Conversely, every partial continuous operation $F : \mathbb{N}^\mathbb{N} \to \mathbb{N}$ with open domain is equal to F_α for some (non-unique) α, as is left for you to check.

For $n \in \mathbb{N}$ and $\alpha \in \mathbb{N}^\mathbb{N}$, write $\langle n \rangle * \alpha$ for the function f defined by $f(0) = n$ and $f(k+1) = \alpha(k)$. We can now define a application on $\mathbb{N}^\mathbb{N}$ as follows:

$\alpha\beta$ is the function $n \mapsto F_\alpha(\langle n \rangle * \beta)$ if for all n, $F_\alpha(\langle n \rangle * \beta)$ is defined; and undefined else.

Lemma 1.4.1 *Suppose $F : \mathbb{N}^\mathbb{N} \times \mathbb{N}^\mathbb{N} \to \mathbb{N}^\mathbb{N}$ is a continuous function of 2 variables. Then there is an element ϕ of $\mathbb{N}^\mathbb{N}$ such that for all $\alpha, \beta \in \mathbb{N}^\mathbb{N}$, $\phi\alpha\beta = F(\alpha, \beta)$.*

Proof. For natural numbers n and k, let U_n^k be the open set

$$\{(\alpha, \beta) \mid F(\alpha, \beta)(n) = k\}$$

Define the function ϕ by the clauses:
$\phi(\langle \rangle) = 0$
$\phi(\langle\langle \rangle\rangle * \tau) = 1$
$\phi(\langle\langle n \rangle * \sigma\rangle * \tau) = 1$ if there is no k such that $U_\tau \times U_\sigma \subseteq U_n^k$
$\phi(\langle\langle n \rangle * \sigma\rangle * \tau) = k + 2$ if there is a (necessarily unique) k such that $U_\tau \times U_\sigma \subseteq U_n^k$.
Then ϕ satisfies the Lemma, as is left to you to check.   ∎

Applying lemma 1.4.1 to the first projection $\mathbb{N}^\mathbb{N} \times \mathbb{N}^\mathbb{N} \to \mathbb{N}^\mathbb{N}$ we see at once that there is $k \in \mathbb{N}^\mathbb{N}$ such that for all α, β, $k\alpha\beta = \alpha$.

The lemma is also useful for showing that an s exists as in 1.1.3. Let us extend the notations $F_\alpha(\beta)$ and $\alpha\beta$ also to codes of finite sequences: if b is a code of a finite sequence, $F_\alpha(b) = k$ if for some (code of) initial segment b' of b, $\alpha(b') = k + 1$, and $\alpha(b'') = 0$ for every proper initial segment b'' of b'. Similarly, we say $\alpha b(n) = k$ if $F_\alpha(\langle n \rangle * b) = k$.

We now define a function $F : \mathbb{N}^\mathbb{N} \times \mathbb{N}^\mathbb{N} \to \mathbb{N}^\mathbb{N}$ as follows:

$F(\alpha, \beta)(\langle\rangle) = 0$

$F(\alpha, \beta)(\langle n \rangle * c) = m + 1$ if and only if there is a $k < \mathrm{lh}(c)$ such that the following are satisfied:

i) $\beta c(0), \dots, \beta c(k - 1)$ are all defined;

ii) $F_\alpha(\langle\langle\rangle\rangle * c), F_\alpha(\langle\langle n \rangle\rangle * c), F_\alpha(\langle\langle n, \beta c(0)\rangle\rangle * c), \dots,$ and $F_\alpha(\langle\langle n, \beta c(0), \dots, \beta c(k - 1)\rangle\rangle * c)$ are all defined;

iii) $F_\alpha(\langle\langle n, \beta c(0), \dots, \beta c(k - 1)\rangle\rangle * c) = m + 1$;

iv) $F_\alpha(\langle\langle n, \beta c(0), \dots, \beta c(i)\rangle\rangle * c) = 0$ for all $i < k - 1$.

$F(\alpha, \beta)(\langle n \rangle * c) = 0$ if no such $k < \mathrm{lh}(c)$ exists.

One can now work out that if $F(\alpha, \beta)(\langle n \rangle * c) = m + 1$, then $\alpha\gamma(\beta\gamma)(n) = m$ for any $\gamma \in U_c$; and conversely if $\alpha\gamma(\beta\gamma)(n) = m$ then there is a c such that $\gamma \in U_c$ and $F(\alpha, \beta)(\langle n \rangle * c) = m + 1$. Hence,

$$F(\alpha, \beta)\gamma \simeq \alpha\gamma(\beta\gamma) \text{ for all } \gamma$$

From the definition of $F(\alpha, \beta)$ it is manifest that F is continuous; by lemma 1.4.1, there is an element $s \in \mathbb{N}^{\mathbb{N}}$ such that for all α, β, $s\alpha\beta = F(\alpha, \beta)$. This s then satisfies the conditions in theorem 1.1.3.

It is easy to see that a partial function $\mathbb{N}^{\mathbb{N}} \rightharpoonup \mathbb{N}^{\mathbb{N}}$ is of the form $\alpha \mapsto \beta\alpha$ for some $\beta \in \mathbb{N}^{\mathbb{N}}$, if and only if its domain is a G_δ set (a countable intersection of open sets) and it is continuous on its domain.

Moreover, every partial function which is continuous on its domain, can be extended to one of this form: see [12].

1.4.4 $\mathcal{K}_2$ generalized

Example $\mathcal{K}_2$ can be generalized. Let κ be a cardinal with the property that $\kappa^{<\kappa} = \kappa$ (for example, under the Continuum Hypothesis this holds for $\kappa = \omega_1$); so there is a bijective coding $\ulcorner \cdot \urcorner$ of functions $f : \lambda \to \kappa$ (with $\lambda < \kappa$) into κ.

Let $A = \kappa^\kappa$. Define a topology on A with basic open sets of the form

$$U_\sigma = \{a \in A \mid \forall \beta < \alpha \, a(\beta) = \sigma(\beta)\}$$

for $\sigma : \alpha \to \kappa$ $(\alpha < \kappa)$.

Then every $a \in A$ defines a partial map $F_a : A \to \kappa$ as follows:
$F_a(b) = \alpha$ if for some $\beta < \kappa$, $a(\ulcorner b{\upharpoonright}\beta\urcorner) = \alpha + 1$ and for all $\gamma < \beta$,
$a(\ulcorner b{\upharpoonright}\gamma\urcorner)$ is a limit ordinal (we see 0 as a limit ordinal!).

Then F_a has open domain and is continuous on its domain, and every
partial function with open domain which is continuous on its domain, is
of the form F_a for some $a \in \kappa$.

Let $\langle \alpha \rangle * b$ be the element of A defined by $\langle \alpha \rangle * b(0) = \alpha$; $\langle \alpha \rangle * b(n+1) =$
$b(n)$ for $n < \omega$; $\langle \alpha \rangle * b(\beta) = b(\beta)$ for $\omega \le \beta < \kappa$.

Then we can define $ab(\alpha)$ as $F_a(\langle \alpha \rangle * b)$; ab is defined if and only if
$ab(\alpha)$ is defined for all $\alpha < \kappa$. The proof that A is a pca follows similar
lines as the proof in example 1.4.3

1.4.5 Sequential computations

Another generalization of $\mathcal{K}_2$ is considered in [173]: here we consider
partial functions from $\mathbb{N}$ to $\mathbb{N}$. Let $\mathcal{B}$ be the set of all those. Topologize
$\mathcal{B}$ by taking as basis the collection of all sets

$$U_p = \{\alpha \in \mathcal{B} \,|\, p \subseteq \alpha\}$$

for some *finite* function p (this is a basis since if $\alpha \in U_p \cap U_q$, then $p \cup q$
is also a finite function, and $\alpha \in U_{p \cup q} = U_p \cap U_q$).

Partial functions from $\mathcal{B}$ to $\mathbb{N}$ can be seen as functions $\mathcal{B} \to N_\perp$,
where $N_\perp = \mathbb{N} \cup \{\perp\}$, $\perp$ a new element. $N_\perp$ is given the topology
$\mathcal{P}(\mathbb{N}) \cup \{N_\perp\}$, and a partial function from $\mathcal{B}$ to $\mathbb{N}$ is called *continuous* if
the corresponding function $\mathcal{B} \to N_\perp$ is continuous.

Every such continuous function F has a *base* B, which is the set of
all finite functions p which are minimal with respect to the property that
$F(p) \in \mathbb{N}$; then $F(\alpha) = k \in \mathbb{N}$ holds iff there is $p \in B$ such that $p \subseteq \alpha$
and $F(p) = k$.

A *sequential tree* is a tree T of finite functions (ordered by inclusion;
the root is the empty function) such that for every $p \in T$ there is a
number n such that all immediate successors q of p in T satisfy $\mathrm{dom}(q) =$
$\mathrm{dom}(p) \cup \{n\}$. A continuous function $F : \mathcal{B} \to N_\perp$ is called *sequential* if
its base is the set of leaves of a sequential tree.

For such an F, $F(\alpha)$ is computed by chasing α through the sequential tree T: start at the root, the empty function. Inductively, in the computation we have arrived at $p \in T$ such that $p \subseteq \alpha$. Let n be such that all immediate successors of p in T have domain $\text{dom}(p) \cup \{n\}$. If $\alpha(n)$ is undefined or $p \cup \{(n, \alpha(n))\} \notin T$, $F(\alpha) = \bot$. Otherwise, repeat with $p \cup \{(n, \alpha(n))\}$. If we arrive at a leaf p of T, $F(\alpha) = F(p)$. An example of a continuous function which is *not* sequential is the function which sends the empty function to $\bot$ and all other functions to 0.

Sequential functions $\mathcal{B} \to \mathbb{N}_\bot$ are encoded by elements of $\mathcal{B}$ as follows. Let $\alpha, \beta \in \mathcal{B}$. A *dialogue* between α and β is a code of a sequence $u = \langle u_0, \ldots, u_k \rangle$ such that for each $i \le k$ there is a $j \in \mathbb{N}$ such that $\alpha(u^{<i}) = 2j$ and $\beta(j) = u_i$ (we write $u^{<i}$ for $\langle u_0, \ldots, u_{i-1} \rangle$; $u^{<0} = \langle \rangle$).

Define $\alpha | \beta = m$ if there is a dialogue u between α and β such that $\alpha(u) = 2m + 1$. It is easy to see that the function $F_\alpha : \beta \mapsto \alpha | \beta$ is sequential, and that every sequential function is of the form F_α for some (non-unique) α.

We now define an application on $\mathcal{B}$. Let α_x denote the partial function $y \mapsto \alpha(\langle x, y \rangle)$. $\alpha\beta$ is the partial function $x \mapsto \alpha_x | \beta$.

Then $\mathcal{B}$ is a total combinatory algebra. This can be seen as follows. First observe that the map $\alpha, \beta \mapsto \alpha\beta$ is recursive in α and β. That is, if we denote by $\varphi_e^{\xi, \eta}$ the partial function computed by the program with code e with partial oracles ξ and η, then there is a program e such that for all $\alpha, \beta \in \mathcal{B}$, $\varphi_e^{\alpha, \beta} = \alpha\beta$. Likewise, for every term $t(x_1, \ldots, x_n)$ there is a program e such that for every n-tuple $\alpha_1, \ldots, \alpha_n$,

$$\varphi_e^{\alpha_1, \ldots, \alpha_n} = t(\alpha_1, \ldots, \alpha_n)$$

The next observation is that for each $n \ge 0$ there is a primitive recursive function T_n such that for all $\alpha_1, \ldots, \alpha_{n+1}$:

$$(\varphi_{T_n(e)}^{\alpha_1, \ldots, \alpha_n})\alpha_{n+1} = \varphi_e^{\alpha_1, \ldots, \alpha_{n+1}}$$

Namely, let $\varphi_{T_n(e)}^{\alpha_1, \ldots, \alpha_n}(\langle x, u \rangle)$ be $2k$ if, in a computation of $\varphi_e^{\alpha_1, \ldots, \alpha_{n+1}}(x)$, after having asked values of α_{n+1} $\text{lh}(u)$ many times and received answers $u_0, \ldots, u_{\text{lh}(u)-1}$, the value of $\alpha_{n+1}(k)$ is asked by the program; $2k+1$ if, in this situation, the program terminates with output k; and undefined in all other cases.

Putting these two observations together, one now shows that for every term $t(x_1, \ldots, x_n)$ there is an α such that for all $\beta_1, \ldots, \beta_n \in \mathcal{B}$, $\alpha\beta_1 \cdots \beta_n = t(\beta_1, \ldots, \beta_n)$; in other words, that $\mathcal{B}$ is combinatory complete.

It was shown in [173] that the extensional type structure of $\mathcal{B}$ is isomorphic to the finite types over N in Ehrhard and Bucciarelli's "hypercoherences" ([29]).

1.4.6   The graph model $\mathcal{P}(\omega)$

Our next example is Scott's *graph model* $\mathcal{P}(\omega)$ (discovered by D.S. Scott in 1969; see [145]).

$\mathcal{P}(\omega)$ is the powerset of $\mathbb{N}$. This is topologized in the following way: $\mathcal{P}(\omega) = \{0,1\}^{\mathbb{N}}$. Give $\{0,1\}$ the Sierpinski topology (the open sets are $\emptyset$, $\{1\}$ and $\{0,1\}$) and $\{0,1\}^{\mathbb{N}}$ the product topology. Basic opens can be identified with sets of the form

$$U_p = \{A \subseteq \mathbb{N} \,|\, p \subseteq A\}$$

for a finite $p \subseteq \mathbb{N}$.

It is easily established that $F : \mathcal{P}(\omega) \to \mathcal{P}(\omega)$ is continuous for this topology, if and only if we have

$$F(A) = \bigcup\{F(p) \,|\, p \subseteq A \text{ finite}\}$$

for every $A \in \mathcal{P}(\omega)$ (in particular, every continuous F is monotone w.r.t. $\subseteq$).

Let us write $[\mathcal{P}(\omega) \to \mathcal{P}(\omega)]$ for the set of such continuous functions. There are maps

$$\text{graph} : \; [\mathcal{P}(\omega)] \to \mathcal{P}(\omega)] \to \mathcal{P}(\omega)$$
$$\text{fun} : \quad \mathcal{P}(\omega) \to [\mathcal{P}(\omega) \to \mathcal{P}(\omega)]$$

such that for every $F \in [\mathcal{P}(\omega) \to \mathcal{P}(\omega)]$, $\text{fun}(\text{graph}(F)) = F$, and for every $A \in \mathcal{P}(\omega)$, $\text{graph}(\text{fun}(A)) \supseteq A$.

The maps graph and fun depend on a bijective coding of finite subsets of $\mathbb{N}$ as numbers: the number n corresponds to the finite set e_n if

$$n = \sum_{i \in e_n} 2^i$$

So $e_0 = \emptyset$, $e_1 = \{0\}$, $e_2 = \{1\}$, $e_3 = \{0,1\}$ etc. One defines

$$\begin{aligned} \text{graph}(F) &= \{\langle n, m \rangle \mid m \in F(e_n)\} \\ \text{fun}(A)(B) &= \{m \mid \exists n \, (e_n \subseteq B \text{ and } \langle n, m \rangle \in A)\} \end{aligned}$$

The relations $\text{fun}(\text{graph}(F)) = F$ and $A \subseteq \text{graph}(\text{fun}(A))$ are left to you to check.

An application map $\mathcal{P}(\omega) \times \mathcal{P}(\omega) \to \mathcal{P}(\omega)$ can now be defined by

$$AB = \text{fun}(A)(B)$$

This function is continuous. On the other hand, for any continuous function $F : (\mathcal{P}(\omega))^n \to \mathcal{P}(\omega)$ there is an $A \in \mathcal{P}(\omega)$ such that for all $B_1, \ldots, B_n$, $AB_1 \cdots B_n = F(B_1, \ldots, B_n)$.

We see that $\mathcal{P}(\omega)$ is a total combinatory algebra. Actually it is a lot more: $\mathcal{P}(\omega)$ is a model of the λ-calculus. However, for our purposes this distinction is not of importance.

1.4.7 Graph models

The example $\mathcal{P}(\omega)$ is one of a range of 'graph models', as studied by Engeler ([40]) and Bethke.

There is the following general construction. Let A be a nonempty set. Define sets $G_n(A)$ inductively by:

$$\begin{aligned} G_0(A) &= A \\ G_{n+1}(A) &= G_n(A) \cup \{(B, b) \mid B \subseteq G_n(A) \text{ finite}, b \in G_n(A)\} \end{aligned}$$

Let $G(A) = \bigcup_{n \in \mathbb{N}} G_n(A)$. For $X, Y \subseteq G(A)$ define:

$$XY = \{b \mid \exists B \subseteq Y \, (B, b) \in X\}$$

Then $\mathcal{P}(G(A))$ is a combinatory algebra with this application map.

1.4.8   Domain models

Another group of combinatory algebras is obtained from a construction
which was also discovered by Scott ([144]).

   A *cpo* is a poset D with a least element $\perp$ which has a least upper
bound $\bigvee X$ for every directed subset X of D (recall that X is directed
if $X \neq \emptyset$ and for every $x, y \in X$ there is $z \in X$ such that $x \leq z$ and
$y \leq z$).

   Such cpos are endowed with the *Scott topology*: a subset $U \subseteq D$ is
open if U is upwards closed and inaccessible for directed joins, that is:
U is open if and only if the following conditions hold:

i) $\forall x \in U \forall y \geq x \, y \in U$

ii)   for every directed $X \subseteq D$, if $\bigvee X \in U$ then $X \cap U \neq \emptyset$

$[D \to D]$ denotes the set of Scott-continuous maps from D to D (it
is easy to see that a map is Scott-continuous iff it is monotone and
preserves least upper bounds of directed subsets). Scott showed that
every cpo D can be embedded in a cpo D_∞ which has the property
that D_∞ is isomorphic to $[D_\infty \to D_\infty]$. It follows that D_∞ has the
structure of a combinatory algebra: if fun : $D_\infty \to [D_\infty \to D_\infty]$ is one
part of the isomorphism, one can define an application map by putting
$ab = \text{fun}(a)(b)$.

   Models of this form are studied in *domain theory*: a good modern
introduction to this topic is the book by Amadio and Curien ([7]).

1.4.9   Relativized models

Many of the preceding examples can be relativized: there is $\mathcal{K}_2^{\mathrm{rec}}$ (the
set of total recursive functions from $\mathbb{N}$ to $\mathbb{N}$ with the application from
$\mathcal{K}_2$ (clearly, if α, β are recursive and $\alpha\beta$ is defined, then $\alpha\beta$ is recursive;
also, recursive choices for k and s are possible), $\mathcal{K}_2^{\mathrm{rec}(F)}$ (functions recur-
sive in F), $\mathcal{B}^{\mathrm{rec}}$ (partial recursive functions), $\mathcal{P}(\omega)^{\mathrm{re}}$ (r.e. subsets of $\mathbb{N}$),
$\mathcal{P}(\omega)^{\mathrm{re}(F)}$, etc.

1.4.10 Term models

I should mention different kinds of *term models*. The terms of the λ-calculus (with the normal application – juxtaposition – map) form a combinatory algebra. We already mentioned the model of strongly normalizing λ-terms as an example of a genuine c-pca. Similarly, there is a term model of 'partial combinatory logic' (for this logic, see [22]). I do not go into details.

1.4.11 Pitts' construction

The following construction occurs in [123], and will be of importance in section 3.8.3.

Suppose A is a pca; by the theory of section 1.3 we have the Curry numerals $\{\bar{n} \mid n \in \mathbb{N}\}$ in A, such that every partial recursive function is represented in A by an element (1.3.6). In particular there is an element $u \in A$ such that, whenever $nm = k$ in $\mathcal{K}_1$, then $u\bar{n}\bar{m} = \bar{k}$ in A. Define a pca $\mathbb{N} \ltimes A$ as follows: its underlying set is the product $\mathbb{N} \times A$, and application is given by

$$(n, a)(n', a') \simeq (nn', a(p\bar{n'}a'))$$

Suppose K_N and S_N satisfy the axioms for k and s in $\mathbb{N}$, and K_A and S_A do so for A. Write

$$y * z \equiv p(u(p(p_0y)(p_0z)))((p_1y)z)$$

Define
$$k = (K_N, \langle x \rangle K_A(p_1x))$$
$$s = (S_N, \langle xyz \rangle (p_1x)z(y * z))$$

Then k and s satisfy the axioms in $\mathbb{N} \ltimes A$, as I leave for you to check.

A generalization of the construction, together with a categorical interpretation, is in [68].

1.4.12 Models of Arithmetic

Of course, every model M of Peano Arithmetic is a pca. One defines '$ab = c$' by

$$M \models \exists y (T(a, b, y) \wedge U(y) = c)$$

1.5   Morphisms and Assemblies

In many accounts of the theory of pcas, the elements k and s required by theorem 1.1.3 form part of the definition of a pca, and are therefore taken as *structure* which should be preserved by morphisms of pcas.

I have chosen to define a pca as a combinatory complete pas. It is true that combinatory completeness follows from existence of k and s, but it also follows from existence of other sets of elements with special properties, and for me the elements k and s (which are non-unique anyway) do not have any distinguished status.

If a pca is defined as a pas together with a *choice* for k and s, and a homomorphism should preserve application and k and s, then there is not an abundance of such homomorphisms. Examples are the inclusion of $\mathcal{K}_2^{\mathrm{rec}}$ into $\mathcal{K}_2$, and similar embeddings of a relativized structure into the original one.

The question of which morphisms to choose in order to organize pcas into a category, should be answered according to the behaviour of the structures, built on pcas, one is interested in. We have already mentioned the set of $\mathcal{P}(A)$-valued predicates on a set X, with its Heyting algebra structure. Closely related to this (a relationship which will be made precise in chapter 2) is the category of *assemblies* on a pca A, which I introduce at this point.

Definition 1.5.1 (Assemblies) Let A be a pca. An *assembly* on A is a pair (X, E) where X is a set, and $E : X \to \mathcal{P}^*(A)$ assigns to any $x \in X$ a nonempty subset $E(x)$ of A.

A *morphism* of assemblies $f : (X, E) \to (Y, F)$ is a function $f : X \to Y$ with the property that there exists an element a of A such that for all $x \in X$ and all $b \in E(x)$, ab is defined, and is an element of $F(f(x))$. Such an element is said to *track* the function f.

The identity function on the set X is tracked by i, and if a tracks $f : (X, E) \to (Y, F)$ and b tracks $g : (Y, F) \to (Z, G)$ then the composition $gf : X \to Z$ is tracked by $\langle x \rangle b(ax)$, so assemblies on A and their morphisms form a category $\mathrm{Ass}(A)$.

In order to relate the pca A to its associated category of assemblies $\mathrm{Ass}(A)$, we have to establish a few easy properties of this category.

Theorem 1.5.2 *The category* Ass(A) *is regular, cartesian closed, and has finite colimits. Moreover, there are regular functors* $\Gamma : \mathrm{Ass}(A) \to$ Set *and* $\nabla : \mathrm{Set} \to \mathrm{Ass}(A)$ *such that* $\Gamma \dashv \nabla$ *and the composite* $\Gamma\nabla$ *is the identity functor on* Set.

Proof. Clearly, the assembly $(\{*\}, E)$ with $E(*) = A$ is a terminal object in Ass(A). The product of two assemblies (X, E) and (Y, F) is $(X \times Y, G)$ with $G(x, y) = \{pab \,|\, a \in E(x), b \in F(y)\}$; the projections are tracked by p_0 and p_1, respectively, and if $f : (Z, G) \to (X, E)$ and $g : (Z, G) \to (Y, F)$ are tracked by a and b then the mediating map $(f, g) : Z \to X \times Y$ is tracked by $\langle x\rangle p(ax)(bx)$. Given two morphisms $f, g : (X, E) \to (Y, F)$, their equalizer is (X', E') where $X' = \{x \in X \,|\, f(x) = g(x)\}$ and E' is the restriction of E to X'. The reader should check this, as well as the statement that a morphism $f : (X, E) \to (Y, F)$ is a regular mono if and only if f is an injective function and $f : (X, E) \to (f(X), F')$ (where F' is the restriction of F to $f(X)$) is an isomorphism.

$(\emptyset, \emptyset)$ is an initial object in Ass(A). The coproduct of two assemblies (X, E) and (Y, F) is the object $(X + Y, G)$ where $X + Y = \{0\} \times X \cup \{1\} \times Y$ is the disjoint union of X and Y, and $G(0, x) = \{p\bar{0}a \,|\, a \in E(x)\}$, $G(1, y) = \{p\bar{1}b \,|\, b \in F(y)\}$ together with coprojections from X and Y (you should find trackings for these maps!). Given two morphisms $f, g : (X, E) \to (Y, F)$, their coequalizer is the map $q : (Y, F) \to (Y', F')$ where Y' is the quotient of Y by the equivalence relation generated by $\{(y, y') \,|\, \exists x \in X \,(f(x) = y \text{ and } g(x) = y')\}$, q is the quotient map, and $F'(\alpha) = \bigcup_{q(y)=\alpha} F(y)$. Again, the reader is invited to check this, as well as the statement that $f : (X, E) \to (Y, F)$ is a regular epi if and only if f is a surjective function and the identity on Y is an isomorphism: $(Y, F') \to (Y, F)$ where $F'(y) = \bigcup_{f(x)=y} E(x)$.

Obviously, a morphism in Ass(A) is mono if and only if it is an injective function, and from the description of regular epis it is easily seen that any morphism f factors as a regular epimorphism followed by a mono. The reader can work out that regular epimorphisms are stable under pullback, so this proves that Ass(A) is a regular category with finite coproducts.

For cartesian closure, for the exponential $(Y, F)^{(X,E)}$ one can take

(Z, G) where

$$Z = \{f : X \to Y \mid f \text{ is a morphism } (X, E) \to (Y, F)\}$$

and $G(f) = \{a \in A \mid a \text{ tracks } f\}$. The evaluation map: $(Z, G) \times (X, E) \to (Y, F)$ is tracked by $\langle w \rangle p_0 w(p_1 w)$ and if $g : (W, H) \times (X, E) \to (Y, F)$ is tracked by a, its exponential transpose $\tilde{g} : (W, H) \to (Z, G)$ is tracked by $\langle wx \rangle a(pwx)$.

The functor $\Gamma : \text{Ass}(A) \to \text{Set}$ sends (X, E) to X and f to f. By the characterizations of finite limits and regular epimorphisms given above, Γ is regular. $\nabla : \text{Set} \to \text{Ass}(A)$ sends a set X to the pair (X, ∇_X) where $\nabla_X(x) = A$ for all $x \in X$. Every function $f : X \to Y$ is then a morphism $\nabla X \to \nabla Y$, tracked by i. Obviously, Γ and ∇ are functors, ∇ is regular, and $\Gamma \nabla$ is the identity on Set. The adjunction $\Gamma \dashv \nabla$ is immediate. ∎

In [99], John Longley has proposed a definition of morphisms between pcas which correlates well with certain functors between the associated categories of assemblies.

Definition 1.5.3 (Longley) Let A and B be pcas. An *applicative morphism* $\gamma : A \to B$ is a function γ which assigns to every $a \in A$ a nonempty subset $\gamma(a)$ of B, in such a way that there exists an element $r \in B$ which satisfies, for every $a, a' \in A$ and every $b \in \gamma(a), b' \in \gamma(a')$:

$$\text{if } aa' \downarrow \text{ then } rbb' \downarrow \text{ and } rbb' \in \gamma(aa')$$

Such a required element r is said to *realize* the morphism γ.

If γ and δ are two applicative morphisms $A \to B$, then we say $\gamma \preceq \delta$ if there is an element $t \in B$ such that for every $a \in A$ and every $b \in \gamma(a)$, $tb \downarrow$ and $tb \in \delta(a)$.

Remark. Before we show that with this definition we obtain a preorder-enriched category PCA, it is useful to make a remark. First of all, observe that if r realizes a morphism $\gamma : A \to B$ and (in B) $r' = \langle x \rangle r(p_0 x)(p_1 x)$ then we have for $b \in \gamma(a), b' \in \gamma(a')$: if $aa' \downarrow$ then $r'(pbb') \in \gamma(aa')$.

Now the pair (A, γ) is an object of $\mathrm{Ass}(B)$. Let Ap be the subassembly of $(A, \gamma) \times (A, \gamma)$ on the domain of the application map of A: Ap is $(\{(a, a') \in A \times A \,|\, aa'{\downarrow}\}, \gamma')$ with

$$\gamma'(a, a') = \{pbb' \,|\, b \in \gamma(a), b' \in \gamma(a')\}$$

We see then that the requirement that γ has a realizer can be restated as follows: the application map $\mathrm{Ap} \to (A, \gamma)$ is a map of assemblies on B.

Moreover, for two applicative morphisms γ and δ from A to B we have $\gamma \preceq \delta$ if and only if the identity map on A is a map in $\mathrm{Ass}(B)$ from (A, γ) to (A, δ).

Proposition 1.5.4 *The relation $\preceq$ between applicative morphisms is a preorder. There is a composition law for applicative morphisms which respects $\preceq$ in both variables, and defines a preorder-enriched category* PCA.

Proof. For a formal definition of the notion 'preorder-enriched category', see subsection 2.1.1. The first assertion is left to the reader to prove. If $\gamma : A \to B$ and $\delta : B \to C$ are applicative morphisms we define

$$\delta\gamma(a) = \bigcup_{b \in \gamma(a)} \delta(b)$$

as the composition of δ and γ. This has a realizer, because if r realizes γ, s realizes δ and $r' \in \delta(r)$, then $\langle xy \rangle s(sr'x)y$ realizes $\delta\gamma$: suppose $c \in \delta\gamma(a)$, $c' \in \delta\gamma(a')$, and $aa'{\downarrow}$. There are $b \in \gamma(a)$, $b' \in \gamma(a')$ such that $c \in \delta(b)$ and $c' \in \delta(b')$. Since r realizes γ, $rbb' \in \gamma(aa')$. Since s realizes δ, $sr'c \in \delta(rb)$; again applying s we get $s(sr'c)c' \in \delta(rbb')$; so $s(sr'c)c' \in \delta\gamma(aa')$.

The identity applicative morphism id on A is the map $a \mapsto \{a\}$, which is realized by $\langle xy \rangle xy$ and satisfies $\gamma \mathrm{id} = \gamma$ and $\mathrm{id}\delta = \delta$ for appropriate γ and δ.

It is trivial to verify that composition is associative, so it remains to prove that it respects $\preceq$. Suppose t realizes $\gamma \preceq \gamma' : A \to B$ and u realizes $\delta \preceq \delta' : B \to C$. If r realizes δ and $t' \in \delta(t)$, then $\langle x \rangle u(rt'x)$ realizes $\delta\gamma \preceq \delta'\gamma'$. ∎

Definition 1.5.5 Given a pair $\iota : A \to B, \gamma : B \to A$ of applicative morphisms, we naturally say that ι is *left adjoint to* γ, or $\iota \dashv \gamma$, if $\iota\gamma \preceq \mathrm{id}_B$ and $\mathrm{id}_A \preceq \gamma\iota$.

Examples. Some examples of applicative morphisms are listed below. It should be stressed that the category PCA is not very well understood at the moment of writing, and only a few nontrivial relations between pcas have been investigated. There is a lot to explore here.

1) Let $\mathbb{I}$ be the trivial pca consisting of one element. For any pca A there is exactly one applicative morphism from A to $\mathbb{I}$; conversely, for every nonempty subset B of A there is an applicative morphism ι_B from $\mathbb{I}$ to A sending the unique element of $\mathbb{I}$ to B, but it is easily seen that any two such applicative morphisms are isomorphic in the preorder $\mathrm{PCA}(\mathbb{I}, A)$. So if $\mathrm{PCA}/\!\!\sim$ denotes the quotient category obtained by identifying isomorphic morphisms, $\mathbb{I}$ is a zero object (both initial and terminal) in $\mathrm{PCA}/\!\!\sim$.

2) There is an applicative morphism $\gamma : \mathcal{K}_2^{\mathrm{rec}} \to \mathcal{K}_1$: define $\gamma(\alpha) = \{e \,|\, \alpha = \varphi_e\}$. Clearly, there is a primitive recursive function F such that for all indices e, e' of total recursive functions and all numbers x: $F(e)e'\!\downarrow$ in $\mathcal{K}_1$ and

$$\varphi_{F(e)e'}(x) \simeq (\varphi_e\varphi_{e'})(x)$$

(the application on the right hand side is in $\mathcal{K}_2$). Any index for such F is then a realizer for γ.

3) For any pca A there is an applicative morphism $\mathcal{K}_1 \to A$. Let $\{\bar{n} \,|\, n \in \mathbb{N}\}$ be the set of Curry numerals in A. By the results in section 1.3, every partial recursive function is represented (for the Curry numerals) by an element of A; in particular the application function $n, m \mapsto \varphi_n(m)$. Any representative for this partial function is a realizer for the applicative morphism $n \mapsto \{\bar{n}\}$.

4) This example was first noted in [11]. There is an applicative morphism from $\mathcal{P}(\omega)$ to $\mathcal{K}_2$: for $A \subseteq \mathbb{N}$ let

$$\gamma(A) = \{\alpha \in \mathcal{K}_2 \,|\, \{k \,|\, k + 1 \in \mathrm{im}(\alpha)\} = A\}$$

To see that this is an applicative morphism, recall that in $\mathcal{P}(\omega)$, AB is defined as $\{n \mid \exists k(\langle k, n\rangle \in A \text{ and } e_k \subseteq B)\}$ (see section 1.4.6). Let $F : \mathbb{N}^{\mathbb{N}} \to \mathbb{N}^{\mathbb{N}}$ be the function defined by:

$F(\alpha)(\langle\rangle) = 0$;

$F(\alpha)(\langle n\rangle * \sigma) = 0$ if $\mathrm{lh}(\sigma) < n$;

$F(\alpha)(\langle n\rangle * \sigma) = m + 2$ if $\mathrm{lh}(\sigma) \geq n$ and m is minimal with the properties that (i) there are $i \leq n$ and $k \leq \sum_{j<n} 2^{(\sigma)_j}$ such that $e_k \subset \{(\sigma)_j - 1 \mid j < n, (\sigma)_j > 0\}$ and $\alpha(i) = \langle k, m\rangle + 1$ and (ii) $F(\alpha)(\langle j\rangle * \sigma^{<j}) \neq m + 2$ for all $j < n$;

$F(\alpha)(\langle n\rangle * \sigma) = 1$ if an m as in the previous clause doesn't exist.

Then F is continuous, and by unravelling the definition one finds that for every $\alpha \in \gamma(A)$ and $\beta \in \gamma(B)$, $F(\alpha)(\beta) \in \gamma(AB)$. By Lemma 1.4.1 there is a δ such that $\delta\alpha = F(\alpha)$ for all α; this is the required realizer for γ.

5) There is also an applicative morphism $\iota : \mathcal{K}_2 \to \mathcal{P}(\omega)$. Define $\iota(\alpha) = \{S(\alpha)\}$ where

$$S(\alpha) = \{\sigma \in \mathbb{N} \mid \forall i < \mathrm{lh}(\sigma)\,(\sigma)_i = \alpha(i)\}$$

The reader is invited to check for himself that ι is realizable.

Let us investigate the compositions $\iota\gamma$ and $\gamma\iota$. Since the map $F : \mathcal{K}_2 \to \mathcal{K}_2$ defined by $F(\alpha)(n) = \bar{\alpha}n + 1$ is continuous, there is $\delta \in \mathcal{K}_2$ such that $\delta\alpha = F(\alpha)$ for all α; this means that δ realizes $\mathrm{id}_{\mathcal{K}_2} \preceq \gamma\iota$.

We also have $\gamma\iota \preceq \mathrm{id}_{\mathcal{K}_2}$. There is an element $\varepsilon \in \mathcal{K}_2$ such that for all $\beta \in \mathcal{K}_2$, $\varepsilon\beta(x)$ is defined iff there is an n satisfying $\beta(n) > 0$ and $\mathrm{lh}(\beta(n) - 1) > x$; and $\varepsilon\beta(x)$ is equal to $(\beta(n) - 1)_x$ for the least such n, if it is defined. Then $\gamma\iota \preceq \mathrm{id}_{\mathcal{K}_2}$ is realized by ε.

There is a third inequality which holds: $\iota\gamma \preceq \mathrm{id}_{\mathcal{P}(\omega)}$. Let

$$B = \{\langle k, m\rangle \mid \exists\sigma \in e_k \exists i < \mathrm{lh}(\sigma)\,(\sigma)_i = m + 1\}$$

Then in $\mathcal{P}(\omega)$, if $A = \{k \mid k + 1 \in \mathrm{im}(\alpha)\}$, then $BS(\alpha) = A$. So B realizes $\iota\gamma \preceq \mathrm{id}_{\mathcal{P}(\omega)}$.

However, $\mathrm{id}_{\mathcal{P}(\omega)} \preceq \iota\gamma$ cannot hold; for this to hold we should have
a $B \subseteq \mathbb{N}$ such that for each $A \in \mathcal{P}(\omega)$, BA would equal $S(\alpha)$ for
some α satisfying the equation $A = \{k \mid k+1 \in \mathrm{im}(\alpha)\}$. But there
is no continuous map $\mathcal{P}(\omega) \to \mathcal{P}(\omega)$ which for each A picks such
an $S(\alpha)$ (recall that continuous maps should be monotone).

1.6   Applicative morphisms and S-functors between categories of assemblies

The material in this section is entirely due to Longley and reworked
from [99].

Recall that the categories $\mathrm{Ass}(A)$ come equipped with a pair of functors $\Gamma_A : \mathrm{Ass}(A) \to \mathrm{Set}$ and $\nabla_A : \mathrm{Set} \to \mathrm{Ass}(A)$.

An S-functor $F : \mathrm{Ass}(A) \to \mathrm{Ass}(B)$ is a functor which is the identity
on the level of sets, so $F(X, E) = (X, E')$ for some E'; and $F(f) = f$.
Longley worked with the concept of Γ-functor: this is a functor $F :$
$\mathrm{Ass}(A) \to \mathrm{Ass}(B)$ such that $\Gamma_B \circ F$ is naturally isomorphic to Γ_A. As
the first part of the following proposition shows, it is no real restriction
to work with S-functors.

Proposition 1.6.1   *i)   Every Γ-functor is naturally isomorphic to an
S-functor;*

*ii)   Every natural transformation between two S-functors consists of
identity functions on the level of sets.*

Proof.   (i) If F is a Γ-functor and (X, E) an object of $\mathrm{Ass}(A)$, let
$\iota : \Gamma_A \to \Gamma_B \circ F$ be a natural isomorphism and $\iota_{(X,E)} : X \to \Gamma_B F(X, E)$
its component at (X, E). Then $F(X, E) = (\Gamma_B(X, E), E')$ for some
E'; define $G(X, E) = (X, E' \circ \iota_{(X,E)})$. It is easy to check that G is an
S-functor and that G is naturally isomorphic to F.

(ii) Suppose $\alpha : F \to G$ is a natural transformation between two
S-functors. Let 1 be the one-element set $\{*\}$ and (X, E) an object of
$\mathrm{Ass}(A)$. Every $x \in X$ determines a unique morphism $\hat{x} : \nabla_A(1) \to$
(X, E) which sends the unique element $*$ of 1 to x. Since F and G are
S-functors, $\alpha_{\nabla_A(1)} : 1 \to 1$ is the identity function. Naturality of α now

gives that $\alpha_{(X,E)}(x) = \alpha_{(X,E)}(F(\hat{x})(*)) = G(\hat{x})(*) = x$. So $\alpha_{(X,E)}$ is the identity function on X. ∎

Theorem 1.6.2   *i)   Every applicative morphism $\gamma : A \to B$ gives rise to a regular S-functor $\gamma^* : \mathrm{Ass}(A) \to \mathrm{Ass}(B)$. Moreover, if also $\delta : A \to B$ then $\gamma \preceq \delta$ implies that there is a (necessarily unique) natural transformation from γ^* to δ^*.*

ii)   Every regular S-functor $F : \mathrm{Ass}(A) \to \mathrm{Ass}(B)$ determines an applicative morphism $\tilde{F} : A \to B$. If G is another such functor and there is a natural transformation $F \to G$, then $\tilde{F} \preceq \tilde{G}$.

iii)   For every $\gamma : A \to B$, γ is equal to $\widetilde{(\gamma^*)}$, and for every regular S-functor $F : \mathrm{Ass}(A) \to \mathrm{Ass}(B)$, F is naturally isomorphic to $(\tilde{F})^*$. The assignment $A \mapsto \mathrm{Ass}(A)$, $\gamma \mapsto \gamma^*$ gives therefore an equivalence of 2-categories between PCA and the sub-2-category of Cat consisting of categories of the form $\mathrm{Ass}(A)$, regular S-functors and natural transformations.

Proof.   (i) Define $\gamma^*(X,E)$ as (X,E_γ) where $E_\gamma(x) = \bigcup_{a \in E(x)} \gamma(a)$, and $\gamma(f) = f$. This is well-defined, because if r realizes γ, t tracks $f : (X,E) \to (Y,E')$ and $t' \in \gamma(t)$, then $\langle y \rangle rt'y$ tracks $f : (X,E_\gamma) \to (Y,E'_\gamma)$ in $\mathrm{Ass}(B)$. Clearly, γ^* is an S-functor from $\mathrm{Ass}(A)$ to $\mathrm{Ass}(B)$.

Let us show that γ^* is regular. The assmbly $\gamma^*(\nabla_A(1))$ is isomorphic to $\nabla_B(1)$ because $\gamma(*)$ is nonempty; so γ^* preserves the terminal object. Given two objects (X,E) and (Y,E') in $\mathrm{Ass}(A)$, their product can be given as the object $(X \times Y, E \wedge E')$ where

$$(E \wedge E')(x,y) = \{p_A ab \,|\, a \in E(x),\ b \in E'(y)\}$$

(We denote the respective pairing and projection operators in A and B by subscripts)
We claim that $\gamma^*(X \times Y, E \wedge E')$ is isomorphic to $(X \times Y, E_\gamma \wedge E'_\gamma)$ via the identity map. One direction is obvious since $(X \times Y, E_\gamma \wedge E'_\gamma)$ is a product in $\mathrm{Ass}(B)$; so it remains to prove that the identity on $X \times Y$ is a morphism: $(X \times Y, E_\gamma \wedge E'_\gamma) \to \gamma^*(X \times Y, E \wedge E')$. Let $p' \in \gamma(p_A)$. Then if $b \in (E_\gamma \wedge E'_\gamma)(x,y)$,

$$r(rp'((p_0)_B b)((p_1)_B b) \in (E \wedge E')_\gamma(x,y)$$

which shows that this map is tracked. We conclude that γ^* preserves finite products. By the characterization of equalizers and regular epimorphisms in categories of assemblies in the proof of theorem 1.5.2, it is obvious that they are preserved by γ^*; so γ^* is a regular functor as desired.

Suppose $\gamma \preceq \delta$ is realized by r. Then for each (X, E) in $\mathrm{Ass}(A)$, the identity function on X is tracked by r as a morphism $(X, E_\gamma) \to (X, E_\delta)$ in $\mathrm{Ass}(B)$. Clearly, these identity functions constitute a natural transformation $\gamma^* \to \delta^*$.

(ii) Suppose $F : \mathrm{Ass}(A) \to \mathrm{Ass}(B)$ is a regular S-functor. Consider the A-assemblies $(A, \{\cdot\})$ and (A', E) where $A' = \{(a, a') \in A \times A \,|\, aa'{\downarrow}\}$ and $E(a, a') = \{paa'\}$. Then (A', E) is a regular subobject of $(A, \{\cdot\}) \times (A, \{\cdot\})$. Since F is a regular S-functor, it follows that if $F(A, \{\cdot\}) = (A, \gamma)$, $F(A', E)$ is isomorphic to (A', E'') where $E''(a, a') = \{p_B bb' \,|\, b \in \gamma(a),\, b' \in \gamma(a')\}$. Now the application map $A' \to A$ is a morphism $(A', E) \to (A, \{\cdot\})$ in $\mathrm{Ass}(A)$, so it must also have a tracking in B as a morphism $(A', E'') \to (A, \gamma)$ in $\mathrm{Ass}(B)$. So there is an element $t \in B$ such that for all $a, a' \in A$ with $aa'{\downarrow}$ and all $b \in \gamma(a), b' \in \gamma(a')$, $t(p_B bb') \in \gamma(aa')$. From such a t one easily gets a realizer for γ as applicative morphism $A \to B$. Set $\tilde{F} = \gamma$.

Now suppose $\alpha : F \to G$ is a natural transformation. By proposition 1.6.1 we know that α is the identity on underlying sets, and we therefore have that the identity on A is a map in $\mathrm{Ass}(B)$ from $(A, \tilde{F})$ to $(A, \tilde{G})$. This means exactly (see also the remark following definition 1.5.3) that $\tilde{F} \preceq \tilde{G}$.

(iii) Clearly, $\gamma^*(A, \{\cdot\}) = (A, \gamma)$, so $\widetilde{(\gamma^*)} = \gamma$. It is also evident that for $\gamma : A \to B$ and $\delta : B \to C$, $(\delta\gamma)^* = \delta^* {\circ} \gamma^*$, and that $(\mathrm{id}_A)^*$ is the identity functor on $\mathrm{Ass}(A)$. We have seen that $\gamma \preceq \delta$ gives a natural transformation $\gamma^* \to \delta^*$, and all required identities follow from the fact that between any two S-functors there is at most one natural transformation. So $\gamma \mapsto \gamma^*$ gives a 2-functor $\mathbf{PCA} \to \mathbf{Cat}$. Its image is contained in the sub-2-category of $\mathbf{Cat}$ on objects of the form $\mathrm{Ass}(A)$, 1-cells the regular S-functors, and 2-cells the natural transformations. By (ii), we know that this is a 2-equivalence once we have proved that for every regular S-functor F, we have that F is naturally isomorphic to $(\tilde{F})^*$. To this end, it is useful to prove a lemma:

Lemma 1.6.3 *For every S-functor $F : \mathrm{Ass}(A) \to \mathrm{Ass}(B)$ the functors $F \circ \nabla_A$ and ∇_B are naturally isomorphic.*

Proof. We prove that for every set X the identity on X is a morphism $\nabla_B(X) \to F(\nabla_A(X))$ in $\mathrm{Ass}(B)$. Since it is always a morphism in the other direction, this gives the required natural isomorphism.

Given X, choose a set Y such that $|Y| > |B| \times |X|$ and let $F(\nabla_A(Y))$ be (Y, E). For $b \in B$ let $Y_b = \{y \in Y \mid b \in E(y)\}$. The $Y \subseteq \bigcup_{b \in B} Y_b$ so it follows that there must be a $b \in B$ such that $|Y_b| \geq |X|$. Let $i : X \to Y_b$ be a 1-1 function; then composing with the inclusion $Y_b \subseteq Y$ we get a map $\nabla_B(X) \to (Y, E)$, tracked by $\langle x \rangle b$. Choose a map $j : Y \to X$ such that $j \circ i = \mathrm{id}_X$. j is then a map $\nabla_A(Y) \to \nabla_A(X)$ hence (applying F) also a map $F(\nabla_A(Y)) \to F(\nabla_A(X))$. Composing, we have id_X as a map $\nabla_B(X) \to F(\nabla_A(X))$, as desired. ∎

Continuing the proof of theorem 1.6.2(iii): it follows from lemma 1.6.3 that if $\eta_{(X,E)} : (X, E) \to \nabla_A(X)$ is the unit at (X, E) of the adjunction $\Gamma \dashv \nabla$, then $F(\eta_{(X,E)}) = \eta_{F(X,E)}$, by uniqueness of natural transformations between S-functors.

Let $\gamma = \tilde{F}$. To show: $\gamma^* = F$.

Call a map $f : (X, E) \to (Y, E')$ of assemblies *cartesian* if there is an isomorphism $g : (Y, E') \to (Z, E'')$ such that the composite gf has the property that $E(x) = E''(gf(x))$ for all $x \in X$. It is easy to convince oneself of the fact that f is cartesian if and only if the naturality square

$$
\begin{array}{ccc}
(X, E) & \xrightarrow{\;f\;} & (Y, E') \\
\eta \downarrow & & \downarrow \eta \\
\nabla(X) & \xrightarrow[\nabla(f)]{} & \nabla(Y)
\end{array}
$$

is a pullback. Therefore, every S-functor preserves cartesian maps.

We now consider two special objects of $\mathrm{Ass}(A)$: El is the object $(\{a, S) \mid a \in S \subseteq A\}, E)$ with $E(a, S) = \{a\}$, and D is the object $(\mathcal{P}^*(A), \mathrm{id})$. There are projections $\pi_1 : \mathrm{El} \to (A, \{\cdot\})$ and $\pi_2 : \mathrm{El} \to D$.

Note that π_1 is cartesian and π_2 is regular epi. Since F preserves cartesian maps and is an S-functor, the two squares

$$
\begin{array}{ccc}
F(\mathrm{El}) & \xrightarrow{F(\pi_1)} & F(A,\{\cdot\}) \\
\downarrow{\scriptstyle \eta} & & \downarrow{\scriptstyle \eta} \\
\nabla_B\Gamma_B F(\mathrm{El}) & \xrightarrow{\nabla_B\Gamma_B F(\pi_1)} & \nabla_B(A)
\end{array}
\qquad \text{and} \qquad
\begin{array}{ccc}
\gamma^*(\mathrm{El}) & \xrightarrow{\gamma^*(\pi_1)} & \gamma^*(A,\{\cdot\}) \\
\downarrow{\scriptstyle \eta} & & \downarrow{\scriptstyle \eta} \\
\nabla_B\Gamma_B\gamma^*(\mathrm{El}) & \xrightarrow{\nabla_B\Gamma_B\gamma^*(\pi_1)} & \nabla_B(A)
\end{array}
$$

are pullback squares. But the bottom rows of these diagrams are the same, and $\gamma^*(A,\{\cdot\}) = (A,\gamma) = F(A,\{\cdot\})$ by definition of γ. It follows that $F(\mathrm{El})$ is isomorphic to $\gamma^*(\mathrm{El})$.

Moreover, we have two commutative squares

$$
\begin{array}{ccc}
F(\mathrm{El}) & \xrightarrow{\eta} & \nabla_B\Gamma_B F(\mathrm{El}) \\
\downarrow{\scriptstyle F(\pi_2)} & & \downarrow{\scriptstyle \nabla_B\Gamma_B F(\pi_2)} \\
F(D) & \xrightarrow{\eta} & \nabla_B\Gamma_B F(D)
\end{array}
\qquad \text{and} \qquad
\begin{array}{ccc}
\gamma^*(\mathrm{El}) & \xrightarrow{\eta} & \nabla_B\Gamma_B\gamma^*(\mathrm{El}) \\
\downarrow{\scriptstyle \gamma^*(\pi_2)} & & \downarrow{\scriptstyle \nabla_B\Gamma_B\gamma^*(\pi_2)} \\
\gamma^*(D) & \xrightarrow{\eta} & \nabla_B\Gamma_B\gamma^*(D)
\end{array}
$$

But $\Gamma_B F(D) = \Gamma_A(D) = \Gamma_B\gamma^*(D)$. Since η is always mono, both $F(\pi_2)$ and $\gamma^*(\pi_2)$ are regular epi. From uniqueness of regular epi-mono factorizations in a regular category, it follows that $F(D)$ is isomorphic to $\gamma^*(D)$.

Let now (X,E) be an arbitrary object of $\mathrm{Ass}(A)$. There is a cartesian morphism $E : (X,E) \to D$ sending x to $E(x)$. This gives us pullback squares

$$
\begin{array}{ccc}
F(X,E) & \xrightarrow{F(E)} & F(D) \\
\downarrow{\scriptstyle \eta} & & \downarrow{\scriptstyle \eta} \\
\nabla_B(X) & \xrightarrow{\nabla_B(E)} & \nabla_B(\mathcal{P}^*(A))
\end{array}
\qquad \text{and} \qquad
\begin{array}{ccc}
\gamma^*(X,E) & \xrightarrow{\gamma^*(E)} & \gamma^*(D) \\
\downarrow{\scriptstyle \eta} & & \downarrow{\scriptstyle \eta} \\
\nabla_B(X) & \xrightarrow{\nabla_B(E)} & \nabla_B(D)
\end{array}
$$

Since $F(D)$ is isomorphic tp $\gamma^*(D)$, we see that $F(X,E) \cong \gamma^*(X,E)$. The isomorphism is natural (it is the identity on underlying sets), so this completes the proof. ∎

1.7 Decidable applicative morphisms and adjoining partial functions to a pca

Let us write T for the Boolean *true*, which is k, and F for *false*$=\bar{k}$. The following definition is also due to Longley.

Definition 1.7.1 Let A and B be pcas with Booleans $\mathsf{T}_A, \mathsf{F}_A$ in A and $\mathsf{T}_B, \mathsf{F}_B$ in B. An applicative morphism $\gamma : A \to B$ is *decidable* if there is an element d in B (a *decider* for γ) which is such that for every $a \in \gamma(\mathsf{T}_A)$, $da\downarrow$ and $da = \mathsf{T}_B$, and for every $a \in \gamma(\mathsf{F}_A)$, $da\downarrow$ and $da = \mathsf{F}_B$.

The name 'decidable' is not very well chosen; a better name would be 'decision-preserving', because an applicative morphism satisfying definition 1.7.1 does not make A decidable in B (for any sensible interpretation of what this might mean); rather, it means that whatever is decidable in A remains so in B. This is articulated in the following theorem by Longley:

Theorem 1.7.2 *An applicative morphism $\gamma : A \to B$ is decidable if and only if the corresponding regular S-functor $\gamma^* : \mathrm{Ass}(A) \to \mathrm{Ass}(B)$ preserves binary coproducts. Moreover this is equivalent to: γ^* preserves the natural numbers object.*

Let us note the following immediate corollary of this theorem:

Corollary 1.7.3 *If $\delta = \gamma\zeta$ is a commutative triangle of applicative morphisms such that δ and ζ are decidable, then so is γ.*

The purpose of this section is to prove that the pca $\mathcal{K}_1^F$ of 'partial recursive application in F', where F is a partial function on the natural numbers, is an example of a construction that can be applied to arbitrary pcas. In order to formulate it properly, we employ the notions of decidable applicative morphism and the idea of a partial function f on A being *representable* w.r.t. an applicative morphism $\gamma : A \to B$, as in the following definition.

Definition 1.7.4 Let $\gamma : A \to B$ be an applicative morphism of pcas and $f : A \rightharpoonup A$ a partial function. We say that f is *representable* w.r.t. γ if there is an element $r_f \in B$ such that for every $a \in \mathrm{dom}(f)$ and every $b \in \gamma(a)$, $r_f b \downarrow$ and $r_f b \in \gamma(f(a))$. We say that f is representable in A if f is representable w.r.t. the identity morphism on A.

The representability of f with respect to γ can also be seen as follows: let $(\mathrm{dom}(f), \gamma)$ be the regular sub-assembly of (A, γ) (as assemblies on B). Then f is representable with respect to γ if and only if f is a map of assemblies: $(\mathrm{dom}(f), \gamma) \to (A, \gamma)$.

Theorem 1.7.5 *For every pca A and every partial endofunction f on A there exist a pca $A[f]$ and a decidable applicative morphism $\iota_f : A \to A[f]$ with the following properties:*

i) f *is representable w.r.t.* ι_f;

ii) *for every decidable applicative morphism $\gamma : A \to B$ such that f is representable w.r.t. γ, there is a decidable applicative morphism $\gamma_f : A[f] \to B$ such that $\gamma_f \iota_f = \gamma$, and γ_f is unique with this property. Moreover, if $\delta : A[f] \to B$ is such that $\delta \iota_f \cong \gamma$, then $\delta \cong \gamma_f$*

Proof. For the construction of $A[f]$, let's agree on some notation for codes of finite sequences (see also subsection 1.3.1): if $u = [u_0, \ldots, u_{n-1}]$ and $i < n$, $u^{<i}$ denotes $[u_0, \ldots, u_{i-1}]$ and $u^{\geq i}$ denotes $[u_i, \ldots, u_{n-1}]$; for $i \leq j < n$, $^i\!\leq\!u^{<j}$ denotes $[u_i, \ldots, u_{j-1}]$. If $u = [u_0, \ldots, u_{n-1}]$ and $v = [v_0, \ldots, v_{m-1}]$, we write $u * v$ for $[u_0, \ldots, u_{n-1}, v_0, \ldots, v_{m-1}]$. Let Not be an element of A such that $\mathsf{NotT} = \mathsf{F}$ and $\mathsf{NotF} = \mathsf{T}$.

The underlying set of $A[f]$ will be A. We define a new application $\cdot^f$ on A as follows. For $a, b \in A$, an *f-dialogue* between a and b is a code of a sequence $u = [u_0, \ldots, u_{n-1}]$ such that for all $i < n$ there is a $v_i \in A$ such that

$$a \cdot ([b] * u^{<i}) = p\mathsf{F}v_i \text{ and } f(v_i) = u_i$$

We say that $a \cdot^f b$ is defined with value c, if there is an f-dialogue u between a and b such that

$$a \cdot ([b] * u) = p\mathsf{T}c$$

We show first, that $(A, \cdot^f)$ is a pca.

Let $K_f = \langle x \rangle p\mathsf{T}(\langle y \rangle p\mathsf{T}x_0)$. Then clearly $K_f \cdot^f a = \langle y \rangle p\mathsf{T}a$ for all $a \in A$, so $(K_f \cdot^f a) \cdot^f b = a$ for all $a, b \in A$.

For the element S_f, by primitive recursion it is possible to construct a term $t(x, y)$ of A such that for all u, the application $t(x, y) \cdot u$ is given by the following instructions:
$t(x, y) \cdot u =$

> xu if $\forall i \leq \mathsf{lh}u \; \mathsf{Not}(p_0(xu^{<i}))$.
>
> If i is minimal such that $p_0(xu^{<i})$, let $\alpha = p_1(xu^{<i})$ and output $y([u_0] * u^{\geq i})$ if $\forall j(i \leq j < \mathsf{lh}u \to \mathsf{Not}p_0(y([u_0] *^{i \leq} u^{<j})))$.
>
> If j is minimal such that $p_0(y([u_0] *^{i \leq} u^{<j}))$, let $\beta = p_1(y([u_0] *^{i \leq} u^{<j}))$ and output $\alpha([\beta] * u^{\geq j})$ if $\forall k(j \leq k < \mathsf{lh}u \to \mathsf{Not}(p_0(\alpha([\beta] *^{j \leq} u^{<k}))))$.
>
> If k is minimal such that $(p_0(\alpha([\beta] *^{j \leq} u^{<k})))$, output $(p_1(\alpha([\beta] *^{j \leq} u^{<k})))$.

Note, that $t(a, b) \cdot^f c \simeq (a \cdot^f c) \cdot^f (b \cdot^f c)$ for all a, b, c. Therefore, let

$$S_f = \langle x \rangle p\mathsf{T}(\langle y \rangle p\mathsf{T}t(x_0, y_0))$$

Then $(S_f \cdot^f a) \cdot^f b = t(a, b)$ for all a and b. This establishes $A[f]$ as a pca.

Note that the combinators K_f and S_f don't really depend on f. This is analogous to the fact that for a coding of Turing machine computations with oracle U, the S_n^m-functions are primitive recursive, and do not depend on U.

The map $\iota_f : A \to A[f]$ given by $a \mapsto \{a\}$ is an applicative morphism $A \to A[f]$. Indeed, if $ab = c$ then $(\langle x \rangle p\mathsf{T}(ax_0)) \cdot^f b = c$; so if $r = \langle yx \rangle p\mathsf{T}(y_0x_0)$ then r realizes ι_f.

The decidability of ι_f is left to the reader.

For the universal property, suppose $\gamma : A \to B$ is a decidable applicative morphism which is realized by r and let d be a decider for γ. Moreover suppose that $\overline{f}$ represents f w.r.t. γ.

Let $\pi_0, \pi_1 \in B$ be such that if $b \in \gamma(a)$ then $\pi_i b \in \gamma(p_i a)$. Similarly, let C and C' in B be such that if $b \in \gamma(a)$ and $v \in \gamma(u)$ then $Cbv \in \gamma([a] * u)$ and $C'bv \in \gamma(u * [a])$.

Now use the fixed point theorem in B to find an element U such that for all b, b', v:

$$
\begin{aligned}
Ubb'v \quad \simeq \quad &\text{If } d(\pi_0(rb(Cb'v))) \\
&\text{then } \pi_1(rb(Cb'v)) \\
&\text{else } Ubb'(C'(\overline{f}(\pi_1(rb(Cb'v)))))v)
\end{aligned}
$$

The reader can check the following: suppose u is an f-dialogue between a and a' in A, $b \in \gamma(a), b' \in \gamma(a')$, $i < \mathsf{lh}u$, $v \in \gamma(u^{<i})$ and $w = C'(\overline{f}(\pi_1(rb(Cb'v))))v$. Then $w \in \gamma(u^{\le i})$ and $Ubb'v = Ubb'w$. Furthermore, if u is such that $a([a'] * u) = p\top c$, then $Ubb'v \in \gamma(c)$.

Therefore, choose $e \in \gamma([\,])$ and let

$$
\rho = \langle xx' \rangle Uxx'e
$$

Then ρ realizes γ as applicative morphism: $A[f] \to B$. We denote this last morphism by γ_f.

Obviously, the diagram

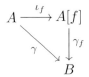

commutes on the nose. Moreover, since $\iota_f(a) = \{a\}$, if $\delta : A[f] \to B$ were such that $\delta\iota_f \cong \gamma_f\iota_f$, then $\delta \cong \gamma_f$. So γ_f is unique with respect to the property that the diagram commutes on the nose, and essentially unique with respect to the property that it commutes up to isomorphism. The decidability of γ_f is a direct consequence of Corollary 1.7.3 and can also be verified directly. ∎

Corollary 1.7.6

i)   *If f is representable in A, then A and $A[f]$ are isomorphic pcas.*

ii)   *If f and g are two partial endofunctions on A, the pcas $A[f][g]$ and $A[g][f]$ are isomorphic; we may therefore write $A[f, g]$.*

iii)   *If $f : \mathbb{N} \to \mathbb{N}$ is a partial function, then $\mathcal{K}_1^f$ is isomorphic to $\mathcal{K}_1[f]$.*

iv) *Every total pca is isomorphic to a nontotal one.*

v) *Every extensional pca is isomorphic to a non-extensional one.*

Proof. The first two statements are immediate from the uniqueness statement in theorem 1.7.5. The third statement is easy.

The fourth statement follows from the fact that $A[f]$ is never total (the element $a = \Lambda^*x.p\bot\bot$ is such that $a \cdot^f b$ is never defined), so if A is total and f is representable in A, then $A \cong A[f]$ by i), so A is isomorphic to the nontotal pca $A[f]$.

For the last statement, let A be extensional. Take any element $a \in A$ and let f be the partial function realized by a. Let α and β be elements of A such that for each u:

$$\begin{aligned} \alpha u &\simeq \mathsf{p}\mathsf{T}(au_0) \\ \beta u &\simeq \mathsf{If}(\mathsf{lh}(u) \leq 1)(\mathsf{p}\mathsf{F}u_0)\mathsf{else}(\mathsf{p}\mathsf{T}u_1) \end{aligned}$$

Then $\alpha[b] \simeq \mathsf{p}\mathsf{T}(ab)$ and $\beta[b] \simeq \mathsf{p}\mathsf{F}b$, so α and β are different elements of A, hence in $A[f]$. But both α and β represent f in $A[f]$, so $A[f]$ is not extensional. But $A[f]$ is isomorphic to A, since f is representable in A. ■

Remarks

1. The construction of $A[f]$ induces a preorder on the set of partial endofunctions of A, which generalizes Turing degrees: let $f \leq_A g$ if and only if f is representable in $A[g]$ (with respect to ι_g). Since the diagram

$$\begin{array}{ccc} A & \longrightarrow & A[g] \\ \downarrow & & \downarrow \\ A[h] & \longrightarrow & A[g,h] \end{array}$$

commutes, it is easy to see that $\leq_A$ is a transitive relation (it is reflexive by Theorem 1.7.5(i)): suppose $f \leq_A g$ and $g \leq_A h$. Then the bottom arrow in the diagram is an isomorphism and the top arrow factors through $\iota_f : A \to A[f]$. It follows that also the map $A \to A[h]$ factors through ι_f; that is, $f \leq_A h$.

2. There is a universal solution to the problem of "making A decidable"; adjoin a function f to A where

$$f(x) = \begin{cases} \top & \text{if } p_0 x = p_1 x \\ \bot & \text{else} \end{cases}$$

3. Every way of organizing mathematical structures into a category, imposes a view on the study of these structures. The properties worth studying must, from this point of view, at least be stable under isomorphism. For example, a definition of 'topology' could be that it studies those properties of spaces which are invariant under homeomorphism. Once we have committed ourselves to Longley's category of applicative morphisms, it follows that 'totality' and 'extensionality' are not really properties of pcas.

1.8   Order-pcas

In this section we discuss a generalization of the notion of pca which was introduced in [171] under the name "$\leq$-pca". A further development appeared in [69], where the structures were called "ordered pcas". However, as we have seen, many pcas have a partial order structure, but for "ordered pcas" the essential feature is that the pca-axioms hold only 'up to order'. Therefore I now believe that the name 'order-pca' is the most appropriate.

Definition 1.8.1 An *order-pas* is a poset $(A, \leq)$ together with a partial map $A \times A \to A$ (written as $(a, b) \mapsto ab$, as before) such that if $ab\downarrow$, $a' \leq a$ and $b' \leq b$ hold, then $a'b'\downarrow$ and $a'b' \leq ab$.

Definition 1.8.2 An order-pas A is called *weakly combinatory complete* if for every term $t(x_1, \ldots, x_n)$ there is an element $a \in A$ such that for every $n + 1$-tuple $a_1, \ldots, a_n$ of elements of A the following statements hold:

i) $aa_1 \cdots a_n\downarrow$

ii)   If $t(a_1, \ldots, a_{n+1})\!\downarrow$ then $aa_1 \cdots a_{n+1}\!\downarrow$ and

$$aa_1 \cdots a_{n+1} \leq t(a_1, \ldots, a_{n+1})$$

Definition 1.8.3 An *order-pca* is weakly combinatory complete order-pas.

The following analogue of Theorem 1.1.3 is straightforward.

Theorem 1.8.4 *Let A be an order-pas. Then A is an order-pca if and only if there are elements k and s in A such that for all $a, b, c \in A$ the following hold:*

i) $sab\!\downarrow$

ii) $kab \leq a$

iii)   *If $ac(bc)\!\downarrow$ then $sabc\!\downarrow$ and $sabc \leq ac(bc)$*

Examples of order-pcas.

1. Of course, every pca is an order-pca with the discrete order. Conversely, an order-pca whose underlying order is discrete is a pca if and only if for every a, b, c: if $sabc\!\downarrow$, then $ac(bc)\!\downarrow$.

2. The original motivating example for the definition was the following: suppose A is a pca. We can define an application map on $\mathcal{P}(A)$ in the following way: for $\alpha, \beta \subseteq A$, say that $\alpha\beta = \{ab \mid a \in \alpha, b \in \beta\}$ if for all $a \in \alpha$ and $b \in \beta$, $ab\!\downarrow$; otherwise, $\alpha\beta$ is undefined.

    Now $\mathcal{P}(A)$ is not a pca with this application map, but if k and s satisfy Theorem 1.1.3 for A, then $\{k\}$ abd $\{s\}$ satisfy Theorem 1.8.4 for $\mathcal{P}(A)$, where $\leq$ is taken to be inclusion between subsets of A.

    You are invited to check for yourself that in this example, $sabc\!\downarrow$ does *not* always imply that $ac(bc)\!\downarrow$.

    Instead of $\mathcal{P}(A)$, one can also take $\mathcal{P}^*(A)$, the set of nonempty subsets of A, or the set of nonempty, finite subsets of A.

3. Any meet-semilattice $(A, \wedge)$ is an order-pca if $\wedge$ is taken as the application map; in fact, any element of A serves both as k and as s. This example shows that Proposition 1.3.1 fails for order-pcas.

4. Given any pas A, one can add an extra element $\bot$, define an order on $A \cup \{\bot\}$ by putting $x \leq y$ iff $x = y$ or $x = \bot$, and extend the application map by putting $\bot y = \bot$. Then $\bot$ serves as k and s.

5. Combining examples 1) and 3): if A is a pca and $(P, \wedge)$ is a semilattice, consider the product $A \times P$ with the pointwise order (A considered with the discrete order). Let $(a,p)(b,q)$ be defined just when $ab{\downarrow}$ in A; in that case, $(a,p)(b,q) = (ab, p \wedge q)$. Actually this is an example of a *product* of order-pcas.

6. Given a pca A, choose k and s in A satisfying 1.1.3. Define a reduction relation $\rightsquigarrow$ on the set $E(A)^c$ of closed terms over A by the clauses:

$$
\begin{array}{llll}
(ab) & \rightsquigarrow & c & \text{if } a, b \in A \text{ and } ab = c \\
(uv) & \rightsquigarrow & (u'v') & \text{if } u \rightsquigarrow u' \text{ and } v \rightsquigarrow v' \\
((ku)v) & \rightsquigarrow & u & \\
(((su)v)w) & \rightsquigarrow & ((uw)(vw)) &
\end{array}
$$

If $\leq$ is the reflexive-transitive closure of the relation $\rightsquigarrow$, and $u \sim v$ iff $u \leq v$ and $v \leq u$, then the quotient $E(A)^c/\sim$ is an order-pca with application $[u][v] = [uv]$, and order $\leq$. Note that the application map is total.

There is an inclusion $i : A \rightarrow E(A)^c/\sim$ by $i(a) = [a]$. Note that i does not necessarily preserve application, but if $ab{\downarrow}$, then $i(a)i(b) \leq i(ab)$.

Let A be an order-pca. There is an analogon of the $\mathcal{P}(A)$-valued predicates of section 1.2. Instead of $\mathcal{P}(A)$, we now take the set $\mathcal{T}(A)$ of downwards closed subsets of A (i.e. those subsets $B \subseteq A$ such that if $b' \leq b$ and $b \in B$, then $b' \in B$). For $\varphi, \psi \in \mathcal{T}(A)^X$ we define the relation $\varphi \leq \psi$ exactly as in 1.2, and we have the corresponding theorem:

Theorem 1.8.5 *If A is an order-pca, then the set $\mathcal{T}(A)^X$, together with the relation $\leq$, is a preordered set whose poset reflection is a Heyting algebra.*

Apart from this, most of the theory of pcas remains valid for order-pcas, provided order is introduced instead of equality. Let us replace the relation $\simeq$ between closed terms by a relation $\preceq$:

$t \preceq s$ means that whenever $s{\downarrow}$, then $t{\downarrow}$ and $t \leq s$.

The property of weak combinatory completeness can then be stated in the following way: for every term $t(\vec{a}, x)$ there is an element $\langle x \rangle t(\vec{a}, x)$ such that for each b, $(\langle x \rangle t(\vec{a}, x))b \preceq t(\vec{a}, b)$.

By a straightfoward adaptation of the methods of section 1.3, we have:

Proposition 1.8.6 (Fixed Points) *There are elements $y, z \in A$ such that:*

i) $yf \preceq f(yf)$

ii) $zf{\downarrow}$ *and* $zfa \preceq f(zf)a$

If we define the Curry numerals $\bar{n}$ just as for pcas, we also obtain

Proposition 1.8.7 (Primitive Recursion) *There is $R \in A$ such that*

i) $Raf\bar{0} \leq a$

ii) $Raf(\overline{n+1}) \preceq f\bar{n}(Raf\bar{n})$

Proposition 1.8.8 *For every partial recursive function F there is an element a_F of A such that, if $f(n_1, \dots, n_k)$ is defined,*

$$a_F \overline{n_1} \cdots \overline{n_k} \leq \overline{F(n_1, \dots, n_k)}$$

We call an order-pca A *trivial* if there is a least element $\perp$ in A. In that case, we necessarily have $\perp a = \perp$ for every $a \in A$, since $\perp a \leq k \perp a \leq \perp$. The reason for calling such A trivial is, that in this case the preorder $\mathcal{T}(A)^X$ is equivalent to 2^X; that is, A induces the same predicates as the trivial pca.

Once we have defined a suitable 2-category of order-pcas, we shall see that an order-pca is trivial if and only if it is equivalent to a one-element (order-)pca.

Of the list of examples, if A is a pca then $\mathcal{P}(A)$ is a trivial order-pca; but if A has more than one element, then $\mathcal{P}^*(A)$ is nontrivial. A meet-semilattice is nontrivial if there is no least element. However, it has a feature in common with trivial order-pcas: it has an element which serves both as k ands s. Such order-pcas will be called *pseudo-trivial.* We define a 2-category similar to Longley's for pcas.

Definition 1.8.9 Let A and B be order-pcas. An *applicative morphism* is a function $f : A \to B$ such that the following two conditions hold:

i)   there exists an element $r \in B$ such that for every $a, a' \in A$: if $aa'\downarrow$ then $rf(a)f(a')\downarrow$ and $rf(a)f(a') \leq f(aa')$.

ii)   there exists an element $u \in B$ such that for every $a, a' \in A$: if $a \leq a'$ then $uf(a)\downarrow$ and $uf(a) \leq f(a')$.

Given two applicative morphisms f and g from A to B we say that $f \leq g$ if there is $b \in B$ such that for all $a \in A$, $bf(a)\downarrow$ and $bf(a) \leq g(a)$.

In order to see that these applicative morphisms compose, suppose that $f : A \to B$ is realized by r and u (satisfying i) and ii) of definition 1.8.9, respectively) and $g : B \to C$ by s and v, define t and w in C by

$$
\begin{aligned}
t &\equiv \langle xy \rangle v(s(sg(r)x)y) \\
w &\equiv \langle x \rangle v(sg(u)x)
\end{aligned}
$$

Then $gf : A \to C$ is realized by t and w, as you can check for yourself.

It is easy to see that the relation $\leq$ between applicative morphisms with the same domain and codomain is a preorder, and that composition of applicative morphisms is order-preserving. Hence, we have a preorder-enriched category which we shall denote by OPCA^+.

In OPCA^+, the one-element pca $1 = \{*\}$ is clearly a terminal object. It is also pseudo-initial: this means that for any order-pca A there is an applicative morphism $1 \to A$, and this applicative morphism is unique up to isomorphism. Indeed, pick an arbitrary $a \in A$ and define $f_a(*) = a$.

Since $kf_a(*)f_a(*) \leq f_a(*)$, k realizes the first requirement for f_a to be applicative; the second one is realized by $i = skk$. And clearly, for any $a, b \in A$, $f_a \leq f_b$ holds.

It is easy to see that if A is a trivial order-pca, then A is equivalent in OPCA$^+$ to the one-element pca 1 via the unique map $! : A \to 1$ and the map $f_\perp : 1 \to A$. Conversely, if $g : 1 \to A$ is part of an equivalence, then we must have $g\circ! \leq \mathrm{id}_A$. So there must be $\rho \in A$ such that for all $a \in A$,

$$\rho(g(*)) \leq a$$

That is, $\rho(g(*))$ is a bottom element of A.

Now suppose that A and B are pcas and $f : A \to B$ is an applicative morphism in Longley's sense (the sense of definition 1.5.3). Then f is a function $A \to \mathcal{P}^*(B)$ and actually, as such, an applicative morphism of order-pcas. This can be expressed in a more elegant way. If A is an order-pca, let $T(A)$ consist of the nonempty, downward closed subsets of A. For two such downsets α, β, we say that $\alpha\beta$ is defined if for all $a \in \alpha$ and $b \in \beta$, $ab\downarrow$ in A; in that case, let $\alpha\beta$ be the downward closure of the set $\{ab \,|\, a \in \alpha, b \in \beta\}$. With the inclusion ordering, $T(A)$ becomes an order-pca. Note that $T(A)$ is trivial precisely when A is trivial.

Proposition 1.8.10 *The operation T on order-pcas has the structure of a 2-monad on the 2-category* OPCA$^+$. *The full sub-2-category of the Kleisli 2-category of this monad on those objects which are pcas, is isomorphic to Longley's 2-category of pcas and applicative morphisms.*

Proof. This was noted in [69]. It is completely straightforward. ∎

Next, we discuss another 2-category of order-pcas: a subcategory of OPCA$^+$. For motivation, let us first extend the definition of assemblies (1.5.1) to the context of order-pcas: if A is an order-pca, an assembly on A is a pair (X, E) where X is a set and E is a function $X \to T(A)$. A morphism of assemblies $(X, E) \to (Y, F)$ on A is a function $f : X \to Y$ for which there exists a tracking, just as in definition 1.5.1.

Theorem 1.6.2 extends to the context of order-pcas, applicative morphisms, and assemblies on order-pcas. This is a routine verification; the only changes that have to be made in the proof are the introduction of some downward closures; e.g. instead of $(A, \{\cdot\})$ we now take

$(A, \downarrow\{\cdot\})$ where the notation $\downarrow\alpha$ stands for the downward closure of a subset $\alpha \subset A$.

Later on, we shall be interested in those regular S-functors which have right adjoints which are also S-functors. For our purposes, it seems most useful to express this in terms of *triposes*, see section 2.5.3.

Definition 1.8.11 Let $f : A \to B$ be an applicative morphism of order-pcas. Then f is called *computationally dense* (cd) if there exists an element $m \in B$ satisfying the following condition:

(cd) $\forall b \in B \exists a \in A \forall a' \in A (b \cdot f(a') \downarrow \Rightarrow aa' \downarrow \land m \cdot f(aa') \leq b \cdot f(a'))$

Roughly, computational density means that computations in B on data from A can, up to order and up to a realizer, already be done in A. Obviously, the identity map on every order-pca is computationally dense; and it is not hard to verify that the cd maps are closed under composition.

We denote by OPCA the 2-category of order-pcas, computationally dense morphisms and inequalities between them. The 2-monad T from proposition 1.8.10 restricts to OPCA, since the components of the natural transformations which make up the monad structure are all computationally dense, and the action of T on morphisms preserves computational density.

Examples of computationally dense morphisms.

1. The unique morphism $A \to 1$ is computationally dense, as is easy to verify.

2. Suppose $\iota : A \to B$ is an applicative morphism of pcas that has a right adjoint $\gamma : B \to A$. Then, considered as map of order-pcas $A \to T(B)$, ι is computationally dense. Let us show this:

   Choose realizers s for γ, t for the inequality $\iota\gamma \preceq \mathrm{id}_B$, and u for the inequality $\mathrm{id}_A \preceq \gamma\iota$.

   We take t for m in (cd). That is, we show that for every $\beta \in T(B)$ there is an $a \in A$ such that

   $(*)$ $\forall a' \in A[\beta(\iota(a'))\downarrow \Rightarrow aa' \downarrow \land t(\iota(aa')) \subseteq \beta(\iota(a'))]$

Given β, let b be any element of $\gamma(\beta) = \bigcup_{b' \in \beta} \gamma(b')$, and put $a \equiv \langle v \rangle sb(uv)$.

Suppose $\beta(\iota(a'))\!\downarrow$. Applying γ we find that

$$s\gamma(\beta)\gamma\iota(a')\!\downarrow \wedge s\gamma(\beta)\gamma\iota(a') \subseteq \gamma(\beta(\iota(a')))$$

so in particular $aa' = sb(ua') \in \gamma(\beta(\iota(a')))$.

Applying ι we see that $\iota(aa') \subseteq \iota\gamma(\beta(\iota(a')))$, hence by choice of t,

$$t(\iota(aa')) \subseteq \beta(\iota(a'))$$

as desired.

3. The applicative morphism $\iota_f : A \to A[f]$ from theorem 1.7.5 is computationally dense. Let m be an element of A such that for every $y \in A$ and every code of a sequence v, $m([y] * v) \simeq yv$.

Given $b \in A$, let $a \in A$ be such that for all $a' \in A$, $aa' \simeq \langle v \rangle b([a'] * v)$. Then aa' is always defined. Moreover,

$$m([aa'] * v) \simeq (aa')v \simeq b([a'] * v)$$

It follows that $m \cdot^f (aa') \simeq b \cdot^f a'$ in $A[f]$.

Chapter 2

Realizability triposes and toposes

2.1 Triposes

In 1979, Martin Hyland discovered the effective topos. The construction was similar to a presentation of the category of sheaves on a complete Heyting algebra that had been given by Dennis Higgs ([64, 65]). Higgs had shown that this category was equivalent to the category of "H-valued sets" for a complete Heyting algebra H (see also [44] for a good exposition). It was Andy Pitts who discovered a common generalization of the two constructions, the notion of a *tripos*, and he laid down its theory in his thesis ([123]). Part of the theory (and restricted to the case where the base category is Set) also appeared in [74]. Most of the material in this chapter is due to Pitts and taken from his thesis.

2.1.1 Preorder-enriched categories

This subsection serves mainly to establish some terminology we shall employ regarding preorder-enriched categories. Although we have already used the term 'preorder-enriched' before (proposition 1.5.4), let us give a definition: A *preorder-enriched category* is a category C together with, for each pair A, B of objects of C, a preorder-structure on the set of arrows $C(A, B)$, such that for every triple A, B, C of objects of C the composition map

$$C(A, B) \times C(B, C) \to C(A, C)$$

is order-preserving.

The paradigmatic example is, of course, the category Preord of pre-ordered sets, where the order on the arrows is taken point-wise. In fact, this category plays the role that the category Set plays in the non-enriched setting. Note that in particular every category in the ordinary sense is preorder-enriched with the discrete ordering.

For many notions of category theory, there is a corresponding 'pseudo' notion in the preorder-enriched case, where roughly 'pseudo' means 'up to isomorphism of arrows'. We have already met the term 'pseudo-initial object': in a preorder-enriched category, an object I is pseudo-initial if for any object Y, there is an arrow $I \to Y$ and moreover all arrows $I \to Y$ are isomorphic. In a similar way, we have pseudo-terminal objects, pseudo-limits and so on.

For a pair of arrows $X \xrightarrow{f} Y$, $Y \xrightarrow{g} X$ in a preorder-enriched category we say that f is left adjoint to g (g is right adjoint to f) if $\mathrm{id}_X \leq gf$ and $fg \leq \mathrm{id}_Y$.

Suppose C and D are preorder-enriched categories; a *pseudofunctor* $F : C \to D$ maps objects X of C to objects $F(X)$ of D, arrows $f : X \to Y$ in C to arrows $F(f) : F(X) \to F(Y)$ in D such that the resulting operation: $C(X, Y) \to D(F(X), F(Y))$ is order-preserving, and moreover satisfies the conditions that for each object X of C, $F(\mathrm{id}_X)$ is isomorphic to $\mathrm{id}_{F(X)}$, and for any two composable arrows f, g in C, $F(gf)$ is isomorphic to $F(g)F(f)$.

If a pseudofunctor is a real functor, we shall speak of an *enriched functor*.

Now suppose F and G are pseudofunctors $C \to D$. A *pseudo-natural transformation* $\Phi : F \Rightarrow G$ assigns to any object X of C an arrow $\Phi_X : F(X) \to G(X)$ in D in such a way, that for every arrow $f : X \to Y$ in C the composites $G(f) \circ \Phi_X$ and $\Phi_Y \circ F(f)$ are isomorphic arrows in D.

The following example of a preordered category is also one we have
already met.

Definition 2.1.1 A *Heyting prealgebra* is a preorder whose poset reflection is a Heyting algebra. That is, considered as a category it is
cartesian closed and has finite coproducts.

A *morphism* of Heyting prealgebras is a functor which preserves
all this structure. Equivalently, it is a map of preorders whose poset
reflection is a Heyting homomorphism.

Clearly, there is a preorder-enriched category Heytpre of Heyting prealgebras, where morphisms $G \to H$ are ordered pointwise.

2.1.2   Triposes: definition and basic properties

Definition 2.1.2 Let C be a category with finite products. A C-*tripos*
P is a pseudofunctor from C^{op} to Heytpre satisfying the following conditions:

i) For every morphism $f : X \to Y$ of C the map $P(f) : P(Y) \to P(X)$
    has both a left adjoint $\exists_f$ and a right adjoint $\forall_f$ in Preord. More-
    over these adjoints satisfy the so-called *Beck-Chevalley condition*:
    if

$$
\begin{array}{ccc}
X & \xrightarrow{\ f\ } & Y \\
g \downarrow & & \downarrow h \\
Z & \xrightarrow[\ k\ ]{} & W
\end{array}
$$

is a pullback square in C, then the composite maps of preorders
$\forall_f \circ P(g)$ and $P(h) \circ \forall_k$ are isomorphic.

ii) For every object X of C there is an object $\pi(X)$ of C and an
    element $\in_X$ of $P(X \times \pi(X))$ with the following property:

    for every object Y of C and every element ϕ of $P(X \times Y)$, there
    is a morphism $\{\phi\} : Y \to \pi(X)$ in C such that in $P(X \times Y)$, ϕ
    is isomorphic to $P(\mathrm{id}_X \times \{\phi\})(\in_X)$. The element $\in_X$ is called a
    membership predicate for X in P.

Given two C-triposes P and Q, a *transformation* is a pseudo-natural transformation $\Phi : P \Rightarrow Q$ where both P and Q are considered as pseudofunctors $C \rightarrow Preord$ (that is, Φ_X is just an order-preserving map, not necessarily a morphism of Heyting algebras). There is an obvious point-wise ordering on transformations ($\Phi \leq \Psi$ iff for each X, $\Phi_X \leq \Psi_X$ pointwise), so C-triposes and transformations form a preorder-enriched category C-Trip.

Remarks

1. Let me reiterate that the left and right adjoints $\exists_f$ and $\forall_f$ are not required to be morphisms of Heyting prealgebras; they are just order-preserving maps.

2. The Beck-Chevalley condition implies a similar condition for $\exists_f$ and $\exists_k$, which is seen by taking left adjoints of both composites.

3. Condition ii) in definition 2.1.2 can often be simplified. If the category C is cartesian closed (which will be the case in almost all our examples), it is equivalent to the following statement:

   ii)$'$ There is a *generic element* in P, that is: there is an object Σ of C and an element σ of $P(\Sigma)$ such that for every object X of C and every $\phi \in P(X)$ there is a morphism $[\phi] : X \rightarrow \Sigma$ such that ϕ and $P([\phi])(\sigma)$ are isomorphic elements of $P(X)$.

   To see that ii) implies ii)$'$: let $\Sigma = \pi(1)$, where 1 is the terminal object of C, and let $\sigma \in P(\pi(1))$ correspond to $\in_1 \in P(1 \times \pi(1))$ under the isomorphism between these two Heyting prealgebras.

   For the converse implication in the case that C is cartesian closed, suppose that σ and Σ are as in ii)$'$. For an object X, form the exponential Σ^X and consider the canonical map ev : $X \times \Sigma^X \rightarrow \Sigma$. Let $\pi(X) = \Sigma^X$, and let $\in_X \in P(X \times \Sigma^X)$ be $P(\mathrm{ev})(\sigma)$.

   If $\phi \in P(X \times Y)$, choose $[\phi] : X \times Y \rightarrow \Sigma$ as in ii)$'$, such that ϕ is isomorphic to $P([\phi])(\sigma)$. By cartesian closure, $[\phi]$ transposes to a map $\widetilde{[\phi]} : Y \rightarrow \Sigma^X$, and $\mathrm{ev} \circ (\mathrm{id}_X \times \widetilde{[\phi]}) = [\phi]$. So if $\{\phi\}$ is defined as $\widetilde{[\phi]}$, then by pseudofunctoriality we have that $P(\mathrm{id}_X \times \{\phi\})(\in_X)$, which is $P(\mathrm{id}_X \times \{\phi\})(P(\mathrm{ev})(\sigma))$, is isomorphic to $P(\mathrm{ev} \circ (\mathrm{id}_X \times \{\phi\}))(\sigma)$, which is $P([\phi])(\sigma)$, which is ϕ as desired.

4. If P and Q are C-triposes and $\sigma \in P(\Sigma)$ is a generic element for P, then clearly for every transformation $\Phi : P \Rightarrow Q$ we have that for any $\phi \in P(X)$, $\Phi_X(\phi)$ is isomorphic to $Q([\phi])(\Phi_\Sigma(\sigma))$; that is, up to isomorphism Φ is determined by $\Phi_\Sigma(\sigma) \in Q(\Sigma)$. We see that the category C-Trip is *essentially locally small*; it is equivalent to a locally small category.

Examples. For the moment, we shall restrict ourselves to noting just two basic types of examples, deferring the treatment of variations to a later stage.

We have seen in Proposition 1.2.1 that if A is a pca, then for any set X the collection $\mathcal{P}(A)^X$ of $\mathcal{P}(A)$-valued predicates on X is a Heyting prealgebra.

Recall the structure: the order is defined by: $\phi \leq \psi$ if there is an element $a \in A$ such that for all $x \in X$ and all $b \in \phi(x)$, $ab\downarrow$ and $ab \in \psi(x)$. Let us say: a realizes $\phi \leq \psi$.

The top element $\top$ is the predicate given by $\top(x) = A$ for all $x \in X$; the bottom element $\bot$ is defined by $\bot(x) = \emptyset$ for all $x \in X$.

For elements ϕ and ψ of $\mathcal{P}(A)^X$, we have

$$
\begin{aligned}
(\phi \wedge \psi)(x) &= \{pab \,|\, a \in \phi(x) \text{ and } b \in \psi(x)\} \\
(\phi \vee \psi)(x) &= \{pka \,|\, a \in \phi(x)\} \cup \{p\bar{k}b \,|\, b \in \psi(x)\} \\
(\phi \Rightarrow \psi)(x) &= \{a \in A \,|\, \forall b \in \phi(x)(ab\downarrow \text{ and } ab \in \psi(x))\}
\end{aligned}
$$

Clearly, if $f : X \to Y$ is a function then there is an operation $\mathcal{P}(A)^f : \mathcal{P}(A)^Y \to \mathcal{P}(A)^X$ by composition with f, and this operation preserves the structure.

$\mathcal{P}(A)^f$ has both adjoints: for $\phi \in \mathcal{P}(A)^X$ define

$$
\begin{aligned}
\exists_f(\phi)(y) &= \{a \in A \,|\, \exists x \in X(f(x) = y \wedge a \in \phi(x))\} \\
\forall_f(\phi)(y) &= \{a \in A \,|\, \forall b \in A \forall x \in X(f(x) = y \Rightarrow ab\downarrow \wedge ab \in \phi(x))\}
\end{aligned}
$$

Specifically, if e realizes $\psi \leq \forall_f(\phi)$ then $\langle a'\rangle ea'k$ realizes $\psi \circ f \leq \phi$; conversely if e' realizes $\psi \circ f \leq \phi$ then $\langle b'\rangle\langle b\rangle e'b'$ realizes $\psi \leq \forall_f(\phi)$.

The Beck-Chevalley condition holds trivially. Furthermore, since the category Set is cartesian closed it suffices to check ii)$'$ in order to see that

$\mathcal{P}(A)^{(-)}$ is a Set-tripos. But for Σ we can take the set $\mathcal{P}(A)$, and for σ the identity map on $\mathcal{P}(A)$.

This tripos is the fundamental one for realizability. It is called the *realizability tripos* on A. For the special case of $A = \mathcal{K}_1$, one speaks of the *effective tripos*.

Of course, if A is an order-pca there is an analogous tripos $\mathcal{T}(A)^{(-)}$.

We shall see later that there are many variations on realizability triposes. Another basic example of a tripos is given by *complete* Heyting algebras: these are Heyting algebras which are complete as posets, i.e. Heyting algebras H such that for every subset $A \subseteq H$, both the join $\bigvee A$ and the meet $\bigwedge A$ of A exist in H. For such H, the functor $H^{(-)}$ also defines a Set-tripos; every H^X is, with pointwise operations, a Heyting algebra and every H^f preserves this structure. Adjoints to H^f are provided by the completeness of H: for $f : X \rightarrow Y$ and $\phi \in H^X$, we put

$$\begin{aligned}
\exists_f(\phi)(y) &= \bigvee \{\phi(x) \mid f(x) = y\} \\
\forall_f(\phi)(y) &= \bigwedge \{\phi(x) \mid f(x) = y\}
\end{aligned}$$

Again, the identity on H is a generic element for this tripos.

Although at first sight, there is a certain similarity between these two triposes (both being of the form $H^{(-)}$ for a Heyting algebra H), we shall see that there are fundamental differences between them.

The following lemma, which we shall refer to as "change of base for triposes" (we change the category on which the tripos is defined), provides an important tool for the construction of new triposes.

Lemma 2.1.3 (Change of Base) *Let* C *and* D *be categories with finite products. Suppose that* $F : D \rightarrow C$ *is a functor which preserves pullbacks and the terminal object, and has a right adjoint* G. *Then composition with* F *defines an enriched functor* F^*: C-Trip→D-Trip.

Proof. It suffices to show that for any C-tripos P the assignment $X \mapsto P(F(X))$ defines a D-tripos F^*P; the rest of the structure is easily checked.

Clearly, $F^*\mathsf{P}$ is a pseudofunctor from D to $\mathsf{Heytpre}$ and item i) of definition 2.1.2 is easily checked; for the Beck-Chevalley condition one only has to use the assumption that F preserves pullbacks.

The only nontrivial part is the verification of item ii). Since F preserves pullbacks and the terminal object, it preserves products; we shall therefore identify $\mathsf{P}(F(X) \times F(Y))$ with $\mathsf{P}(F(X \times Y))$.

Given an object X of D, let $\rho(X) = G(\pi(F(X)))$. Let $\varepsilon_{\pi(F(X))}$ be the counit of the adjunction $F \dashv G$ at $\pi(F(X))$.

Define δ_X as $\mathsf{P}[\mathrm{id}_{F(X)} \times \varepsilon_{\pi(F(X))}](\in_{F(X)})$; this is an element of $\mathsf{P}(F(X \times G(\pi(F(X)))))$. Here $\in_{F(X)}$ is the membership predicate for $F(X)$ w.r.t. P.

Suppose ϕ is an element of $F^*\mathsf{P}(X \times Y) = \mathsf{P}(F(X) \times F(Y))$. There is a map $\{\phi\} : F(Y) \to \pi(F(X))$ in C such that ϕ is isomorphic to $\mathsf{P}(\mathrm{id}_{F(X)} \times \{\phi\})(\in_{F(X)})$. Let $\widetilde{\{\phi\}} : Y \to \rho(X)$ be the transpose of $\{\phi\}$ across the adjunction $F \dashv G$. We have the following chain of isomorphisms:

$$
\begin{aligned}
F^*\mathsf{P}(\mathrm{id}_X \times \widetilde{\{\phi\}})(\delta_X) &\simeq \\
\mathsf{P}(\mathrm{id}_{F(X)} \times F(\widetilde{\{\phi\}}))(\mathsf{P}[\mathrm{id}_{F(X)} \times \varepsilon_{\pi(F(X))}](\in_{F(X)})) &\simeq \\
\mathsf{P}(\mathrm{id}_{F(X)} \times (\varepsilon_{\pi(F(X))} \circ F(\widetilde{\{\phi\}})))(\in_{F(X)}) &= \\
\mathsf{P}(\mathrm{id}_{F(X)} \times \{\phi\})(\in_{F(X)}) &\simeq \\
\phi &
\end{aligned}
$$

So $\delta_X \in F^*\mathsf{P}(X \times \rho(X))$ is a membership predicate for $F^*\mathsf{P}$. ∎

Lemma 2.1.3 will often be applied in the case where F is the inverse image part of a geometric morphism between toposes.

Notational convention. When we are working in the context of one tripos only, we shall make notation less cumbersome by writing f^* instead of $\mathsf{P}(f)$ for the action of the tripos on morphisms.

2.1.3 Interpretation of languages in triposes

Let P be a C-tripos. We define a C-*typed relational language* as a set of relation symbols R together with a *type*; the type of a relation symbol is a finite sequence $(X_1, \ldots, X_n)$ of objects of C. We also allow the empty sequence ( ) as a type; a relation symbol of this type will be seen as a propositional constant. We write X instead of (X).

Given a C-typed relational language $\mathcal{L}$, we define the set of $\mathcal{L}$-*terms* as follows:

i)   We assume that for every object X of C there is given an infinite set of variables $x_1^X, x_2^X, \ldots$ of type X; these are $\mathcal{L}$-terms of type X.

ii) If $t_1, \ldots, t_n$ are $\mathcal{L}$-terms of types $X_1, \ldots, X_n$ respectively, and $f : X_1 \times \cdots \times X_n \to Y$ is a morphism of C, then $f(t_1, \ldots, t_n)$ is an $\mathcal{L}$-term of type Y.

Next, we define $\mathcal{L}$-*formulas*:

i) $\bot$ and $\top$ are formulas (to be thought of as *false* and *true*, respectively).

ii) If R is a relation symbol of type $(X_1, \ldots, X_n)$ and $t_1, \ldots, t_n$ are $\mathcal{L}$-terms of type $X_1, \ldots, X_n$ respectively, then $R(t_1, \ldots, t_n)$ is a formula.

iii) If ϕ and ψ are formulas then so are $\phi \wedge \psi$, $\phi \vee \psi$, $\phi \to \psi$ and $\neg \phi$.

iv) If ϕ is a formula and x is a variable, then $\forall x \phi$ and $\exists x \phi$ are formulas.

Given a language $\mathcal{L}$, an *interpretation* of $\mathcal{L}$ in P assigns to every relation symbol R of type $(X_1, \ldots, X_n)$ an element $[R]$ of the Heyting prealgebra $\mathsf{P}(X_1 \times \cdots \times X_n)$.

Once an interpretation of $\mathcal{L}$ in P is specified, we define for each formula ϕ with free variables $x_1^{X_1}, \ldots, x_n^{X_n}$ an element $[\phi]$ of $\mathsf{P}(X_1 \times \cdots \times X_n)$. If ϕ has no free variables, $[\phi]$ will be an element of $\mathsf{P}(1)$, where 1 stands for a specified terminal object of C (of course, to be precise the definition is relative to a *choice* of product $X_1 \times \cdots \times X_n$ for every n-tuple of objects of C). The definition goes as follows.

$\bot$ and $\top$ are the bottom and top element of $\mathsf{P}(1)$.

First one defines for every term t of type X with variables $x_1^{X_1}, \ldots, x_n^{X_n}$, a morphism

$$[t] : X_1 \times \cdots \times X_n \to X$$

by letting $[x^X]$ be the identity arrow on X, and, inductively, letting $[f(t_1, \ldots, t_n)]$ be defined from the $[t_i]$ by composition with f. Then, if ϕ is the formula $R(t_1, \ldots, t_n)$, where R is of type $(X_1, \ldots, X_n)$ and $y_1^{Y_1}, \ldots, y_m^{Y_m}$ are the variables appearing in ϕ, the t_i define a morphism

$$Y_1 \times \cdots \times Y_m \xrightarrow{[\vec{t}]} X_1 \times \cdots X_n$$

and we put $[\phi] = [\vec{t}]^*([R]) \in \mathsf{P}(Y_1 \times \cdots \times Y_m)$.

For the propositional connectives, suppose we have defined $[\phi] \in \mathsf{P}(X_1 \times \cdots \times X_n)$ and $[\psi] \in \mathsf{P}(Y_1 \times \cdots \times Y_m)$. If $Z_1, \ldots, Z_k$ is a list of the types of all free variables in $\phi \wedge \psi$, there are evident projections

$$p_1 : Z_1 \times \cdots \times Z_k \to X_1 \times \cdots \times X_n$$
$$p_2 : Z_1 \times \cdots \times Z_k \to Y_1 \times \cdots \times Y_m$$

determined by the inclusions of $X_1, \ldots, X_n$ and $Y_1 \ldots, Y_m$ in the list $Z_1, \ldots, Z_k$.

We let $[\phi \wedge \psi]$ be $p_1^*([\phi]) \wedge p_2^*([\psi])$ (here the $\wedge$ in the RHS refers to the meet operation in the Heyting algebra, of course). The definition for $\vee$ and $\to$ is similar, and for $\neg$ we use the negation operator in the relevant Heyting prealgebra.

For the quantifiers $\exists x$ and $\forall x$ we use the left and right adjoints $\exists_\pi$ and $\forall_\pi$ to the Heyting homomorphism π^*, for a suitable projection π. Suppose $[\phi] \in \mathsf{P}(X_1 \times \cdots \times X_n)$ has been defined, and the free variables in ϕ are $x_1^{X_1}, \ldots, x_n^{X_n}$. For $1 \le i \le n$ let π^i be the projection from $X_1 \times \cdots \times X_n$ to $X_1 \times \cdots \widehat{X_i} \times \cdots \times X_n$ (X_i omitted). Then we put $[\exists x_i \phi] = \exists_{\pi^i}([\phi])$ and $[\forall x_i \phi] = \forall_{\pi^i}([\phi])$.

However, we also have to consider the case of $\exists x \phi$ where x does not occur in ϕ. Suppose x is of type X and $x_1^{X_1}, \ldots, x_n^{X_n}$ are the free variables in ϕ. Let $\pi : X \times X_1 \times \cdots \times X_n \to X_1 \times \cdots \times X_n$ be the projection. We set $[\exists x \phi] = \exists_\pi(\pi^*([\phi]))$ and $[\forall x \phi] = \forall_\pi(\pi^*([\phi]))$.

This finishes the definition of $[\phi]$. If ϕ is a sentence (no free variables), then $[\phi]$ is an element of $\mathsf{P}(1)$ (1 is also the "empty product").

Remark Suppose X is an object for which the Heyting prealgebra is trivial (i.e. $\bot \simeq \top$). Then this will hold also for any Y such that there is a morphism $f : Y \to X$ in C, because the Heyting homomorphism

f^* preserves both $\bot$ and $\top$. In particular it holds for $X \times Y$. If x is a variable of type X, then $[\exists x \phi] \simeq \bot$ in $\mathsf{P}(Y)$ for every ϕ, because $\exists_\pi$, being a left adjoint, preserves the bottom element. Similarly, $[\forall x \phi] \simeq \top$. The type X is like the empty set.

A converse to this is also valid: if, for example $[\forall x \bot]$ is the top element of $\mathsf{P}(1)$ and x is of type X, then $\mathsf{P}(X)$ is trivial; for $[\forall x \bot] = \forall_\pi(\pi^*(\bot))$ for the unique map $\pi : X \to 1$. Hence in $\mathsf{P}(X)$ we have

$$\bot \simeq \pi^*(\bot) \simeq \pi^*(\forall_\pi(\pi^*(\bot))) \simeq \pi^*(\top) \simeq \top$$

Definition 2.1.4 Let ϕ be a sentence in a C-typed relational language $\mathcal{L}$, and let $[\cdot]$ an interpretation of $\mathcal{L}$ in P. Then, relative to $[\cdot]$, we say that ϕ is *true in* P, or $\mathsf{P} \models \phi$, if $[\phi]$ is the top element of $\mathsf{P}(1)$.

The following lemma is used in the proof of the Soundness Theorem (2.1.6) below. Suppose that $\psi(x, \vec{y})$ is an $\mathcal{L}$-formula; let X be the type of x, Y the product of the types of the variables in $\vec{y}$. Suppose t is a term of type X; we consider the substitution instance $\psi(t, \vec{y})$. Let Z be the product of the types of the variables which are free in $\psi(t, \vec{y})$. There is an evident projection $\pi : Z \to Y$ and a morphism $[t] : Z \to X$.

Lemma 2.1.5 (Substitution Lemma) *In the above situation,*

$$[\psi(t, \vec{y})] \simeq \langle [t], \pi \rangle^*([\psi])$$

Proof. By induction on ψ. The only nontrivial step is the one for the quantifiers. Suppose $\psi \equiv \exists w \psi'(w, x, \vec{y})$. For simplicity of notation and without real loss of generality, assume $\vec{y}$ is a single variable y of type Y, and $t = t(x, y)$. We have $[t] : X \times Y \to X$, $\pi : X \times Y \to Y$, $\pi' : W \times X \times Y \to X \times Y$ and $s = \mathrm{id}_W \times \langle [t], \pi \rangle : W \times X \times Y \to W \times X \times Y$. These maps fit into a pullback diagram

$$
\begin{array}{ccc}
W \times X \times Y & \xrightarrow{\ s\ } & W \times X \times Y \\
{\scriptstyle \pi'}\Big\downarrow & & \Big\downarrow{\scriptstyle \pi'} \\
X \times Y & \xrightarrow[\langle [t], \pi \rangle]{} & X \times Y
\end{array}
$$

By induction hypothesis $[\psi'(w, t(x, y), y)] \simeq s^*([\psi'])$, so

$$[\psi(t(x, y), y)] \simeq \exists_{\pi'}(s^*([\psi']))$$

By the Beck-Chevalley condition, the RHS is isomorphic to

$$\langle [t], \pi \rangle^* (\exists_{\pi'}([\psi']))$$

which is $\langle [t], \pi \rangle^*([\psi])$, as desired. The induction step for $\forall$ is analogous. ∎

Theorem 2.1.6 (Soundness Theorem) *Suppose ϕ is a sentence in a C-typed relational language $\mathcal{L}$. If ϕ is provable in intuitionistic logic without equality, then $\mathsf{P} \models \phi$ for every C-tripos P and every interpretation $[\cdot]$ of $\mathcal{L}$ in P.*

Proof. This is proved by induction on proofs in a formal system, for example natural deduction. By way of example we shall look at the rule of $\exists$-elimination. Basically this rule says that for a formula $\psi(x, y)$ with free variables x^X, y^Y, and an arrow $f : Y \to X$ in C, $\psi(f(y), y)$ entails $\exists x \psi(x, y)$; therefore $[\psi(f(y), y)] \leq [\exists x \psi(x, y)]$ should hold.

By the Substitution Lemma (2.1.5), $[\psi(f(y), y)] \simeq \langle f, \mathrm{id}_Y \rangle^*([\psi])$. So we need to prove that $\langle f, \mathrm{id}_Y \rangle^*([\psi]) \leq \exists_\pi([\psi])$, where $\pi : X \times Y \to Y$ is the second projection.

Now the composite $\pi \circ \langle f, \mathrm{id}_Y \rangle : Y \to Y$ is the identity on Y, hence $\exists_{\pi \circ \langle f, \mathrm{id}_Y \rangle}$ is isomorphic to the identity on $\mathsf{P}(Y)$, so

$$\langle f, \mathrm{id}_Y \rangle^*([\psi]) \simeq \exists_\pi(\exists_{\langle f, \mathrm{id}_Y \rangle}(\langle f, \mathrm{id}_Y \rangle^*([\psi])))$$

Since $\exists_{\langle f, \mathrm{id}_Y \rangle}(\langle f, \mathrm{id}_Y \rangle^*([\psi])) \leq [\psi]$ by adjointness, and $\exists_\pi$ is order preserving, the required inequality follows. ∎

2.1.4 A few useful facts

In this subsection I collect a few useful facts that don't seem to have a natural place elsewhere. We work in a C-tripos P.

1. If $i : U \to X$ is a monomorphism in C, then for any $\phi \in \mathsf{P}(U)$, $i^*\exists_i(\phi) \simeq \phi$.

   (Note that this is equivalent to the statement that $\exists_i : \mathsf{P}(U) \to \mathsf{P}(X)$ reflects the order)

   Proof: by elementary category theory, i is a monomorphism if and only if the square

$$
\begin{array}{ccc}
U & \xrightarrow{\ \mathrm{id}\ } & U \\
{\scriptstyle \mathrm{id}}\downarrow & & \downarrow{\scriptstyle i} \\
U & \xrightarrow[\ i\ ]{} & X
\end{array}
$$

   is a pullback. Applying the Beck-Chevalley condition to this pullback and $\phi \in \mathsf{P}(U)$, we get $i^*\exists_i(\phi) \simeq \exists_{\mathrm{id}}(\mathrm{id})^*(\phi) \simeq \phi$, as claimed.

2. For any map $X \xrightarrow{i} Y$, $\psi \in \mathsf{P}(X)$ and $\phi \in \mathsf{P}(Y)$, we have

$$\exists_i(\psi \wedge i^*(\phi)) \simeq (\exists_i\psi) \wedge \phi$$

   (Sometimes, this is called the "Frobenius condition") Proof: since i^* commutes with $\wedge$, and $\exists_i \dashv i^*$, we have $\psi \wedge i^*(\phi) \leq i^*\exists_i(\psi) \wedge i^*(\phi) \simeq i^*(\exists_i\psi \wedge \phi)$, hence

$$\exists_i(\psi \wedge i^*\phi) \leq \exists_i\psi \wedge \phi$$

   For the converse inequality we use that i^* also commutes with Heyting implication; we have a chain of equivalences

$$
\begin{aligned}
\exists_i\psi \wedge \phi \leq \exists_i(\psi \wedge i^*\phi) &\iff \\
\exists_i\psi \leq \phi \to \exists_i(\psi \wedge i^*\phi) &\iff \\
\psi \leq i^*\phi \to i^*\exists_i(\psi \wedge i^*\phi) &\iff \\
\psi \wedge i^*\phi \leq i^*\exists_i(\psi \wedge i^*\phi) &
\end{aligned}
$$

   and the last inequality is a consequence of the adjunction $\exists_i \dashv i^*$.

3. For an object X of C let $\delta_X : X \to X \times X$ be the diagonal embedding. Let $\phi \in \mathsf{P}(X)$; we write $\sim_\phi$ for a binary relation symbol which is interpreted by $\exists_\delta(\phi)$. Then:

i) $\mathsf{P} \models \forall xy (x \sim_\phi y \rightarrow y \sim_\phi x)$

ii) $\mathsf{P} \models \forall xyz (x \sim_\phi y \wedge y \sim_\phi z \rightarrow x \sim_\phi z)$

iii) $\mathsf{P} \models \forall x (x \sim_\phi x \leftrightarrow \phi(x))$

Proof: for i), we have to show that $\exists_\delta(\phi) \leq \mathrm{tw}^*(\exists_\delta(\phi))$ in $\mathsf{P}(X)$, where $\mathrm{tw} : X \times X \rightarrow X \times X$ is the twist map; but this is immediate from the adjunction $\exists_\delta \dashv \delta^*$, since $\delta \circ \mathrm{tw} = \delta$.

For ii): the transitivity statement comes down to

$(*)$ $\pi_{12}^*(\exists_\delta(\phi)) \wedge \pi_{23}^*(\exists_\delta(\phi)) \leq \pi_{13}^*(\exists_\delta(\phi))$

in $\mathsf{P}(X \times X \times X)$, where $\pi_{ij} : X \times X \times X \rightarrow X \times X$ are projections. Observe that the square

$$
\begin{array}{ccc}
X \times X & \xrightarrow{\;\pi_1 \times \pi_1 \times \pi_2\;} & X \times X \times X \\
{\scriptstyle \pi_1}\downarrow & & \downarrow{\scriptstyle \pi_{12}} \\
X & \xrightarrow{\qquad \delta \qquad} & X \times X
\end{array}
$$

is a pullback in C. Using the Beck-Chevalley condition and the $\wedge, \rightarrow$ adjunction, $(*)$ is equivalent to

$$\exists_{\pi_1 \times \pi_1 \times \pi_2}(\pi_1^*(\phi)) \leq \pi_{23}^*(\exists_\delta(\phi)) \rightarrow \pi_{13}^*(\exists_\delta(\phi))$$

But since $\pi_{23} \circ (\pi_1 \times \pi_1 \times \pi_2) = \pi_{13} \circ (\pi_1 \times \pi_1 \times \pi_2) = \mathrm{id}_{X \times X}$, we see that the RHS of this inequality is isomorphic to $\exists_\delta(\phi) \rightarrow \exists_\delta(\phi)$, which is isomorphic to $\top_{X \times X}$.

For iii), we have to show that $\phi \simeq \delta^*(\exists_\delta(\phi))$, which follows from item 1 since δ is always mono.

4. For the relation $\sim_\phi$ of item 3 and any element $\psi \in \mathsf{P}(X)$ such that $\psi \leq \phi$, we have

$$\mathsf{P} \models \forall xy (\psi(x) \wedge x \sim_\phi y \rightarrow \psi(y))$$

Proof: this amounts to proving the inequality

$$\exists_\delta(\phi) \wedge \pi_1^*(\psi) \leq \pi_2^*(\psi)$$

where, as usual, π_1 and π_2 are the two projections $X \times X \to X$. Since $\pi_i \circ \delta = \mathrm{id}_X$, we have $\psi \simeq (\pi_i \circ \delta)^*(\psi) \simeq \delta^*(\pi_i^*(\psi))$ for $i = 1, 2$; in particular, $\exists_\delta(\psi) \leq \pi_i^*(\psi)$ follows by adjointness.

By the Frobenius condition (item 2),

$$\exists_\delta(\phi) \wedge \pi_1^*(\psi) \simeq \exists_\delta(\phi \wedge \delta^*(\pi_1^*(\psi))) \simeq \exists_\delta(\phi \wedge \psi) \simeq \exists_\delta(\psi)$$

Hence $\exists_\delta(\phi) \wedge \pi_1^*(\psi) \simeq \exists_\delta(\psi) \leq \pi_2^*(\psi)$ as desired.

5. For an object X of C, let $\sim_X$ be the relation $\sim_\phi$ from item 3, with $\phi \equiv \top_X$, the top element of $\mathsf{P}(X)$. For any morphism $f : X \to Y$ in C and $\phi \in \mathsf{P}(X)$, we have

$$\exists_f(\phi) \simeq \exists_{\pi_Y}((f \times \mathrm{id}_Y)^*(\sim_Y) \wedge \pi_X^*(\phi))$$

where π_X and π_Y are the projections from $X \times Y$. Note, that the RHS is $[\exists x(f(x) \sim y \wedge \phi(x))]$. The statement means that the left adjoints $\exists_f$ can be defined from the $\exists_\pi$ and the $\exists_\delta$.

Proof: we observe that

$$
\begin{array}{ccc}
X & \xrightarrow{\ f\ } & Y \\
{\scriptstyle \langle \mathrm{id}_X, f \rangle} \downarrow & & \downarrow {\scriptstyle \delta_Y} \\
X \times Y & \xrightarrow[f \times \mathrm{id}_Y]{} & Y \times Y
\end{array}
$$

is a pullback diagram in C. Hence, by the Beck-Chevalley condition,

$$(f \times \mathrm{id}_Y)^*(\sim_Y) \simeq (f \times \mathrm{id}_Y)^* \exists_{\delta_Y}(\top_Y) \simeq$$
$$\exists_{\langle \mathrm{id}_X, f \rangle}(f^*(\top_Y)) \simeq \exists_{\langle \mathrm{id}_X, f \rangle}(\top_X)$$

Therefore we need to show that

$$\exists_f(\phi) \simeq \exists_{\pi_Y}(\exists_{\langle \mathrm{id}_X, f \rangle}(\top_X) \wedge \pi_X^*(\phi))$$

Now for an arbitrary element $\psi \in \mathsf{P}(Y)$ we have the following equivalences:

$$
\begin{aligned}
\exists_{\pi_Y}(\exists_{\langle \mathrm{id}_X, f \rangle}(\top_X) \wedge \pi_X^*(\phi)) &\leq \psi &\Leftrightarrow \\
\exists_{\langle \mathrm{id}_X, f \rangle}(\top_X) \wedge \pi_X^*(\phi) &\leq \pi_Y^*(\psi) &\Leftrightarrow \\
\exists_{\langle \mathrm{id}_X, f \rangle}(\top_X) &\leq \pi_X^*(\phi) \to \pi_Y^*(\psi) &\Leftrightarrow \\
\top_X &\leq \langle \mathrm{id}_X, f \rangle^*(\pi_X^*(\phi) \to \pi_Y^*(\psi)) &\Leftrightarrow \\
\top_X &\leq \phi \to f^*(\psi) &\Leftrightarrow \\
\phi &\leq f^*(\psi) &\Leftrightarrow \\
\exists_f(\phi) &\leq \psi &
\end{aligned}
$$

from which the desired isomorphism follows.

6. A category of P-proto-assemblies on C. For this example, we assume that C has pullbacks.

Define a P-proto-assembly to be a pair (X, ϕ) where X is an object of C and $\phi \in \mathsf{P}(X)$.

A morphism of P-proto-assemblies $(X, \phi) \to (Y, \psi)$ is an equivalence class of pairs (U, f) where U is a subobject of X (represented by a mono $U \xrightarrow{i} X$ say), and $f : U \to Y$ is a morphism in C for which the inequality $\phi \leq \exists_i(f^*(\psi))$ holds in $\mathsf{P}(X)$. Two such pairs (U, f) and (U', f') will be called equivalent if f and f' agree on the intersection $U \cap U'$.

Note that if (U, f) and (U', f') are equivalent and f'' is the restriction of f to $U \cap U'$, then also the pair $(U \cap U', f'')$ has the required property: we have a pullback diagram

$$
\begin{array}{ccc}
U \cap U' & \xrightarrow{\;j\;} & U \\
{\scriptstyle j'}\downarrow & & \downarrow{\scriptstyle i} \\
U' & \xrightarrow[\;i'\;]{} & X
\end{array}
$$

Since $\phi \leq \exists_i(f^*\psi) \leq \exists_i(\top_U)$, by property 2 we have

$$
\phi \simeq \phi \wedge \exists_i(\top_U) \simeq \exists_i(i^*\phi \wedge \top_U) \simeq \exists_i(i^*\phi)
$$

Therefore, using the Beck-Chevalley condition and the given property of ψ once more,

$$\phi \leq \exists_i i^* (\exists_{i'} f'^* \psi) \simeq \exists_i \exists_j (j'^* (f'^* \psi)) \simeq \exists_{ij} (f''^* \psi)$$

Morphisms of P-proto-assemblies are composed as follows: given (U, f) representing $(X, \phi) \to (Y, \psi)$ and (V, g) representing $(Y, \psi) \to (Z, \chi)$, form a pullback

$$\begin{array}{ccccc}
W & \xrightarrow{\ k\ } & U & \xrightarrow{\ i\ } & X \\
{\scriptstyle f'}\downarrow & & \downarrow{\scriptstyle f} & & \\
V & \xrightarrow{\ j\ } & Y & & \\
{\scriptstyle g}\downarrow & & & & \\
Z & & & &
\end{array}$$

and consider (W, gf'). This does indeed represent a morphism $(X, \phi) \to (Z, \chi)$, for

$$\phi \leq \exists_i f^* \psi \leq \exists_i f^* \exists_j g^* \chi \simeq \exists_i \exists_k f'^* g^* \chi \simeq \exists_{ik} (gf')^* \chi$$

The verification that composition is associative is left to the reader.

2.2   The tripos-to-topos construction

Let P be a tripos on a category C with finite products. We define a category C[P] of *partial equivalence relations over* P, as follows.

     An *object* of C[P] is a pair $(X, \sim)$ where X is an object of C and $\sim$ is an element of $P(X \times X)$, such that

$$\mathsf{P} \models \forall xy (x \sim y \to y \sim x)$$
$$\mathsf{P} \models \forall xyz (x \sim y \wedge y \sim z \to x \sim z)$$

both hold. We call $\sim$ an *equality predicate* for X.

     A *morphism*: $(X, \sim) \to (Y, \sim)$ of C[P] is an isomorphism class of elements F of $P(X \times Y)$ that are *functional relations*, that is: such that the following statements hold:

$$\begin{array}{ll}
\mathsf{P} \models \forall xy(F(x,y) \to x \sim x \wedge y \sim y) & F \text{ is } strict \\
\mathsf{P} \models \forall xx'yy'(F(x,y) \wedge x \sim x' \wedge y \sim y' \to F(x',y')) & F \text{ is } relational \\
\mathsf{P} \models \forall xyy'(F(x,y) \wedge F(x,y') \to y \sim y') & F \text{ is } single\text{-}valued \\
\mathsf{P} \models \forall x(x \sim x \to \exists y F(x,y)) & F \text{ is } total
\end{array}$$

It is a useful remark that two functional relations F, G in $\mathsf{P}(X \times Y)$ are isomorphic as soon as either $F \leq G$ or $G \leq F$ holds.

Theorem 2.2.1 (Pitts) $\mathsf{C}[\mathsf{P}]$ *is an elementary topos.*

Proof. First, we shall see that $\mathsf{C}[\mathsf{P}]$, with the given definition of morphism, is a category. If $F \in \mathsf{P}(X \times Y)$ and $G \in \mathsf{P}(Y \times Z)$ represent morphisms $f : (X, \sim) \to (Y, \sim)$ and $g : (Y, \sim) \to (Z, \sim)$ respectively, we define the composition $gf : (X, \sim) \to (Z, \sim)$ to be represented by

$$\exists_{\pi_{13}}(\pi_{12}^*(F) \wedge \pi_{23}^*(G))$$

where $\pi_{12} : X \times Y \times Z \to X \times Y$, $\pi_{23} : X \times Y \times Z \to Y \times Z$, and $\pi_{13} : X \times Y \times Z \to X \times Z$ are projections. Note, that this is

$$[\exists y(F(x,y) \wedge G(y,z))]$$

Now it is an elementary exercise in many-sorted intuitionistic logic to verify that composition is associative, and that the morphism $(X, \sim) \to (X, \sim)$ represented by $\sim$ itself, acts as an identity on $(X, \sim)$. Thus, $\mathsf{C}[\mathsf{P}]$ is a category. Let us examine some structure of this category.

$\mathsf{C}[\mathsf{P}]$ has finite limits. For a terminal object in $\mathsf{C}[\mathsf{P}]$, let I be any weak terminal object in C, and consider the object $(I, \top_{I \times I})$ of $\mathsf{C}[\mathsf{P}]$. For any object $(X, \sim)$ let $F \in \mathsf{P}(X \times I)$ be given by $\pi_X^* \delta^*(\sim)$ in $\mathsf{P}(X \times I)$ (this is $[x \sim x]$, so $\mathsf{P} \models F(x,i) \leftrightarrow x \sim x$). Clearly, this relation is strict, relational and single-valued; and it is total since if $f : X \to I$ is a morphism in C, $\mathsf{P} \models \forall x(x \sim x \to F(x, f(x)))$, hence $\mathsf{P} \models \forall x(x \sim x \to \exists i F(x,i))$. Clearly, the morphism $(X, \sim) \to (I, \top_{I \times I})$ represented by F is unique.

$\quad \mathsf{C}[\mathsf{P}]$ has binary products: for $(X, \sim)$ and $(Y, \sim)$ take $(X \times Y, \sim)$ where

$$(x,y) \sim (x',y') \leftrightarrow (x \sim x') \wedge (y \sim y')$$

The projections are evident.

C[P] has equalizers: given two morphisms $(X, \sim) \to (Y, \sim)$ represented by F and G, construct the equalizer as $(X, \approx)$ where

$$x \approx x' \leftrightarrow x \sim x' \wedge \exists y (F(x, y) \wedge G(x, y))$$

C[P] is cartesian closed. In order to form the exponential $(Y, \sim)^{(X, \sim)}$, consider $\pi(X \times Y)$ (the carrier object for the membership predicate, see definition 2.1.2) and the membership predicate $\in_{X \times Y}$ in $\mathsf{P}(X \times Y \times \pi(X \times Y))$. Using a variable F of type $\pi(X \times Y)$ and writing $\in_{X \times Y}$ as a binary predicate (i.e., write $(x, y) \in_{X \times Y} F$, etc.), we define 4 elements of $\mathsf{P}(\pi(X \times Y))$:

$$
\begin{aligned}
E_1 &\equiv [\forall xy((x, y) \in_{X \times Y} F \to x \sim x \wedge y \sim y)] \\
E_2 &\equiv [\forall x x' y y'((x, y) \in_{X \times Y} F \wedge x \sim x' \wedge y \sim y' \to (x'y') \in_{X \times Y} F)] \\
E_3 &\equiv [\forall x y y'((x, y) \in_{X \times Y} F \wedge (x, y') \in_{X \times Y} F \to y \sim y')] \\
E_4 &\equiv [\forall x(x \sim x \to \exists y(x, y) \in_{X \times Y} F)]
\end{aligned}
$$

Let $E(F) \equiv E_1(F) \wedge E_2(F) \wedge E_3(F) \wedge E_4(F)$. Define:

$$F \sim G \quad \equiv \quad [E(F) \wedge \forall xy((x, y) \in_{X \times Y} F \leftrightarrow (x, y) \in_{X \times Y} G)]$$

Then the object $(\pi(X \times Y), \sim)$ is the required exponential: the evaluation map

$$(X, \sim) \times (\pi(X \times Y), \sim) \to (Y, \sim)$$

is represented by $\in_{X \times Y}$.

Before showing that C[P] has a subobject classifier, it is useful to have an explicit description of pullbacks, subobjects and images in the category.

Given morphisms $(X, \sim) \to (Z, \sim)$ and $(Y, \sim) \to (Z, \sim)$ represented by F and G, and $(X \times Y, \sim)$ is the object given by

$$(x, y) \sim (x', y') \leftrightarrow x \sim x' \wedge y \sim y' \wedge \exists z(F(x, z) \wedge G(y, z))$$

then

$$
\begin{array}{ccc}
(X \times Y, \sim) & \longrightarrow & (X, \sim) \\
\downarrow & & \downarrow {\scriptstyle F} \\
(Y, \sim) & \xrightarrow{\quad G \quad} & (Z, \sim)
\end{array}
$$

is a pullback diagram in $\mathsf{C}[\mathsf{P}]$ (we have left the evident projections un-specified).

Using this description it is not hard to verify that a functional relation $F \in \mathsf{P}(X \times Y)$ represents a monomorphism: $(X, \sim) \to (Y, \sim)$ if and only if

$$\mathsf{P} \models \forall x x' y (F(x, y) \wedge F(x', y) \to x \sim x')$$

In this case, the object $(X, \sim)$ is isomorphic to the object $(Y, \sim_F)$ where $\sim_F$ is the interpretation of the formula $y \sim y' \wedge \exists x F(x, y)$: clearly, $(Y, \sim_F)$ is a subobject of $(Y, \sim)$ and the morphism represented by F factors through $(Y, \sim_F)$; and the inverse $(Y, \sim_F) \to (X, \sim)$ of this factorization is represented by $t^* F$ where $t : Y \times X \to X \times Y$ is the twist map. We see, that every mono into $(Y, \sim)$ is isomorphic to one of the form $(Y, \approx) \to (Y, \sim)$ where $x \approx x' \leftrightarrow (x \sim x' \wedge P(x))$ for some *strict relation* P on $(Y, \sim)$: an element $P \in \mathsf{P}(Y)$ is a strict relation on $(Y, \sim)$ if

$$\mathsf{P} \models \forall y (P(y) \to y \sim y)$$
$$\mathsf{P} \models \forall y y' (P(y) \wedge y \sim y' \to P(y'))$$

both hold. Subobjects of $(Y, \sim)$ are therefore in 1-1 correspondence with isomorphism classes of strict relations on $(Y, \sim)$.

Following [83] we call a map a *cover* if it does not factor through a proper subobject of its codomain. Clearly, every map in $\mathsf{C}[\mathsf{P}]$ factors as a cover followed by a monomorphism: if F represents a map $(X, \sim) \to (Y, \sim)$ the strict relation $[\exists x F(x, y)]$ on $(Y, \sim)$ corresponds to the least subobject of $(Y, \sim)$ through which F factors. This subobject is called the *image* of F.

Finally, we remark that if F represents a map $f : (X, \sim) \to (Y, \sim)$ and the strict relation P on $(Y, \sim)$ corresponds to a subobject , then the inverse image of this subobject under f (represented by the pullback along f of any mono representing it) corresponds to the strict relation $[\exists y (F(x, y) \wedge P(y))]$ on $(X, \sim)$. Using this, it follows at once that *covers are stable under pullback*, and hence that $\mathsf{C}[\mathsf{P}]$ is a *regular category*. Of course, this follows from the claim that $\mathsf{C}[\mathsf{P}]$ is a topos; but it seems easier to establish these facts about subobjects, pullbacks and covers first.

Now we show that $\mathsf{C}[\mathsf{P}]$ has a subobject classifier. Consider the object $\Sigma = \pi(1)$ of C, and the element $\sigma = \in_1$ of $\mathsf{P}(\Sigma)$. For any object X of C and any $\phi \in \mathsf{P}(X)$, there is a morphism $\{\phi\} : X \to \Sigma$ such that $\phi \simeq \{\phi\}^*(\sigma)$ in $\mathsf{P}(X)$. There is an element $\Rightarrow$ of $\mathsf{P}(\Sigma \times \Sigma)$, given by $\pi_1^*(\sigma) \to \pi_2^*(\sigma)$. Note, that for $\phi, \psi \in \mathsf{P}(X)$, $(\phi \to \psi) \simeq \langle\{\phi\}, \{\psi\}\rangle^*(\Rightarrow)$. Let tw $: \Sigma \times \Sigma \to \Sigma \times \Sigma$ be the twist map, and define $\Leftrightarrow$ as $\Rightarrow \wedge \mathrm{tw}^*(\Rightarrow)$. Then $(\Sigma, \Leftrightarrow)$ is an object of $\mathsf{C}[\mathsf{P}]$.

There is a morphism $t : 1 \to (\Sigma, \Leftrightarrow)$ (denoting the terminal object of $\mathsf{C}[\mathsf{P}]$ by 1), given by the element $[p \Leftrightarrow \top]$ of $\mathsf{P}(\Sigma)$. We claim that t is a subobject classifier in $\mathsf{C}[\mathsf{P}]$. Indeed, if $\phi \in \mathsf{P}(X)$ is a strict relation of $(X, \sim)$, there is a morphism $\chi_\phi : (X, \sim) \to (\Sigma, \Leftrightarrow)$ represnted by the element

$$[x \sim x \wedge (\{\phi\}(x) \Leftrightarrow p)]$$

of $\mathsf{P}(X \times \Sigma)$. The reader is invited to convince himself that the pullback of t along χ_ϕ is isomorphic to ϕ (considered as mono into $(X, \sim)$), and that χ_ϕ is unique with this property. This establishes that $\mathsf{C}[\mathsf{P}]$ is a topos, as claimed.

In any topos, a map is a cover if and only if it is an epimorphism. We see therefore, that a functional relation $F \in \mathsf{P}(X \times Y)$ represents an epimorphism $(X, \sim) \to (Y, \sim)$ if and only if

$$\mathsf{P} \models \forall y(y \sim y \to \exists x F(x, y))$$

∎

Remark. Soon after the definition of a tripos was written down, Pitts ([124]) realized that in order that $\mathsf{C}[\mathsf{P}]$ be a topos, it is not necessary that P be a tripos. Instead of the existence of a *morphism* $\{\phi\}$ as in definition 2.1.2ii), it is enough to require that

$$\mathsf{P} \models \forall y \exists p \forall x(\phi(x, y) \leftrightarrow x \in_X p)$$

where p is a variable of type $\pi(X)$ (see also [125]). However, this extra generality will not be of any use to us.

Remark. If the pseudofunctor P satisfies only part i) of definition 2.1.2, one can still form the category $\mathsf{C}[\mathsf{P}]$. By inspection of the proof of theorem 2.2.1, one sees that in this case the category $\mathsf{C}[\mathsf{P}]$ still has the "first-order part" of the properties derived there: that is, it is a regular Heyting category: i.e., for every object the subobject lattice is a Heyting algebra, the pullback operations are Heyting homomorphisms and have both a left and a right adjoint.

2.3 Internal logic of C[P] reduced to the logic of P

We have seen that in P we can interpret many-sorted predicate logic without equality. The internal logic of a topos is formulated *with* equality; which is basically what we added (in the form of equality predicates) in the passage from P to C[P]. It will therefore not be too big a surprise to discover that the logic of C[P] can be reduced to that of P, much in the spirit of Scott's "logic of identity and existence" ([147]).

Suppose we are given a many-sorted first-order language $\mathcal{L}$ with relation symbols, function symbols, equality. An interpretation of $\mathcal{L}$ in C[P] consists of the following data:

- for every sort σ of $\mathcal{L}$, an object $[\![\,\sigma\,]\!] = (X, \sim)$ of C[P];

- for every relation symbol R of $\mathcal{L}$ of type $(\sigma_1, \ldots, \sigma_n)$, a subobject $[\![\,R\,]\!]$ of $[\![\,\sigma_1\,]\!] \times \cdots \times [\![\,\sigma_n\,]\!]$;

- for every function symbol f of $\mathcal{L}$ of type $(\sigma_1, \ldots, \sigma_n \to \tau)$, an arrow $[\![\,f\,]\!] : [\![\,\sigma_1\,]\!] \times \cdots \times [\![\,\sigma_n\,]\!] \to [\![\,\tau\,]\!]$ in C[P].

Once such an interpretation is given, terms and formulas of $\mathcal{L}$ acquire meaning in C[P] in a standard way. First, every term t of $\mathcal{L}$ of type $(\sigma_1, \ldots, \sigma_n \to \tau)$ is interpreted as a morphism $[\![\,t\,]\!] : [\![\,\sigma_1\,]\!] \times \cdots \times [\![\,\sigma_n\,]\!] \to [\![\,\tau\,]\!]$ by the usual inductive clauses (cf. section 2.1.3); then, every formula φ with free variables of sorts $\sigma_1, \ldots, \sigma_n$, a subobject $[\![\,\varphi\,]\!]$ of $[\![\,\sigma_1\,]\!] \times \cdots \times [\![\,\sigma_n\,]\!]$ is assigned.

Suppose φ is the formula $t = s$, where t and s are of the same sort τ. Let $X = \mathrm{dom}([\![\,t\,]\!]), Y = \mathrm{dom}([\![\,s\,]\!])$. There are evident projections π_X and π_Y from the product $[\![\,\sigma_1\,]\!] \times \cdots \times [\![\,\sigma_n\,]\!]$ to X and Y respectively; now $[\![\,\varphi\,]\!]$ is defined as the equalizer of $[\![\,t\,]\!] \circ \pi_X$ and $[\![\,s\,]\!] \circ \pi_Y$. Convince yourself that if $[\![\,t\,]\!]$ is represented by F and $[\![\,s\,]\!]$ by G, then $[\![\,t = s\,]\!]$ is represented by the strict relation $[\exists y(F(\vec{x}, y) \wedge G(\vec{x}, y))]$.

Note: we use single brackets $[\ ]$ for the interpretation of logic in P, and double brackets $[\![\ ]\!]$ for the logic in $\mathsf{C[P]}$.

If φ is a formula $R(t_1, \ldots, t_n)$ where R is a relation symbol of $\mathcal{L}$ and the t_i terms of type τ_i, and φ contains variables of sorts $\sigma_1, \ldots, \sigma_k$, then the t_i determine a map $[\![\,t\,]\!] : [\![\,\sigma_1\,]\!] \times \cdots \times [\![\,\sigma_k\,]\!] \to [\![\,\tau_1\,]\!] \times \cdots \times [\![\,\tau_n\,]\!]$, and $[\![\,\varphi\,]\!]$ is obtained by pulling back the subobject $[\![\,R\,]\!]$ of $[\![\,\tau_1\,]\!] \times \cdots \times [\![\,\tau_n\,]\!]$ along $[\![\,t\,]\!]$.

For the logical structure, we use the Heyting algebra structure on the lattice of subobjects of any object of a topos, as well as the left and right adjoints to the operation on subobjects defined by pulling back along a projection.

Explicitly, suppose two subobjects of $(X, \sim)$ are represented by strict relations (for $\sim$) R and S on X. Then $[R \wedge S]$ and $[R \vee S]$, formed in $\mathsf{P}(X)$, are also strict relations, which represent, respectively, the meet and join of the given subobjects. Heyting implication is represented by $[x \sim x \wedge (R(x) \to S(x))]$.

For the quantifiers, if $[\![\,\varphi\,]\!]$ has been defined as subobject of

$$(Y, \sim) \times (X, \sim)$$

and is represented by the strict relation $R_\varphi \in \mathsf{P}(Y \times X)$, then $[\![\,\exists y \varphi\,]\!]$ is represented by $[\exists y R_\varphi] \in \mathsf{P}(X)$, and $[\![\,\forall y \varphi\,]\!]$ by

$$[x \sim x \wedge \forall y (y \sim y \to R_\varphi)]$$

This defines the internal, first-order logic of $\mathsf{C[P]}$. But every topos admits interpretations of higher-order logic too (see, e.g., [95]). The higher-order aspect is taken care of by the *sorts* of the language, that is: the objects of $\mathsf{C[P]}$: for every object $(X, \sim)$ there is a *power object* $\mathcal{P}(X, \sim) = \Omega^{(X, \sim)}$, where Ω is the subobject classifier. The object $\mathcal{P}(X, \sim)$ is isomorphic to $(\pi(X), \sim)$ where

$$R \sim S \quad \equiv \quad [\forall x(x \in_X R \to x \sim x) \wedge \forall xy(x \in_X R \wedge x \sim y \to y \in_X R) \wedge \\ \forall x(x \in_X R \leftrightarrow x \in_X S)]$$

We shall paraphrase the first two conjuncts by "R is a strict relation for $\sim$" For any subobject R of $(X, \sim) \times (Y, \sim)$, represented by a strict relation $R \in \mathsf{P}(X \times Y)$, there is a map $(Y, \sim) \to \mathcal{P}(X, \sim)$, represented by

$$F_R(y, S) \quad \equiv \quad [\text{``}S \text{ is a strict relation for } \sim\text{''} \land y \sim y \\ \forall x (R(x, y) \leftrightarrow x \in_X S)]$$

This assignment is part of a natural bijection between morphisms

$$(Y, \sim) \to \mathcal{P}(X, \sim)$$

and subobjects of $(X, \sim) \times (Y, \sim)$. Clearly now, we can interpret a higher-order language with quantifiers $\exists X$ etc. intending to run over subsets of the sort σ, by letting them run over $\mathcal{P}(\llbracket \sigma \rrbracket)$.

The internal logic is particularly useful for part of the topos structure of C[P]. For example, for every object $(X, \sim)$ there is a *partial map classifier*: that is, an object $\widetilde{(X, \sim)}$ and a morphism $\eta : (X, \sim) \to \widetilde{(X, \sim)}$ with the property that for every monomorphism $(Y, \sim) \overset{m}{\to} (Z, \sim)$ and every morphism $(Y, \sim) \overset{f}{\to} (X, \sim)$ (this data determines a *partial map* from $(Z, \sim)$ to $(X, \sim)$), there is a unique morphism $\tilde{f} : (Z, \sim) \to \widetilde{(X, \sim)}$ which makes the diagram

$$
\begin{array}{ccc}
(Y, \sim) & \overset{m}{\longrightarrow} & (Z, \sim) \\
{\scriptstyle f} \downarrow & & \downarrow {\scriptstyle \tilde{f}} \\
(X, \sim) & \underset{\eta}{\longrightarrow} & \widetilde{(X, \sim)}
\end{array}
$$

into a pullback.

Constructively as well as classically, $\widetilde{(X, \sim)}$ is "the set of those subsets of $(X, \sim)$ which have at most one element" and "$f(\tilde{z}) = \{f(y) \mid m(y) = z\}$"; so, $\widetilde{(X, \sim)}$ is the subobject of $\mathcal{P}(X, \sim)$ represented by the strict relation

$$[R \sim R \land \forall xy (x \in_X R \land y \in_X R \to x \sim y)]$$

The map η is represented by

$$H(x, R) \quad \equiv \quad [R \sim R \land x \sim x \land \forall y (y \in_X R \leftrightarrow x \sim y)]$$

If $m : (Y, \sim) \to (Z, \sim)$ is represented by M and $f : (Y, \sim) \to (X, \sim)$ is represented by F, then $\tilde{f}$ is represented by

$$\tilde{F}(z, R) \equiv [z \sim z \wedge R \sim R \wedge \forall x (x \in_X R \leftrightarrow \exists y (M(y, z) \wedge F(y, x)))]$$

Another part of the topos structure are the Σ- and Π-functors. Recall that in every topos $\mathcal{E}$, for every object X we can form the *slice category* $\mathcal{E}/X$ whose objects are maps in $\mathcal{E}$ with codomain X, and whose maps are commutative triangles. For every morphism $f : Y \to X$ we have the functor $f^* : \mathcal{E}/X \to \mathcal{E}/Y$ obtained by pulling back alog f. The functor f^* has both a left adjoint Σ_f and a right adjoint Π_f. Σ_f is given by composition with f, but the definition of Π_f is more intricate.

As usual, it is useful to write out such a functor in the case of $\mathcal{E} = \mathrm{Set}$. Given a function $Z \xrightarrow{g} X$ as object of Set/X, and $f : Y \to X$, an arrow from $f^*(Z \xrightarrow{g} X)$ to $(W \xrightarrow{k} Y)$ is a Y-indexed sequence $\{\phi_y : y \in Y\}$ of partial maps $Z \rightharpoonup W$ such that for each y the domain of ϕ_y is $g^{-1}(f(y))$ and for all $z \in \mathrm{dom}(\phi_y)$, $k(\phi_y(z)) = y$. This means that we have for each $z \in Z$ a partial map $\psi_z : Y \rightharpoonup W$ such that the domain of ψ_z is $f^{-1}(g(z))$ and for all $y \in \mathrm{dom}(\psi_z)$, $k(\psi_z(y)) = y$; simply put $\psi_z(y) = \phi_y(z)$.

So if V is the set of all pairs (x, F_x) with $x \in X$ and F_x a partial map $Y \rightharpoonup W$ satisfying $\mathrm{dom}(F_x) = f^{-1}(x)$ and $k(F_x(y)) = y$ for all $y \in f^{-1}(x)$, and $\pi : V \to X$ is the projection, it follows that there is a natural 1-1 correspondence between maps from $f^*(Z \xrightarrow{g} X)$ to $(W \xrightarrow{k} Y)$ in Set/Y, and maps from $(Z \xrightarrow{g} X)$ to $(V \xrightarrow{\pi} X)$ in Set/X; hence, $\Pi_f(W \xrightarrow{k} Y)$ must be isomorphic to $V \xrightarrow{\pi} X$.

So in $\mathsf{C[P]}$, if $f : (Y, \sim) \to (X, \sim)$ is represented by F and

$$k : (W, \sim) \to (Y, \sim)$$

is represented by K, the domain of $\Pi_f(k)$ can be given as $(X \times \pi(Y \times W), \sim)$ with

$$(x, R) \sim (x', S) \equiv [x \sim x' \wedge \forall yw (R(y, w) \leftrightarrow S(y, w)) \wedge E(R)]$$

where $E(R)$ expresses that R represents a partial map $(Y, \sim) \to (Z, \sim)$ etc.

2.4 The 'constant objects' functor

As we have seen in item 3 of section 2.1.4, for every object X of C the element $\exists_\delta(\top_X)$ is an equality predicate on X, and from item 4 in the same section it follows that every element of $\mathsf{P}(X)$ is relational for $\exists_\delta(\top_X)$. It is also trivially strict, for the assertion that $\mathsf{P} \models \psi(x) \rightarrow \exists_\delta(\top_X)$ means that $\psi \leq \delta^*(\exists_\delta(\top_X))$, which is immediate.

For every object X of C we have therefore an object

$$\nabla(X) \;=\; (X, \exists_\delta(\top_X))$$

of $\mathsf{C}[\mathsf{P}]$, and for every arrow $f : X \rightarrow Y$ in C we have an element $\exists_{\langle \mathrm{id}_X, f\rangle}(\top_X)$ of $\mathsf{P}(X \times Y)$, which is a strict relation for both $\exists_\delta(\top_X)$ and $\exists_\delta(\top_Y)$; we claim that it represents an arrow $\nabla(X) \rightarrow \nabla(Y)$ in $\mathsf{C}[\mathsf{P}]$.

It is total, because

$$[\exists y(\exists_{\langle \mathrm{id}_X, f\rangle}(\top_X)(x,y))] \simeq \exists_{\pi_X}\exists_{\langle \mathrm{id}_X, f\rangle}(\top_X) \simeq \exists_{\mathrm{id}_X}(\top_X) \simeq \top_X$$

Next, we observe that $\exists_{\langle \mathrm{id}_X, f\rangle}(\top_X)$ is isomorphic to $(f \times \mathrm{id})^*(\exists_\delta(\top_Y))$ by applying the Beck-Chevalley condition to the pullback diagram

$$
\begin{array}{ccc}
X & \xrightarrow{\;\langle \mathrm{id}_X, f\rangle\;} & X \times Y \\
{\scriptstyle f}\big\downarrow & & \big\downarrow{\scriptstyle f \times \mathrm{id}_Y} \\
Y & \xrightarrow{\quad \delta \quad} & Y \times Y
\end{array}
$$

Now to see that the relation is single-valued, we need to show that

$$(1)\quad \pi_{12}^*(\exists_{\langle \mathrm{id}_X, f\rangle}(\top_X)) \wedge \pi_{13}^*(\exists_{\langle \mathrm{id}_X, f\rangle}(\top_X)) \leq \pi_{23}^*(\exists_\delta(\top_Y))$$

in $\mathsf{P}(X \times Y \times Y)$, where $\pi_{12}, \pi_{13} : X \times Y \times Y \rightarrow X \times Y$ and $\pi_{23} : X \times Y \times Y \rightarrow Y \times Y$ are projections.

We have a pullback diagram

$$
\begin{array}{ccc}
X \times Y & \xrightarrow{\qquad\qquad f\pi_1 \qquad\qquad} & Y \\
{\scriptstyle \langle \pi_1, f\pi_1, \pi_2\rangle}\big\downarrow & & \big\downarrow{\scriptstyle \delta} \\
X \times Y \times Y \xrightarrow{\;\pi_{12}\;} X \times Y & \xrightarrow{\;f\times \mathrm{id}\;} & Y \times Y
\end{array}
$$

so using the Beck-Chevally condition and some elementary adjunctions, we see that (1) above is equivalent to

(2) $\exists_{\langle \pi_1, f\pi_1, \pi_2 \rangle}(\top_{X \times Y}) \leq \pi^*_{13}(\exists_{\langle \mathrm{id}_X, f \rangle}(\top_X)) \rightarrow \pi^*_{23}(\exists_\delta(\top_Y))$

and hence to

(3) $\top_{X \times Y} \leq \exists_{\langle \mathrm{id}_X, f \rangle}(\top_X) \rightarrow (f \times \mathrm{id})^*(\exists_\delta(\top_Y))$

which reduces to

(4) $\top_X \leq \langle f, f \rangle^*(\exists_\delta(\top_Y))$

and this last one follows easily, since $\langle f, f \rangle = \delta f$.

So for every arrow $f : X \rightarrow Y$ in C we have defined an arrow $\nabla(f) : \nabla(X) \rightarrow \nabla(Y)$ in $\mathsf{C}[\mathsf{P}]$, which is represented by $\exists_{\langle \mathrm{id}_X, f \rangle}(\top_X)$. Moreover, this assignment is functorial: we have $\exists_{\langle \mathrm{id}, \mathrm{id} \rangle}(\top) \simeq \exists_\delta(\top)$ in $\mathsf{P}(X \times X)$ so both represent the identity arrow on $\nabla(X)$; and since $\langle \mathrm{id}, g \rangle \langle \mathrm{id}, f \rangle = \langle \mathrm{id}, gf \rangle$ it is also clear that composition is respected. We have a functor $\nabla : \mathsf{C} \rightarrow \mathsf{C}[\mathsf{P}]$.

Proposition 2.4.1 *The functor* $\nabla : \mathsf{C} \rightarrow \mathsf{C}[\mathsf{P}]$ *preserves finite limits.*

Proof. Since $\delta_1 : 1 \rightarrow 1 \times 1 \simeq 1$ is te identity (modulo the isomorphism $1 \simeq 1 \times 1$), ∇ preserves the terminal object.

For binary products, we have to see that in $\mathsf{P}(X \times Y \times X \times Y)$, $\exists_{\delta_{X \times Y}}(\top_{X \times Y})$ is isomorphic to $\pi^*_{13}(\exists_{\delta_X}(\top_X)) \wedge \pi^*_{24}(\exists_{\delta_Y}(\top_Y))$. Now

$$\exists_{\delta_{X \times Y}}(\top_{X \times Y}) \leq \pi^*_{13}(\exists_{\delta_X}(\top_X)) \wedge \pi^*_{24}(\exists_{\delta_Y}(\top_Y))$$

is equivalent to

$$\top_{X \times Y} \leq \pi^*_1 \delta^* \exists_\delta(\top_X) \wedge \pi^*_2 \delta^* \exists_\delta(\top_Y)$$

which is true since the RHS is isomorphic to $\top_{X \times Y}$. The converse inequality is equivalent to

$$\pi^*_{13}(\exists_\delta(\top_X)) \leq \pi^*_{24}(\exists_{\delta_Y}(\top_Y)) \rightarrow \exists_{\delta_{X \times Y}}(\top_{X \times Y})$$

The left hand side is isomorphic to $\exists_{\langle \pi_1, \pi_2, \pi_1, \pi_3 \rangle}(\top_{X \times Y})$ by an application of the Beck-Chevalley condition which should by now be familiar to you;

and similarly, $\langle \pi_1, \pi_2 \rangle^*(\exists_{\delta_Y}(\top_Y)) \simeq \exists_{\langle \pi_1, \pi_2, \pi_2 \rangle}(\top_{X \times Y})$. The inequality reduces to

$$\top_{X \times Y} \leq \langle \pi_1, \pi_2, \pi_1, \pi_2 \rangle^*(\exists_{\delta_{X \times Y}}(\top_{X \times Y}) \simeq \delta^*(\exists_{\delta_{X \times Y}}(\top_{X \times Y}))$$

which is true. This proves preservation of binary products.

Suppose that $D \xrightarrow{e} A \xrightarrow[g]{f} B$ is an equalizer diagram in C. We show that its ∇-image is an equalizer in $\mathsf{C}[P]$. Since ∇ is a functor, the image of $\nabla(e)$ is contained in the equalizer of $\nabla(f)$ and $\nabla(g)$. We show the converse inclusion, as well as that $\nabla(e)$ is mono.

That the equalizer of $\nabla(f)$ and $\nabla(g)$ is contained in the image of $\nabla(e)$, is expressed by the inequality

$$\exists_{\langle \mathrm{id}, f \rangle}(\top_X) \wedge \exists_{\langle \mathrm{id}, g \rangle}(\top_X) \leq \pi_1^*(\exists_e(\top_E))$$

in $\mathsf{P}(E \times X)$. Equivalently,

$$\langle \mathrm{id}, f \rangle^*(\exists_{\langle \mathrm{id}, g \rangle}(\top_X)) \leq \exists_e(\top_E)$$

using that $\langle \mathrm{id}, f \rangle^*(\pi_1^*(\exists_e(\top_E))) \simeq \exists_e(\top_E)$. Now since e is an equalizer of f and g, the diagram

$$
\begin{array}{ccc}
E & \xrightarrow{\ e\ } & X \\
{\scriptstyle e} \downarrow & & \downarrow {\scriptstyle \langle \mathrm{id}, g \rangle} \\
X & \xrightarrow[\langle \mathrm{id}, f \rangle]{} & X \times Y
\end{array}
$$

is a pullback in C, whence we obtain that $\langle \mathrm{id}, f \rangle^*(\exists_{\langle \mathrm{id}, g \rangle}(\top_X)) \simeq \exists_e(\top_E)$, so the desired inequality follows.

For $\nabla(e)$ to be a monomorphism, we need to see that

$$(*) \quad \pi_{13}^*(\exists_{\langle \mathrm{id}, e \rangle}(\top_E)) \wedge \pi_{23}^*(\exists_{\langle \mathrm{id}, e \rangle}(\top_E)) \leq \pi_{12}^*(\exists_\delta(\top_E))$$

in $\mathsf{P}(E \times E \times X)$. Using the pullback diagram

$$
\begin{array}{ccc}
E \times E & \xrightarrow{\langle \pi_1, \pi_2, e\pi_1 \rangle} & E \times E \times X \\
{\scriptstyle \pi_1} \downarrow & & \downarrow {\scriptstyle \pi_{13}} \\
E & \xrightarrow[\langle \mathrm{id}, e \rangle]{} & E \times X
\end{array}
$$

we can rewrite $(*)$ to

$$\langle \pi_2, e\pi_1 \rangle^*(\exists_{\langle \text{id}, e \rangle}(\top_E)) \leq \langle \pi_1, \pi_2 \rangle^*(\exists_\delta(\top_E))$$

Now both sides are isomorphic to $\exists_\delta(\top_E)$ by elementary applications of the Beck-Chevalley condition, which we leave to you. ∎

The functor ∇ is an important instrument for the analysis of the topos $\mathsf{C}[\mathsf{P}]$. We shall see that $\mathsf{C}[\mathsf{P}]$ is, in a sense, "generated by subobjects of ∇'s" (corollary 2.4.5 below).

First, we focus on subobjects of objects of the form $\nabla(X)$. The following proposition is easy.

Proposition 2.4.2 *An object of* $\mathsf{C}[\mathsf{P}]$ *admits a monomorphism into some object* $\nabla(X)$ *if and only if it is isomorphic to an object of the form* $(X, \sim_\phi)$ *for some* $\phi \in \mathsf{P}(X)$, *where* $\sim_\phi$ *is as in item 3 of section 2.1.4.*

Proof. Every subobject of $\nabla(X) = (X, \exists_\delta(\top_X))$ is determined by an element of $\mathsf{P}(X)$ (which is automatically a strict relation for $\exists_\delta(\top)$, as we have seen), and is thus isomorphic to $(X, \sim)$ where

$$\mathsf{P} \models \forall x x'(x \sim x' \leftrightarrow \phi(x) \wedge \exists_\delta(\top)(x, x'))$$

That is, $\sim$ is $\pi_1^*(\phi) \wedge \exists_\delta(\top)$. But it is easy to see that this is isomorphic to $\exists_\delta(\phi)$: $\exists_\delta(\phi) \leq \pi_1^*(\phi) \wedge \exists_\delta(\top)$ because $\phi \leq \delta^* \pi_1^*(\phi) \wedge \delta^* \exists_\delta(\top) \simeq \phi$, and conversely $\exists_\delta(\top) \leq \pi_1^*(\phi) \rightarrow \exists_\delta(\phi)$ because the RHS is isomorphic to $\phi \rightarrow \phi$. ∎

The full subcategory of $\mathsf{C}[\mathsf{P}]$ on the sub-∇'s (subobjects of objects $\nabla(X)$) is regular: it inherits the regular structure of $\mathsf{C}[\mathsf{P}]$, because it is closed under subobjects, and so the inclusion of it in $\mathsf{C}[\mathsf{P}]$ is a regular functor. We shall call it the category of P-*assemblies* on C, and write $\mathrm{Ass}_\mathsf{C}(\mathsf{P})$.

Proposition 2.4.3 *Every object of* $\mathsf{C}[\mathsf{P}]$ *is a quotient of a* P-*assembly on* C.

Proof. This means that for every object $(X, \sim)$ there is an epimorphism $(Y, \sim_\phi) \rightarrow (X, \sim)$ in $\mathsf{C}[\mathsf{P}]$. But this is immediate: take $Y = X$ and $\phi = \delta^*(\sim)$. ∎

The category $\mathrm{Ass}_\mathsf{C}(\mathsf{P})$ is in general not *exact*: it does not admit quotients of equivalence relations. Now for every regular category $\mathcal{C}$, there is a so-called *ex/reg completion* of $\mathcal{C}$, denoted $\mathcal{C}_{\text{ex/reg}}$, together with a regular functor $\mathcal{C} \xrightarrow{\eta} \mathcal{C}_{\mathrm{ex/reg}}$, such that $\mathcal{C}_{\mathrm{ex/reg}}$ is exact, and composition with η induces an equivalence of categories

$$\mathrm{REG}(\mathcal{C}, \mathcal{D}) \simeq \mathrm{REG}(\mathcal{C}_{\mathrm{ex/reg}}, \mathcal{D})$$

for every exact category $\mathcal{D}$ (here $\mathrm{REG}(\mathcal{C}, \mathcal{D})$ is the category of regular functors $\mathcal{C} \to \mathcal{D}$ and natural transformations).

The construction is simple. The objects of $\mathcal{C}_{\mathrm{ex/reg}}$ are pairs (X, E) where X is an object of $\mathcal{C}$ and E is an *equivalence relation* on X in $\mathcal{C}$, that is: E is a subobject of $X \times X$ with the property that for every object Y of $\mathcal{C}$, the relation $\sim$ between morphisms $Y \to X$ given by

$$f \sim g \;\;\text{iff}\;\; \langle f, g \rangle : Y \to X \times X \;\;\text{factors through } E$$

is an equivalence relation on $\mathcal{C}(Y, X)$.

The morphisms $(X, E) \to (X', E')$ in $\mathcal{C}_{\mathrm{ex/reg}}$ are *functional relations* from E to E', that is: subobjects F of $X \times X'$ satisfying the following four conditions:

  i) $\pi_{13}^*(F) \cap \pi_{12}^*(E) \leq \pi_{23}^*(F)$ in $\mathrm{Sub}_{\mathcal{C}}(X \times X \times Y)$
  ii) $\pi_{12}^*(F) \cap \pi_{23}^*(E') \leq \pi_{13}^*(F)$ in $\mathrm{Sub}_{\mathcal{C}}(X \times Y \times Y)$
  iii) $\pi_{12}^*(F) \cap \pi_{13}^*(F) \leq \pi_{23}^*(E')$ in $\mathrm{Sub}_{\mathcal{C}}(X \times Y \times Y)$
  iv) The composite $F \to X \times X' \xrightarrow{\pi_X} X$ is regular epi

In this context, the notation π^* refers to pullback of subobjects.

Conditions i) and ii) say that F respects the equivalence relations E and E' (is "relational"), iii) that "F is single-valued w.r.t. E'", and iv) that F is "total".

Given functional relations F from (X, E) to (X', E') and G from (X', E') to (X'', E'') the composition $G \circ F$, as subobject of $X \times X''$, is the image of the subobject $\pi_{12}^*(F) \cap \pi_{23}^*(G)$ of $X \times X' \times X''$ under the projection $\pi_{13} : X \times X' \times X'' \to X \times X''$. It is a nice exercise in the logic of regular categories to show that this is a functional relation, and that this composition is associative. But the analogy with the construction of C[P] is obvious.

The functor $\eta : \mathcal{C} \to \mathcal{C}_{\mathrm{ex/reg}}$ sends X to (X, Δ_X) (where Δ_X is the diagonal subobject of $X \times X$), and $f : X \to Y$ to the subobject

$X \overset{\langle \mathrm{id}, f \rangle}{\to} X \times Y$. For more information on $\mathcal{C}_{\mathrm{ex/reg}}$, the reader is referred to [48]. The following lemma characterizes these ex/reg completions.

Lemma 2.4.4 *Let* $\mathcal{C} \overset{\Phi}{\to} \mathcal{D}$ *be a regular functor from a regular category* $\mathcal{C}$ *to an exact category* $\mathcal{D}$. *Then the following two conditions are equivalent:*

i) *There is an equivalence of categories* $\mathcal{K} : \mathcal{C}_{\mathrm{ex/reg}} \to \mathcal{D}$ *such that the triangle*

commutes up to isomorphism;

ii) Φ *is full and faithful, surjective on subobjects (every subobject of* $\Phi(X)$ *in* $\mathcal{D}$ *is the* Φ*-image of a subobject of* X *in* $\mathcal{C}$*), and every object of* $\mathcal{D}$ *is a quotient of some object in the image of* Φ.

Proof. For i) $\Rightarrow$ ii) it suffices to see that η has the properties mentioned in ii), since they are clearly stable under equivalences.

Now in $\mathcal{C}_{\mathrm{ex/reg}}$, a functional relation $F : (X, E) \to (X', E')$ is mono if and only if the inequality

$$\pi_{13}^*(F) \cap \pi_{23}^*(F) \leq \pi_{12}^*(E)$$

holds between subobjects of $X \times X \times X'$. If $E' = \Delta_{X'}$, then there is a unique morphism $f : X \to X'$ in $\mathcal{C}$ such that F, as subobject of $X \times X'$, is the image of the composite map

$$E \to X \times X \overset{\mathrm{id} \times f}{\to} X \times X'$$

The conditions that F is relational for E and that F is monic now imply that the kernel pair of f is exactly E. Since E is a kernel pair, it has a coequalizer Y in the regular category $\mathcal{C}$. It follows that (X, E) is isomorphic to $\eta(Y)$ in $\mathcal{C}_{\mathrm{ex/reg}}$. This shows that η is surjective on subobjects and at the same time that η is faithful (because η is a regular functor); and from the first part of the argument it follows easily that η is full.

Finally, in $\mathcal{C}_{\text{ex/reg}}$ every object (X, E) is a quotient of $\eta(X)$ by E which is a regular epimorphism: $(X, \Delta_X) \to (X, E)$.

For ii) $\Rightarrow$ i) suppose $\Phi : \mathcal{C} \to \mathcal{D}$ satisfies the conditions in ii). Let (X, E) be an object of $\mathcal{C}_{\text{ex/reg}}$. Because Φ is left exact, $\Phi(E)$ is an equivalence relation on $\Phi(X)$ in $\mathcal{D}$. By exactness of $\mathcal{D}$, choose a quotient $\mathcal{K}(X, E)$ for this. If $F : (X, E) \to (X', E')$ is a morphism in $\mathcal{C}_{\text{ex/reg}}$, then $\Phi(F)$ determines a morphism $\Phi(X) \to \Phi(X')/\Phi(E) \equiv \mathcal{K}(X, E)$ in $\mathcal{D}$, whose kernel pair contains $\Phi(E)$; hence it factors uniquely through a morphism $\mathcal{K}(F) : \mathcal{K}(X, E) \to \mathcal{K}(X', E')$. This is clearly functorial.

$\mathcal{K}$ is full and faithful: suppose $f : \mathcal{K}(X, E) \to \mathcal{K}(X', E')$ is an arrow in $\mathcal{D}$. Consider the pullback

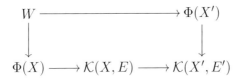

in $\mathcal{D}$. Then W is a subobject of $\Phi(X \times X')$; since Φ is surjective on subobjects there is a unique subobject F of $X \times X'$ in $\mathcal{C}$ such that $W \simeq \Phi(F)$. Then F is a functional relation from E to E': this follows because Φ, being regular and full and faithful, reflects inequalities between subobjects and regular epimorphisms. Hence, we have a unique arrow $F : (X, E) \to (X', E')$ in $\mathcal{C}_{\text{ex/reg}}$ such that $f = \mathcal{K}(F)$.

Moreover, since every object A of $\mathcal{D}$ is covered by some $\Phi(X)$, and the kernel pair of this cover is of the form $\Phi(E)$ for an equivalence relation E on X, A is isomorphic to $\mathcal{K}(X, E)$. Thus $\mathcal{K}$ is essentially surjective, and therefore an equivalence. ∎

Corollary 2.4.5 $\mathsf{C}[\mathsf{P}]$ *is equivalent to* $(\mathrm{Ass}_{\mathsf{C}}(\mathsf{P}))_{\text{ex/reg}}$.

Of course, in order to prove this fact, it was not necessary to state and derive Lemma 2.4.4; one could have done this directly, for the construction of $\mathsf{C}[\mathsf{P}]$ is virtually identical to that of $(\mathrm{Ass}_{\mathsf{C}}(\mathsf{P}))_{\text{ex/reg}}$. But the Lemma is useful for other purposes too.

Corollary 2.4.5 was first *explicitly* stated in the paper [31]; however, at least implicitly it is in Pitts' thesis (his proposition 3.8 is a very close approximation of the result).

Instead of studying subobjects of objects $\nabla(X)$, the P-assemblies, we can also consider *quotients* of them. We shall call such objects *uniform*: $(X, \sim)$ is uniform if and only if there is an epimorphism $\nabla(Y) \to (X, \sim)$ for some Y.

In the generality we are discussing at the moment, there is not much to say about uniform objects, although they turn out to be of importance in the study of realizability toposes. We limit ourselves here to two propositions: one characterizing uniform objects, and one giving a closure property for them.

Proposition 2.4.6 *An object of* C[P] *is uniform if and only if it is isomorphic to an object* $(X, \sim)$ *for which* $\mathsf{P} \models \forall x (x \sim x)$.

Proof. First, if $\mathsf{P} \models \forall x (x \sim x)$ then $\sim$ is total as relation from $(X, \exists_\delta(\top))$ to $(X, \sim)$ and hence represents a cover of $(X, \sim)$ by $\nabla(X)$.

Conversely, suppose that F is a functional relation from $\nabla(Y)$ to $(X, \sim)$ which represents a cover. Then we can define an equality predicate on Y by

$$y \approx y' \;\equiv\; [\exists x (F(y, x) \wedge F(y', x))]$$

Then F is also a functional relation from $(Y, \approx)$ to $(X, \sim)$, and it is easily seen that F represents an isomorphism between these two objects. Moreover, since F is total for $\exists_\delta(\top_Y)$, it follows at once that

$$\mathsf{P} \models \forall y (y \approx y)$$

∎

The following proposition was first, for the special case of the effective topos, formulated in [169].

Proposition 2.4.7 *If* $(X, \sim)$ *is uniform then so is* $\mathcal{P}(X, \sim)$.

Proof. Without loss of generality, assume $\mathsf{P} \models \forall x (x \sim x)$. It is then not hard to see that $\mathcal{P}(X, \sim)$ is isomorphic to the object $(\pi(X), \approx)$ where

$$R \approx S \;\equiv\; [\forall x x' (x \sim x' \to (x \in_X R \leftrightarrow x' \in_X S))]$$

since every R is automatically strict for $\sim$, and $R \approx R$ is P-equivalent to saying that R is relational for $\sim$.

Now consider the element $Z \in \mathsf{P}(\pi(X) \times X)$ defined by

$$[Z(R, x)] \equiv [\exists x'(x \sim x' \wedge x' \in_X R)]$$

By the generic property of $\pi(X)$ there is an arrow $\zeta : \pi(X) \to \pi(X)$ in C such that

$$\mathsf{P} \models \forall R \forall x (Z(R, x) \leftrightarrow x \in_X \zeta(R))$$

Now define $[R \approx' S] \equiv [\zeta(R) \approx \zeta(S)]$. One can prove by logic:

i) $\mathsf{P} \models \forall R (\zeta(R) \approx \zeta(R))$

ii) $\mathsf{P} \models \forall R (R \approx R \to R \approx \zeta(R))$

From this it follows that $\mathsf{P} \models \forall R (\zeta(R) \approx' \zeta(R))$, so $(\pi(X), \approx')$ is uniform; and $(\pi(X), \approx')$ is easily seen to be isomorphic to $(\pi(X), \approx)$.   ∎

Example. In virtually every example of interest, the functor ∇ is faithful. For realizability triposes on Set, ∇ is even full and faithful. That this is not always the case, is shown by the following example, which is inspired by the theory of forcing in Set Theory.

Let A and B be two infinite sets. Consider the poset P of partial injective functions $A \rightharpoonup B$ with finite domain, ordered by reverse inclusion (so $q \leq p$ iff the function q extends p). Let $\mathcal{B}$ be the collection of those downwards closed subsets U of P that satisfy the following condition:

For every $p \in P$, if $\forall q \leq p \exists r \leq q(r \in U)$, then $p \in U$

$\mathcal{B}$ is ordered by inclusion. It is not hard to check that $\mathcal{B}$ is a complete Boolean algebra: the top element is P, the bottom element is $\emptyset$, binary meet is given by intersection, and for a collection $\{U_i \mid i \in I\}$ of elements of $\mathcal{B}$, the join is given by

$$\bigvee_{i \in I} U_i = \{p \in P \mid \forall q \leq p \exists r \leq q \exists i \in I (r \in U_i)\}$$

The poset P has a top element, the empty function $\langle \rangle$, so for $U \in \mathcal{B}$ it holds that U is the top element if and only if $\langle \rangle \in U$.

We consider the tripos $\mathsf{P} = \mathcal{B}^{(-)}$ on Set. We claim that in Set$[\mathsf{P}]$, the objects $\nabla(A)$ and $\nabla(B)$ are isomorphic. Clearly, if A and B have different cardinalities, this shows that ∇ cannot be full.

Indeed, define $F : A \times B \to \mathcal{B}$ by

$$F(a,b) = \{p \in P \,|\, a \in \mathrm{dom}(p) \text{ and } p(a) = b\}$$

Note, that this is an element of $\mathcal{B}$, so $F \in \mathsf{P}(A \times B)$, hence F is a strict relation from $\nabla(A)$ to $\nabla(B)$. F is total, because for every $a \in A$, every $p \in P$ has an extension q with $a \in \mathrm{dom}(q)$ (recall that A and B were assumed to be infinite); that means that for every $a \in A$, $\langle \rangle \in [\exists b F(a,b)]$.

F is single-valued because if $p \in F(a,b) \cap F(a,b')$, the requirement that p is a function forces that $b = b'$. So F represents a morphism $\nabla(A) \to \nabla(B)$ in Set$[\mathsf{P}]$. This morphism is monic: if $p \in F(a,b) \cap F(a',b)$ then since P consists of *injective* functions, $a = a'$ holds.

Finally, F represents also an epimorphism: for every $b \in B$, every $p \in P$ has an extension q with $b \in \mathrm{ran}(q)$; that is, $\langle \rangle \in [\exists a F(a,b)]$. We cocclude that F represents an isomorphism, as claimed.

2.5   Geometric morphisms

2.5.1   Geometric morphisms of toposes

An important tool in the study of toposes is the notion of *geometric morphism*. Recall that for toposes $\mathcal{E}$ and $\mathcal{F}$, a geometric morphism $f : \mathcal{E} \to \mathcal{F}$ consists of an adjoint pair of functors $f^* \dashv f_*$ where $f_* : \mathcal{E} \to \mathcal{F}$, $f^* : \mathcal{F} \to \mathcal{E}$, and f^* preserves finite limits. The functor f_* is called the *direct image* and f^* is the *inverse image* of f. We write $f = (f_*, f^*)$.

There is an extensive theory of geometric morphisms, which I shall not review here. The interested reader is referred to the monumental work [83]. However, it will be useful to go over a few elements.

The basic example of a geometric morphism is given by considering slices of a topos $\mathcal{E}$: for every object X of $\mathcal{E}$, the slice category $\mathcal{E}/X$ is a topos. Given an arrow $f : Y \to X$ in $\mathcal{E}$, then as we recalled in section 2.3, the pullback functor $f^* : \mathcal{E}/X \to \mathcal{E}/Y$ has both adjoints. It also preserves finite limits, so we have a geometric morphism (Π_f, f^*) : $\mathcal{E}/Y \to \mathcal{E}/X$. This is actually an example of an *essential* geometric morphism, which is one for which the inverse image functor has a left adjoint.

There are many 'factorization theorems' about geometric morphisms. They state that every geometric morphism $\mathcal{E} \xrightarrow{f} \mathcal{F}$ factors aa a composite

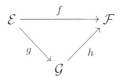

with g and h of certain specified types. I state and briefly explain two of these theorems.

Definition 2.5.1 Let $f : \mathcal{E} \to \mathcal{F}$ be a geometric morphism of toposes. Then f is called a *surjection* or *surjective geometric morphism* if f^* is faithful, and f is called an *inclusion* or *geometric inclusion* if f_* is full and faithful.

Happily, this terminology is in harmony with our basic example: if $f : Y \to X$ is an arrow in $\mathcal{E}$, then (Π_f, f^*) is surjective as geometric morphism precisely when f is an epimorphism in $\mathcal{E}$; and it is an inclusion precisely when f is mono.

Surjections and inclusions arise naturally by two basic constructions of new toposes from old ones.

It is a theorem in topos theory that given a comonad G on a topos $\mathcal{E}$ for which the underlying functor preserves finite limits, the category $\mathcal{E}_G$ of coalgebras for G is a topos. Moreover, the canonical adjunction $U \dashv C$ (where $C : \mathcal{E} \to \mathcal{E}_G$ is the cofree comonad functor, and U is the forgetful functor) defines a geometric morphism $\mathcal{E} \to \mathcal{E}_G$: U preserves finite limits because G does. Clearly, the forgetful functor U is faithful, so this is a surjection. Conversely, every surjection arises in this way.

Another way to construct new toposes from old ones is by considering *universal closure operations* on a topos $\mathcal{E}$: a universal closure operation cl on a left exact category $\mathcal{E}$ gives for every object X of $\mathcal{E}$ a closure operation (in the lattice-theoretic sense) cl_X on $Sub(X)$: that is, for every subobject A of X we should have $A \leq \mathsf{cl}_X(A) = \mathsf{cl}_X(\mathsf{cl}_X(A))$. Moreover, this system of closure operations should be stable under pullback in the sense that for any morphism $u : Y \to X$ and every subobject A of X, we have $\mathsf{cl}_Y(f^*(A)) = f^*(\mathsf{cl}_X(A))$.

Given such a universal closure operation, we call a subobject A of X *dense* if $\mathsf{cl}_X(A) = X$. X is a *sheaf* for cl if for every dense mono $U \xrightarrow{m} Y$ and every arrow $f : U \to X$ there is a unique arrow $\bar{f} : Y \to X$ such that $\bar{f}m = f$.

The full subcategory $\mathcal{E}_{\mathsf{cl}}$ of $\mathcal{E}$ on the sheaves for cl is a topos, and the inclusion functor has a finite-limit preserving left adjoint. Therefore, the embedding of $\mathcal{E}_{\mathsf{cl}}$ into $\mathcal{E}$ defines a geometric inclusion of toposes. Conversely, if $\mathcal{E} \to \mathcal{F}$ is a geometric inclusion, there is a unique universal closure operation cl on $\mathcal{F}$ and an equivalence $\mathcal{E} \simeq \mathcal{F}_{\mathsf{cl}}$ such that the diagram

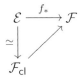

commutes up to isomorphism.

In our basic example of slice categories $\mathcal{E}/X$, we can use the factorization $f = mc$ of any arrow $f : Y \to X$ as epi followed by mono, to factor the geometric morphism (Π_f, f^*) as surjection followed by inclusion.

This factorization holds more generally.

Proposition 2.5.2 *Every geometric morphism factors as a surjection followed by an inclusion. The factorization is essentially unique.*

For a proof, see [83]. However, the factorization has an easy description, which I want to outline. Given $f : \mathcal{E} \to \mathcal{F}$, the composition $f^* f_*$ is a comonad G on $\mathcal{E}$ which preserves finite limits, and $\mathcal{E} \to \mathcal{E}_G$ is the 'surjective part' of the factorization.

For the inclusion part, f induces a universal closure operation on $\mathcal{F}$ as follows. Given a mono $U \to X$ representing a subobject A, the subobject $\mathsf{cl}_X(A)$ is represented by $\bar{U} \to X$, where $\bar{U}$ is such that the square

$$\begin{array}{ccc} \bar{U} & \longrightarrow & X \\ \downarrow & & \downarrow{\scriptstyle \eta} \\ f_*f^*(U) & \longrightarrow & f_*f^*(X) \end{array}$$

is a pullback diagram (η denotes the unit of the adjunction $f^* \dashv f_*$). It is not hard to check that this is indeed a universal closure operation cl. $\mathcal{F}_{\mathsf{cl}} \to \mathcal{F}$ is the 'inclusion part' of f. Note that $\mathcal{E}_G \simeq \mathcal{F}_{\mathsf{cl}}$.

There is another factorization that I mention, although it will play no further role in this book: the *hyperconnected-localic* factorization. Let $\Omega_{\mathcal{E}}$, $\Omega_{\mathcal{F}}$ denote the respective subobject classifiers in $\mathcal{E}$, $\mathcal{F}$. There is a canonical map $f_*(\Omega_{\mathcal{E}}) \to \Omega_{\mathcal{F}}$ in $\mathcal{F}$: it classifies the subobject $f_*(\mathrm{true}) : 1 \simeq f_*(1) \to f_*(\Omega_{\mathcal{E}})$. The geometric morphism f is called *hyperconnected* if this map is an isomorphism. This is equivalent to: f^* is full and faithful, and its image is closed under subobjects in $\mathcal{E}$.

A geometric morphism f is *localic* if for every object X of $\mathcal{E}$ there is a diagram

$$\begin{array}{ccc} A & \overset{m}{\longrightarrow} & f^*(Y) \\ {\scriptstyle e}\downarrow & & \\ X & & \end{array}$$

with m mono and e epi (X is said to be a *subquotient* of $f^*(Y)$).

Proposition 2.5.3 *Every geometric morphism factors, essentially uniquely, as a hyperconnected one followed by a localic one.*

Locale is another word for 'complete Heyting algebra' (well... not *just* another word. The theory of locales aims to study those aspects of topology that do not refer to the points of a space, and the morphisms of locales are therefore not Heyting maps. For an introduction to locale theory, which is also very fundamental for topos theory, see [81], [86], the already cited [83] and the more recent [176]). The construction of the category of sheaves on a locale can be performed for any 'internal locale' L in a topos $\mathcal{E}$, giving rise to the topos $\mathrm{sh}_{\mathcal{E}}(L)$ and a localic geometric morphism $\mathrm{sh}_{\mathcal{E}}(L) \to \mathcal{E}$. For any geometric morphism $f : \mathcal{E} \to \mathcal{F}$, $f_*(\Omega_{\mathcal{E}})$

is an internal locale in $\mathcal{F}$, and the hyperconnected-localic factorization of f is given by

$$\mathcal{E} \to \mathrm{sh}_{\mathcal{F}}(f_*(\Omega_{\mathcal{E}})) \to \mathcal{F}$$

For future reference I record here the definitions of two other types of geometric morphisms we shall encounter.

Definition 2.5.4

i)   A geometric morphism $f : \mathcal{E} \to \mathcal{F}$ is *open* if f^* preserves universal quantification: if, for an arrow $u : X \to Y$ in $\mathcal{F}$, $\forall_u : \mathrm{Sub}_{\mathcal{F}}(X) \to \mathrm{Sub}_{\mathcal{F}}(Y)$ denotes the right adjoint to pulling back along u, then

$$f^*(\forall_u(A)) = \forall_{f^*(u)}(f^*(A))$$

ii)   A geometric morphism $f : \mathcal{E} \to \mathcal{F}$ is *local* if f_* has a full and faithful right adjoint.

Since for every geometric morphism f the inverse image part f^*, being a left exact left adjoint, preserves existential quantification, union and intersection of subobjects, f is open if and only if f^* preserves first-order logic, that is: f^* is a Heyting functor.

2.5.2   Geometric morphisms of triposes

Definition 2.5.5 Let P and Q be C-triposes. A *geometric morphism* P $\to$ Q is an adjoint pair $\Phi^+ \dashv \Phi_+$ of transformations, with $\Phi_+ : $ P $\to$ Q, $\Phi^+ : $ Q $\to$ P, such that for every C-object X the preorder-map $\Phi_X^+ :$ Q$(X) \to$ P(X) preserves finite meets. We write $\Phi = (\Phi_+, \Phi^+)$.

Remark. From the adjunction it follows that Φ^+ commutes, up to isomorphism, with the left adjoints $\exists_f$: if for $f : X \to Y$ in C, $\exists_f^{\mathsf{P}} \dashv$ P(f) and $\exists_f^{\mathsf{Q}} \dashv$ Q(f), then $\Phi_Y^+ \circ \exists_f^{\mathsf{Q}} \simeq \exists_f^{\mathsf{P}} \circ \Phi_X^+$. This is seen by taking right adjoints. Transformations with these properties of Φ^+, i.e. which preserve finite meets in each component and commute with $\exists_f$, will be called *regular*.

Given a geometric morphism $\Phi : \mathsf{P} \to \mathsf{Q}$, it is a consequence of the fact that Φ^+ preserves finite meets, that if $(X, \sim)$ is an object of $\mathsf{C}[\mathsf{Q}]$ then $(X, \Phi_{X \times X}^+(\sim))$ is an object of $\mathsf{C}[\mathsf{P}]$. Moreover, since Φ^+ preserves existential quantification, it is also true that if $F \in \mathsf{Q}(X \times Y)$ represents a morphism $(X, \sim) \to (Y, \sim)$ in $\mathsf{C}[\mathsf{Q}]$, then $\Phi_{X \times Y}^+(F)$ represents a morphism $(X, \Phi_{X \times X}^+(\sim)) \to (Y, \Phi_{Y \times Y}^+(\sim))$ in $\mathsf{C}[\mathsf{P}]$. We have therefore a functor $\Phi^* : \mathsf{C}[\mathsf{Q}] \to \mathsf{C}[\mathsf{P}]$. Again using the fact that Φ^+ is regular, we also see that the diagram

commutes, where ∇_P and ∇_Q denote the constant object functors.

Proposition 2.5.6 Φ^* *preserves finite limits.*

Proof. This follows easily from the description of finite limits in the proof of 2.2.1, and the regularity of Φ^+. ∎

We wish to prove that the functor Φ^* has a right adjoint. The problem to overcome is that for a functional relation F from $(X, \sim)$ to $(Y, \sim)$, $\Phi_+(F)$ is only a partial functional relation (it is a single-valued strict relation from $(X, \Phi_+(\sim))$ to $(Y, \Phi_+(\sim))$). Therefore first we look at objects $(X, \sim)$ which do have the property that whenever Φ is a finite-meet preserving transformation of triposes and F is a functional relation into $(X, \sim)$, $\Phi(F)$ is a functional relation into $(X, \Phi(\sim))$. Such objects are called *weakly complete*. Given an arbitrary object $(X, \sim)$ of $\mathsf{C}[\mathsf{P}]$, consider the object $(\pi(X), \sim_S)$ where $\sim_S$ is defined as follows: put

$$[S(U)] \equiv [\exists x (x \sim x \land \forall x'(x' \in_X U \leftrightarrow x \sim x'))]$$
$$[U \sim_S V] \equiv [S(U) \land \forall x (x \in_X U \leftrightarrow x \in_X V)]$$

The object $(\pi(X), \sim_S)$ is the subobject of $\mathcal{P}(X, \sim)$ consisting of the singleton subsets of $(X, \sim)$ (in the logic of $\mathsf{C}[\mathsf{P}]$), and hence isomorphic to $(X, \sim)$.

Lemma 2.5.7 *The object $(\pi(X), \sim_S)$ is weakly complete.*

Proof. Let Φ be a finite-meet preserving transformation of triposes and F a functional relation from $(Y, \sim)$ to $(\pi(X), \sim_S)$. We need to prove that $\Phi(F)$ is total.

Let $\check{F} \in \mathsf{P}(Y \times X)$ be defined by

$$[\check{F}(y, x)] \equiv [\exists U (F(y, U) \wedge x \in_X U)]$$

Then $\check{F}$ is a functional relation from $(Y, \sim)$ to $(X, \sim)$. By the defining property of $\pi(X)$, there is an arrow $u : Y \to \pi(X)$ in C such that

$$\mathsf{P} \models \forall yx (\check{F}(y, x) \leftrightarrow x \in_X u(y))$$

It is now easy to see that

$$\mathsf{P} \models \forall y (y \sim y \to F(y, u(y)))$$

that is, $\sim \leq \langle \mathrm{id}_Y, u \rangle^*(F)$. Since Φ is a transformation of triposes, we have that $\Phi(\sim) \leq \langle \mathrm{id}_Y, u \rangle^*(\Phi(F))$; it follows that

$$\mathsf{Q} \models \forall y (\Phi(y \sim y) \to \exists U \Phi(F)(y, U))$$

so $\Phi(F)$ is total, as desired.   ∎

Theorem 2.5.8

i)   *Let $\Phi = (\Phi_+, \Phi^+) : \mathsf{P} \to \mathsf{Q}$ be a geometric morphism of triposes, and $\Phi^* : \mathsf{C[Q]} \to \mathsf{C[P]}$ be the functor constructed from Φ as above. Then Φ^* has a right adjoint. Thus every geometric morphism of triposes induces a geometric morphism on the toposes whose inverse image part preserves constant objects.*

ii)   *Conversely, every geometric morphism $\mathsf{C[P]} \to \mathsf{C[Q]}$ whose inverse image preserves constant objects is induced by an essentially unique geometric morphism of triposes.*

Proof. i) The functor $\Phi_* : \mathsf{C}[\mathsf{P}] \to \mathsf{C}[\mathsf{Q}]$ is defined as follows: on objects $(X, \sim)$ we put $\Phi_*(X, \sim) = (\pi(X), \Phi_+(\sim_S))$ where $(\pi(X), \sim_S)$ is the object of singletons of $(X, \sim)$. Given an arrow $f : (X, \sim) \to (Y, \sim)$, let $F \in \mathsf{P}(\pi(X) \times \pi(Y))$ represent the composite map

$$(\pi(X), \sim_S) \overset{\sim}{\to} (X, \sim) \overset{f}{\to} (Y, \sim) \overset{\sim}{\to} (\pi(Y), \sim_S)$$

We let $\Phi_*(f)$ be the arrow in $\mathsf{C}[\mathsf{Q}]$ represented by $\Phi_+(F)$. This is well-defined by Lemma 2.5.7.

Note that if $f : (X, \sim) \to (Y, \sim)$ and $g : (Y, \sim) \to (Z, \sim)$ are represented by functional relations F and G respectively, the composition gf is represented by $[x \sim x \wedge \forall y(F(x,y) \to G(y,z))]$. Hence if $\Phi_+(F)$ and $\Phi_+(G)$ are functional relations, then since Φ_+, being a right adjoint, commutes with universal quantifiers,

$$\begin{aligned}
\Phi_+([x \sim x \wedge \forall y(F(x,y) \to G(y,z))]) \;\;&\simeq\\
\Phi_+([x \sim x]) \wedge \forall y \Phi_+([F(x,y) \to G(y,z)]) \;\;&\leq\\
\Phi_+([x \sim x]) \wedge [\forall y((\Phi_+F)(x,y) \to (\Phi_+G)(y,z))]
\end{aligned}$$

Since both sides of the inequality are functional relations, it is in fact an isomorphism, and we conclude that the defined action of Φ_* on arrows preserves composition. It also trivially preserves identities, so Φ_* is a functor.

To prove the adjunction $\Phi^* \dashv \Phi_*$, it seems easiest to construct, for objects $(X, \sim)$ of $\mathsf{C}[\mathsf{P}]$ and $(Y, \sim)$ of $\mathsf{C}[\mathsf{Q}]$, a natural bijection between maps $\Phi^*(Y, \sim) \to (\pi(X), \sim_S)$ in $\mathsf{C}[\mathsf{P}]$ and maps $(Y, \sim) \to \Phi_*(X, \sim)$ in $\mathsf{C}[\mathsf{Q}]$. Since the isomorphism $(X, \sim) \to (\pi(X), \sim_S)$ is natural in $(X, \sim)$, this suffices.

Given a functional relation F from $\Phi^*(Y, \sim) = (Y, \Phi^+(\sim))$ to $(\pi(X), \sim_S)$, $\Phi_+(F)$ is a functional relation from $(Y, \Phi_+\Phi^+(\sim))$ to $(\pi(X), \Phi_+(\sim_S)) = \Phi_*(X, \sim)$, by lemma 2.5.7. There is also an obvious morphism $(Y, \sim) \to (Y, \Phi_+\Phi^+(\sim))$ represented by

$$H(y, y') \equiv [y \sim y \wedge \Phi_+\Phi^+(y \sim y')]$$

The morphism $(Y, \sim) \to \Phi_*(X, \sim)$ corresponding to F is given by the composition of these two maps; it is easily checked that this is represented by

$$\tilde{F}(y, R) \equiv [y \sim y \wedge (\Phi_+F)(y, R)]$$

Conversely, if G is a functional relation from $(Y, \sim)$ to $\pi(X), \Phi_+(\sim_S))$, then $\Phi^+ G$ is one from $(Y, \Phi^+(\sim))$ to $(\pi(X), \Phi^+ \Phi_+(\sim_S))$. There is a functional relation K from $(\pi(X), \Phi^+ \Phi_+(\sim_S))$ to $(\pi(X), \sim_S)$ given by

$$K(R', R) \equiv [\Phi^+ \Phi_+(R' \sim_S R') \wedge R' \sim_S R]$$

The morphism $\Phi^*(Y, \sim) \to (\pi(X), \sim_S)$ corresponding to G is the composite of these two, and represented by

$$\overline{G}(y, R) \equiv [\Phi^+(y \sim y) \wedge \forall R'(\Phi^+ G(y, R) \to R' \sim_S R)]$$

Then

$$\begin{aligned} \widetilde{\overline{G}} &\equiv [y \sim y \wedge \Phi_+ \Phi^+(y \sim y)] \wedge \Phi_+([\forall R'(\Phi^+ G(y, R') \to R' \sim_S R)]) \\ &\simeq [y \sim y \wedge \forall R' \Phi_+([\Phi^+ G(y, R') \to R' \sim_S R])] \\ &\simeq [y \sim y \wedge \forall R'(G(y, R') \to \Phi_+(R' \sim_S R))] \\ &\simeq G(y, R) \end{aligned}$$

In this sequence one uses respectively: that Φ_+ commutes with universal quantification, that for an adjunction $\Phi^+ \dashv \Phi_+$ between Heyting pre-algebras one has $\Phi_+(\Phi^+ a \to b) \simeq a \to \Phi_+ b$, and that G is a functional relation.

Similarly we have

$$\begin{aligned} \widetilde{\overline{F}}(y, R) &\equiv [\Phi^+(y \sim y) \wedge \forall R'(\Phi^+(y \sim y \wedge \Phi_F(y, R')) \to R' \sim_S R)] \\ &\simeq [\Phi^+(y \sim y) \wedge \forall R'(\Phi^+ \Phi_+ F(y, R') \to R' \sim_S R)] \end{aligned}$$

From this it is easy to see that $\mathsf{Q} \models F(y, R) \to \overline{F}(y, R)$. Since both are functional relations, they are isomorphic. This proves the desired adjunction.

ii) Now suppose $(\Phi^* \dashv \Phi_*) : \mathsf{C[P]} \to \mathsf{C[Q]}$ is a geometric morphism such that the functors ∇_P and $\Phi^* \circ \nabla_\mathsf{Q}$ are naturally isomorphic. Then Φ^* sends Q-assemblies to P-assemblies. For every C-object X and every $\phi \in \mathsf{Q}(X)$, choose $\psi = \Phi_X^+(\phi) \in \mathsf{P}(X)$ such that the P-assembly $\Phi^*(X, \sim_\phi)$ is isomorphic to $(X, \sim_\psi)$. This requirement determines ψ up to isomorphism, and we have a transformation Φ^+ of triposes. Moreover, Φ^+ is regular. Now the fact that Φ^* coincides with the functor obtained from Φ^+ in the way described before, follows from the characterization of $\mathsf{C[P]}$ as ex/reg completion of $\mathrm{Asm}_\mathsf{C}(\mathsf{P})$ (Corollary 2.4.5).

Since Φ^* preserves finite limits, Φ^+ preserves binary meets in each fibre: for $\phi, \psi \in \mathsf{Q}(X)$, the diagram

$$
\begin{array}{ccc}
(X, \sim_{\phi \wedge \psi}) & \longrightarrow & (X, \sim_\phi) \\
\downarrow & & \downarrow \\
(X, \sim_\psi) & \longrightarrow & \nabla_\mathsf{Q}(X)
\end{array}
$$

is a pullback in $\mathsf{C[Q]}$; hence $\Phi^+(\phi \wedge \psi) \simeq \Phi^+(\phi) \wedge \Phi^+(\psi)$. And also, Φ^+ preserves the top element.

We have to prove that Φ^+ has a right adjoint. Let $\psi \in \mathsf{P}(X)$. Let $\mu : \nabla_\mathsf{Q}(X) \to \Phi_*(\nabla_\mathsf{P}(X))$ be the transpose (under $\Phi^* \dashv \Phi^*$) of the isomorphism $\Phi^*(\nabla_\mathsf{Q}(X)) \to \nabla_\mathsf{P}(X)$.

Define $\Phi_+(\psi)$ in $\mathsf{Q}(X)$ by the requirement that the square

$$
\begin{array}{ccc}
(X, \sim_{\Phi_+(\psi)}) & \longrightarrow & \Phi_*(X, \sim_\psi) \\
\downarrow & & \downarrow \\
\nabla_\mathsf{Q}(X) & \longrightarrow & \Phi_*(\nabla_\mathsf{P}(X))
\end{array}
$$

be a pullback in $\mathsf{C[Q]}$ (Note that the right hand side vertical in the diagram is always a monomorphism, so this definition makes sense). For arbitrary $\phi \in \mathsf{Q}(X)$ we then have the following equivalences:

$\Phi^+(\phi) \leq \psi$ in $\mathsf{P}(X)$

$\Leftrightarrow$ the map $(X, \sim_{\Phi^+(\phi)}) \to \nabla_\mathsf{P}(X)$ factors through $(X, \sim_\psi)$

$\Leftrightarrow$ the map $\Phi^*(X, \sim_\phi) \to \Phi^*(\nabla_\mathsf{Q}(X)) \xrightarrow{\sim} \nabla_\mathsf{P}(X)$ factors through $(X, \sim_\psi)$

$\Leftrightarrow$ the map $(X, \sim_\phi) \to \nabla_\mathsf{Q}(X) \to \Phi_*(\nabla_\mathsf{P}(X))$ factors through $\Phi_*(X, \sim_\psi)$

$\Leftrightarrow$ $\phi \leq \Phi_+(\psi)$ in $\mathsf{Q}(X)$.

So Φ^+ has a right adjoint Φ_+ as desired. ∎

2.5.3   Geometric morphisms between realizability triposes on Set

We consider now the realizability triposes $\mathcal{T}(A)^{(-)}$ on Set, for order-pcas A. The following theorem is very similar to the situation of section 1.5, and parts i) and ii) appeared essentially in [123].

Theorem 2.5.9

i)   *Every applicative morphism $A \xrightarrow{\gamma} T(B)$ of order-pcas induces a regular transformation γ^* of triposes: $\mathcal{T}(A)^{(-)} \to \mathcal{T}(B)^{(-)}$. Moreover, if $\gamma \preceq \delta$ then $\gamma^* \leq \delta^*$ pointwise.*

ii) *Conversely, every regular transformation of triposes $\mathcal{T}(A)^{(-)} \to \mathcal{T}(B)^{(-)}$ is induced in this way by an essentially unique applicative morphism $A \xrightarrow{\gamma} T(B)$. Hence, the 2-category of realizability triposes on Set, regular transformations, and order-relations between them is biequivalent to the Kleisli 2-category of the 2-monad T on OPCA$^+$.*

iii) *Suppose $A \xrightarrow{\gamma} T(B)$ is an applicative morphism. Then the induced transformation γ^* has a right adjoint if and only if γ is computationally dense. Hence the 2-category of realizability triposes on Set, geometric morphisms and order-relations between their inverse image parts, is biequivalent to the opposite of the Kleisli 2-category of the 2-monad T on OPCA.*

Proof. i) The transformation γ^* is given by composition with the function $\mathcal{T}(A) \to \mathcal{T}(B)$ which sends α to $\bigcup_{a \in \alpha} \gamma(a)$. Clearly, if $\gamma \preceq \delta$ is realized by r, then for each set X and each $\phi \in \mathcal{T}(A)^X$, the inequality $\gamma_X^*(\phi) \leq \delta_X^*(\phi)$ is also realized by r. It is also easy to see that γ^* is order-preserving.

Existential quantification in realizability triposes is given by unions, so γ^* preserves this. Because γ takes values in the *nonempty* downsets of B, it follows that γ^* preserves the top element of each $\mathcal{T}(A)^X$.

In order to see that $\gamma^*(\phi) \wedge \gamma^*(\psi) \leq \gamma^*(\phi \wedge \psi)$ (the converse inequality follows by monotonicity of γ^*), let p be the pairing combinator in A and fix $q \in \gamma(p)$. Then if $a_1 \in \phi$, $a_2 \in \psi$, $pa_1a_2 \in \phi \wedge \psi$ so if $b_1 \in$

$\gamma^*(\phi)$, $b_2 \in \gamma^*(\psi)$ we have $r(rqb_1)b_2 \in \gamma^*(\phi \wedge \psi)$. Therefore the element $\langle x \rangle r(rq(p_0 x))(p_1 x)$ realizes $\gamma^*(\phi) \wedge \gamma^*(\psi) \leq \gamma^*(\phi \wedge \psi)$ for all ϕ and ψ.

ii) Conversely, suppose $\lambda : \mathcal{T}(A)^{(-)} \to \mathcal{T}(B)^{(-)}$ is a regular transformation. Let $d : A \to \mathcal{T}(A)$ be such that $d(a) = {\downarrow}(a)$. Then $l = \lambda_A(d)$ is a function from A to $\mathcal{T}(B)$. We shall see that actually, $l : A \to T(B)$, l is an applicative morphism and that λ is induced by l in the way of part i).

Let $E = \{(a, \sigma) \in A \times \mathcal{T}(A) \mid a \in \sigma\}$ with projections $\pi_1 : E \to A$ and $\pi_2 : E \to \mathcal{T}(A)$. Then $\mathrm{id}_{\mathcal{T}(A)} \in \mathcal{T}(A)^{\mathcal{T}(A)}$ is isomorphic to $\exists_{\pi_2}(\pi_1^*(d))$. Because λ commutes with $\exists$ and is a transformation of triposes we see that $\lambda_{\mathcal{T}(A)}(\mathrm{id}_{\mathcal{T}(A)}) \simeq \exists_{\pi_2}(\pi_1^*(l))$. It follows that, up to isomorphism, for arbitrary $\phi \in \mathcal{T}(A)^X$ and $x \in X$,

$$\lambda_X(\phi)(x) = \bigcup_{a \in \phi(x)} l(a)$$

so λ is induced by l in the sense of i).

Next, we prove that $l(a) \neq \emptyset$ for $a \in A$, as well as that l satisfies the second requirement for being an applicative morphism. First consider the element ϕ_a of $\mathcal{T}(A)^1$, $\phi_a(*) = {\downarrow}a$. In $\mathcal{T}(A)^1$, $\phi_a \simeq \top$ so in $\mathcal{T}(B)^1$, $\lambda_1(\phi_a) \simeq \top$, which means that

(1) $\bigcup \{l(a') \mid a' \leq a\} \neq \emptyset$

Then, look at $O = \{(a, b) \mid a \leq b\}$ with projections $\pi_1, \pi_2 : O \to A$. Clearly, $i = skk \in A$ realizes $\pi_1^*(d) \leq \pi_2^*(d)$. It follows that $\pi_1^*(l) \leq \pi_2^*(l)$ in $\mathcal{T}(B)^O$; so there is an element $m \in B$ such that for all $a \leq b$ in A, $m \in l(a) \Rightarrow l(b)$. Together with (1) this shows that $l(a)$ is nonempty for all $a \in A$. Moreover, it follows that for $M = {\downarrow}m$ in $T(B)$ we have

$$a \leq b \;\Rightarrow\; M{\cdot}l(a) \leq l(b)$$

so l satisfies the second requirement for being an applicative morphism.

As to the first requirement, let $\Delta = \{(a, a') \in A \times A \mid aa'{\downarrow}\}$, and $\phi \in \mathcal{T}(A)^\Delta$ be given by $\phi(a, a') = {\downarrow}aa'$. Then $\pi_1^*(d) \wedge \pi_2^*(d) \leq \phi$ in $\mathcal{T}(A)^\Delta$. Since λ preserves $\wedge$, $\pi_1^*(l) \leq \pi_2^*(l) \leq \lambda_\Delta(\phi)$. It follows that there is a $t \in B$ such that for all $a, a' \in A$ with $aa'{\downarrow}$, and all $b \in l(a), b' \in l(a')$, $tbb'{\downarrow}$

and $tbb' \in \bigcup_{a'' \leq aa'} l(a'')$. So $m(tbb') \in l(aa')$. Therefore, $r = \langle xy \rangle m(txy)$ satisfies the first requirement for l to be an applicative morphism.

iii) Suppose the applicative morphism $\gamma : A \to T(B)$ induces the regular transformation $\lambda : \mathcal{T}(A)^{(-)} \to \mathcal{T}(B)^{(-)}$ as in i). Let $m \in T(B)$ satisfy the computational density for γ, that is: for all $\beta \in T(B)$ there is an $a \in A$ such that

$$\forall a' \in A (\beta \cdot \gamma(a')\downarrow \Rightarrow aa'\downarrow \wedge m\gamma(aa') \leq \beta \cdot \gamma(a'))$$

Let r, u satisfy i) and ii) of the definition of applicative morphism for γ. Define $\hat{\lambda} : \mathcal{T}(B) \to \mathcal{T}(A)$ by

$$\hat{\lambda}(\beta) = \downarrow\{a \in A \mid m\gamma(a) \leq \beta\}$$

We show that $\hat{\lambda}$ (or more precisely, the transformation determined by $\hat{\lambda}$) is a right adjoint for λ.

Let $\alpha \in \mathcal{T}(A)$. For $a \in \alpha$ we have in $T(B)$ that $i\gamma(\alpha) \subseteq \bigcup_{a' \in \alpha} \gamma(a') = \lambda(\alpha)$. Applying computational density to i we find an $\bar{a} \in A$ such that for all $a \in \alpha$, $\bar{a}a\downarrow$ and $m\gamma(\bar{a}a) \leq i\gamma(a) \subseteq \lambda(\alpha)$; that is, $\bar{a}\alpha \subseteq \hat{\lambda}\lambda(\alpha)$. This shows that the identity transformation is $\leq \hat{\lambda}\lambda$. On the other hand, since $\lambda\hat{\lambda}(\beta) = \bigcup_{m\gamma(a) \subseteq \beta} \gamma(a)$, clearly $m \cdot \lambda\hat{\lambda}(\beta) \subseteq \beta$. This shows that $\lambda\hat{\lambda} \leq \mathrm{id}$, so $\hat{\lambda}$ is a right adjoint for λ.

Conversely, suppose that λ has a right adjoint $\hat{\lambda}$. Using $\lambda\hat{\lambda} \leq \mathrm{id}$ we find an clement m of $T(B)$ such that for all $\beta \in T(B)$, $m \cdot \lambda\hat{\lambda}(\beta) \subseteq \beta$.

To show that m satisfies computational density for γ, let $\beta \in T(B)$. Consider $D = \{a \in A \mid \beta \cdot \gamma(a)\downarrow\}$, let $j : D \to A$ be the inclusion, and again let $d(a) = \downarrow(a)$. We find a realizer α for $\lambda(j^*(d)) \leq \phi$, where $\phi(a) = \downarrow\beta \cdot \gamma(a)$. Hence $j^*(d) \leq \hat{\lambda}(\phi)$, so $\lambda(j^*(d)) \leq \lambda\hat{\lambda}(\phi)$. Therefore if $\beta \cdot \gamma(a)\downarrow$ then $\alpha a\downarrow$ and $m \cdot (\alpha a) \leq \beta \cdot \gamma(a)$, as desired.   ∎

Notation If A is an order-pca, and $\mathcal{T}(A)^{(-)}$ its associated realizability tripos on Set, we shall denote the topos $\mathrm{Set}[\mathcal{T}(A)^{(-)}]$ by $\mathsf{RT}(A)$, and we speak about the *realizability topos on* A.

Examples.

i)   In examples 4 and 5 of section 1.5 we have seen that there are applicative morphisms $\iota : \mathcal{K}_2 \to \mathcal{P}(\omega)$ and $\gamma : \mathcal{P}(\omega) \to \mathcal{K}_2$, such that $\iota \dashv \gamma$ and $\gamma\iota \simeq \mathrm{id}_{\mathcal{K}_2}$.

Therefore, by Example 2 at the end of section 1.8, ι is computationally dense. So also the composition of ι with the canonical map
$\mathcal{P}(\omega) \to T(\mathcal{P}(\omega))$. Theorem 2.5.9 gives that we have a geometric
morphism of triposes

$$T(\mathcal{P}(\omega))^{(-)} \to T(\mathcal{K}_2)^{(-)}$$

which in turn induces a geometric morphism from the realizability
topos on $\mathcal{P}(\omega)$ to the one on $\mathcal{K}_2$. From $\gamma\iota \simeq \mathrm{id}_{\mathcal{K}_2}$ it follows that
the transformation induced by ι reflects the preorder on predicates.
From this it is easy to deduce that the induced functor

$$\mathsf{RT}(\mathcal{K}_2) \to \mathsf{RT}(\mathcal{P}(\omega))$$

which is the inverse image of the geometric morphism, is faithful.
We conclude that this geometric morphism is a surjection.

ii) For another example of a surjection arising in this way, consider the
function $\iota : \mathcal{K}_1 \to \mathcal{K}_2^{\mathrm{rec}}$ defined by $\iota(n) = \lambda x.n$ (the function with
constant value n). In the other direction, let $\gamma : \mathcal{K}_2^{\mathrm{rec}} \to \mathcal{P}(\mathcal{K}_1)$
be given by $\gamma(\alpha) = \{e \,|\, \varphi_e = \alpha\}$ I leave it to you to work out
that ι and γ give applicative morphisms of pcas. The inequalities
$\mathrm{id}_{\mathcal{K}_1} \preceq \gamma\iota$ and $\iota\gamma \preceq \mathrm{id}_{\mathcal{K}_2^{\mathrm{rec}}}$ hold, so $\iota \dashv \gamma$ and we have a geometric
morphism $\mathsf{RT}(\mathcal{K}_2^{\mathrm{rec}}) \to \mathsf{RT}(\mathcal{K}_1)$, just as in the previous example.
Also in this case one can see that in fact we have that $\gamma\iota \simeq \mathrm{id}_{\mathcal{K}_1}$,
so this is also a surjection.

2.5.4 Inclusions of triposes and toposes

In section 2.5.1 it was mentioned that geometric inclusions into a topos
$\mathcal{E}$ correspond to universal closure operations on $\mathcal{E}$: for every object X
an operation cl_X on $\mathrm{Sub}(X)$ satisfying $A \le \mathsf{cl}_X(A) = \mathsf{cl}_X(\mathsf{cl}_X(A))$, as well
as stability under pullback: for $f : Y \to X$ and $A \in \mathrm{Sub}(X)$, we have
$\mathsf{cl}_Y(f^*(A)) = f^*(\mathsf{cl}_X(A))$.

   If $1 \xrightarrow{t} \Omega$ is the subobject classifier in $\mathcal{E}$, then every $A \in \mathrm{Sub}(X)$ is
$\phi_A^*(t)$ for a unique $\phi_A : X \to \Omega$, so $\mathsf{cl}_X(A) = \phi_A^*(\mathsf{cl}_\Omega(t))$; that is to say,
the whole closure operation is determined once we know the subobject

$J = \mathsf{cl}_\Omega(t)$ of Ω, or, equivalently, its classifying map $j : \Omega \to \Omega$. Clearly, if $A = \phi_A^*(t)$ then $\mathsf{cl}_X(A) = (j\phi_A)^*(t) = \phi_A^*(J)$.

In the internal logic of $\mathcal{E}$ the map j satisfies the following axioms:

i) $j(t) = t$

ii) $jj = j$

iii) $j(a \wedge b) = j(a) \wedge j(b)$

Such a map $j : \Omega \to \Omega$ in a topos is called a *local operator*.

We wish to have a closer look at local operators in toposes of the form $\mathsf{C}[\mathsf{P}]$. Here Ω is the object $(\Sigma, \Leftrightarrow)$ with map $1 \xrightarrow{t} \Omega$ represented by $[p \Leftrightarrow \top]$ (see the proof of theorem 2.2.1). A local operator is a functional relation $J \in \mathsf{P}(\Sigma \times \Sigma)$ (w.r.t. $\Leftrightarrow$), satisfying the obvious conditions. But since $\mathsf{P} \models x \leftrightarrow (x \Leftrightarrow \top)$ (where x is a variable of type Σ, it is not hard to infer from the axioms i)-iii) that

$$\mathsf{P} \models J(x, y) \leftrightarrow (y \Leftrightarrow J(x, \top))$$

so J is determined by the element τ of $\mathsf{P}(\Sigma)$ given by $\tau(x) \equiv [J(x, \top)]$.

The element τ in turn determines, up to isomorphism, a transformation $\Phi_j : \mathsf{P} \to \mathsf{P}$ of triposes, by $\Phi_j(\phi) = [\phi]^*(\tau)$. The transformation Φ_j has te same properties as the local operator j we started with, that is: it is order-preserving, inflationary, idempotent and it preserves finite meets. We call such Φ_j a *closure transformation* on P.

So every universal closure operation in $\mathsf{C}[\mathsf{P}]$, equivalently: local operator in $\mathsf{C}[\mathsf{P}]$, determines a closure transformation on P; conversely, it is easy to retrieve the local operator from the closure transformation.

Now suppose that $\Phi : \mathsf{P} \to \mathsf{P}$ is a closure transformation. For every C-object X let

$$Q(X) = \{\phi \in \mathsf{P}(X) \,|\, \Phi_X(\phi) \simeq \phi\}$$

Then $Q(X)$ is a Heyting pre-algebra: clearly, it inherits finite meets from $\mathsf{P}(X)$, but also, if $\psi \in Q(X)$ then $\phi \to \psi$ is an element of $Q(X)$ for every $\phi \in \mathsf{P}(X)$: we have that $\phi \wedge \Phi_X(\phi \to \psi) \leq \Phi_X(\psi) \simeq \psi$, so $\Phi_X(\phi \to \psi) \leq \phi \to \psi$. Finally, if ϕ and ψ are elements of $Q(X)$ and $\phi \vee_\mathsf{P} \psi$ denotes their join in $\mathsf{P}(X)$, then $\Phi_X(\phi \vee_\mathsf{P} \psi)$ is their join in $Q(X)$.

For any C-morphism $f : X \to Y$, the map $\mathsf{P}(f) : \mathsf{P}(Y) \to \mathsf{P}(X)$ restricts to a map $\mathsf{Q}(f) : \mathsf{Q}(Y) \to \mathsf{Q}(X)$, because Φ is a transformation. For the right adjoint $\forall_f$ to $\mathsf{P}(f)$ we have that if $\phi \in \mathsf{Q}(X)$ then $\forall_f(\phi) \in \mathsf{Q}(Y)$. This is seen as follows: applying $\mathsf{P}(f) \dashv \forall_f$ and $\phi \in \mathsf{Q}(X)$, we see that $\Phi_X(\mathsf{P}(f)(\forall_f(\phi))) \leq \phi$, that is: $\mathsf{P}(f)(\Phi_Y(\forall_f(\phi))) \leq \phi$. Applying the adjunction once again we find $\Phi_Y(\forall_f(\phi)) \leq \forall_f(\phi)$, as desired. Therefore $\mathsf{Q}(f)$ has a right adjoint. The Beck-Chevalley condition clearly holds. Similar to the case of disjunction, composing Φ with the left adjoint $\exists_f$ to $\mathsf{P}(f)$ gives a left adjoint to $\mathsf{Q}(f)$.

Finally, if $\in_X$ in $\mathsf{P}(X \times \pi(X))$ is a membership predicate for P, then $\Phi_{X \times \pi(X)}(\in_X)$ is one for Q. We have verified that Q is a C-tripos.

Clearly, the embedding $\mathsf{Q} \to \mathsf{P}$ is a transformation of triposes. Now $\Phi : \mathsf{P} \to \mathsf{P}$ takes values in Q (since Φ is idempotent), and is a left adjoint for the embedding. Since we have already seen that it preserves finite meets, we have a geometric morphism of triposes.

Definition 2.5.10 Let Q and P be C-triposes. A geometric morphism $\Phi = (\Phi_+, \Phi^+) : \mathsf{Q} \to \mathsf{P}$ is an *inclusion of triposes* if Φ_+ is full and faithful (in other words, reflects as well as preserves the preorder); equivalently, the transformation $\Phi^+ \Phi_+ : \mathsf{Q} \to \mathsf{Q}$ is isomorphic to the identity.

Suppose $\Phi : \mathsf{Q} \to \mathsf{P}$ is an inclusion of C-triposes. Then the geometric morphism $(\Phi_*, \Phi^*) : \mathsf{C}[\mathsf{Q}] \to \mathsf{C}[\mathsf{P}]$ is an inclusion of toposes: in the notation of the proof of theorem 2.5.8, we have that

$$\Phi^* \Phi_*(X, \sim) = (\pi(X), \Phi^+ \Phi_+(\sim_S)) \cong (\pi(X), \sim_S) \cong (X, \sim)$$

so Φ_* is full and faithful.

We summarize our reasonings in this section in the following theorem:

Theorem 2.5.11 *Let P be a C-tripos.*

i) *Every inclusion of toposes into $\mathsf{C}[\mathsf{P}]$ is, up to equivalence, of the form $\mathsf{C}[\mathsf{Q}] \overset{\Phi}{\to} \mathsf{C}[\mathsf{P}]$ for a C-tripos Q and an inclusion of triposes $\mathsf{Q} \to \mathsf{P}$.*

ii) *Inclusions into P correspond, up to equivalence, to closure transformations on P.*

In the case of an inclusion of triposes $Q \to P$ we shall call Q a *subtripos* of P.

2.6 Examples of triposes and inclusions of triposes

2.6.1 Sublocales

If $P = \mathcal{H}^{(-)}$ for a complete Heyting algebra (or *locale*) $\mathcal{H}$, subtriposes of P correspond to *sublocales* of $\mathcal{H}$, that is: locales $\mathcal{K} \subseteq \mathcal{H}$ such that the inclusion has a left adjoint preserving finite meets.

2.6.2 Order-pcas

Consider a geometric morphism $\mathcal{T}(B)^{(-)} \to \mathcal{T}(A)^{(-)}$ induced by a computationally dense morphism $\gamma : A \to T(B)$ of order-pcas. The following lemma provides some simplification in the characterization of precisely when the geometric morphism is an inclusion.

Lemma 2.6.1 *Every computationally dense morphism $A \to T(B)$ is isomorphic to a computationally dense morphism which preserves the order.*

Proof. Set $\gamma'(a) = \bigcup_{a' \le a} \gamma(a')$. This is clearly order preserving. If u is such that $a' \le a \Rightarrow u\gamma(a') \subseteq \gamma(a)$ then u realizes $\gamma' \preceq \gamma$; the converse inequality is realized by i. If r realizes γ as applicative morphism then $r' = \langle xy \rangle r(ux)(uy)$ does it for γ', and if m realizes the computational density for γ then $m' = \langle x \rangle m(ux)$ does it for γ', as you can verify yourself. ∎

Proposition 2.6.2 *Suppose $\gamma : A \to T(B)$ is an order preserving computationally dense morphism. Then the induced geometric morphism $\mathcal{T}(B)^{(-)} \to \mathcal{T}(A)^{(-)}$ is an inclusion if and only if there is an element $e \in B$ such that*

(in) $\forall b \in B \exists a \in A \, (eb \in \gamma(a) \wedge m\gamma(a) \subseteq {\downarrow}b)$

where m realizes the computational density of γ.

In particular, if $g : A \to B$ is a function between pcas such that $a \mapsto \{a\}$ is a computationally dense applicative morphism, then we get an inclusion of triposes if there is an $e \in B$ such that

(in)' $\forall b \in B \exists a \in A \, (eb = g(a) \wedge mg(a) = b)$

Proof. Let Φ_γ be the induced geometric morphism. Then it is easily verified that for all $\beta \in T(B)$,

$$(\Phi_\gamma)^+ (\Phi_\gamma)_+ (\beta) = \bigcup \{\gamma(a) \mid m\gamma(a) \subseteq \beta\}$$

so the element e satisfies (in) if and only it is an element of

$$\bigcap \{\beta \Rightarrow (\Phi_\gamma)^+ (\Phi_\gamma)_+ (\beta) \mid \beta \in T(B)\}$$

The formula for the unordered case follows at once. ∎

2.6.3 Set as a subtopos of $RT(A)$

Let us look at the trivial order-pca $\mathbb{I} = \{*\}$. $\mathcal{T}(\mathbb{I})$ has exactly two elements. $\mathcal{T}(\mathbb{I})^X$ can be identified with the power set of X via $\phi \mapsto \{x \in X \mid * \in \phi(x)\}$; we have $\phi \leq \psi$ if and only if $\phi \subseteq \psi$ (modulo this identification).

An object $(X, \sim)$ of $RT(\mathbb{I})$ can be seen as a set X together with a partial equivalence relation on X; i.e. a symmetric and transitive, not necessarily reflexive relation. A functional relation $F : (X, \sim) \to (Y, \sim)$ is a relation which respects the equivalence relations and relates to each x in the domain of the equivalence relation on X, up to equivalence exactly one y. That means that F can be identified with a function:

$$\{x \in X \mid x \sim x\}/\sim \; \to \; \{y \in Y \mid y \sim y\}/\sim$$

We see, that there is an equivalence of categories between $RT(\mathbb{I})$ and Set.

Let A be an order-pca. The unique applicative morphism $A \to \mathbb{I}$ is computationally dense as we saw in Example 1 at the end of section 1.8.

It also satisfies the condition (in) from proposition 2.6.2, as is trivial to check; thus it gives rise to a geometric inclusion

$$\mathsf{Set} \;\rightarrow\; \mathsf{RT}(A)$$

The inverse image functor $\Gamma : \mathsf{RT}(A) \rightarrow \mathsf{Set}$ sends $(X, \sim)$ to the quotient $\{x \in X \mid [x \sim x] \neq \emptyset\}/ \approx$, where $\approx$ is the equivalence relation:

$$x \approx x' \text{ iff } [x \sim x'] \neq \emptyset$$

Γ has a right adjoint ∇: $\nabla(X) = (X, \sim_\nabla)$ where

$$[x \sim_\nabla y] \;=\; \{a \in A \mid x = y\}$$

For a function $f : X \rightarrow Y$, $\nabla(f)$ is the functional relation

$$[\nabla(f)(x, y)] \;=\; \{a \in A \mid f(x) = y\}$$

We observe that this functor ∇ is the 'constant objects' functor of section 2.4. For realizability toposes, this functor is the direct image functor of a geometric inclusion. This is diametrically opposed to the case for complete Heyting algebras: there, ∇ is *inverse* image part of a unique geometric morphism to Set.

Another example: let A be a pca and consider the construction $\mathbb{N} \ltimes A$ of 1.4.11. There is a map $\mathbb{N} \ltimes A \rightarrow A$, sending (n, a) to $p\bar{n}a$. It is easily checked that this is a computationally dense morphism satisfyng (in)$'$, and so it gives rise to a geometric inclusion of $\mathsf{RT}(A)$ into $\mathsf{RT}(\mathbb{N} \ltimes A)$. For the significance of this inclusion, see section 3.8.3 below.

2.6.4   Relative recursion

Next, let us look at the construction $A[f]$ of section 1.7. There was an applicative morphism $\iota_f : A \rightarrow A[f]$, and in Example 3 of section 1.8 we noted that it is computationally dense. We therefore have a geometric morphism

$$\mathsf{RT}(A[f]) \rightarrow \mathsf{RT}(A)$$

Let us see that this geometric morphism is an inclusion (for $A = \mathcal{K}_1$, this was first shown by Hyland in [70] and the corresponding closure transformation was explicitly described in [121]). In fact, we can easily check condition $(in)'$ of proposition 2.6.2 for ι_f.

Let $e \in A$ be $\langle x \rangle p\mathsf{T}(\langle v \rangle p\mathsf{T}(p_0 x))$. Then for every $a \in A$, $e[a] = p\mathsf{T}(\langle v \rangle p\mathsf{T}(p_0 a))$, so

$$c \cdot^f a = \langle v \rangle p\mathsf{T}(p_0[a])$$

and $m([c \cdot^f a]) = (c \cdot^f a)[\,] = p\mathsf{T}a$. Therefore $m \cdot^f (c \cdot^f a) = a$. This proves $(in)'$.

2.6.5 Order-pcas with the pasting property

Not all geometric inclusions into realizability triposes arise from computationally dense morphisms of order-pcas. In this and the following examples, we shall sketch a number of important 'realizability-like' triposes which are subtriposes of realizability triposes, but not themselves of that form (the *proof* that they are not of that form has to be deferred until later, when we know more about the structure of toposes of the form $\mathsf{RT}(A)$).

Our first example is a construction that can often be performed on triposes on order-pcas. Let us say that an order-pca A has the *pasting property* if the underlying order has pushouts (i.e., if $a, b \in A$ have a common lower bound, then $a \vee b$ exists) and application preserves these in the sense that if a, b have a common lower bound then $ca\downarrow, cb\downarrow$ implies $c(a \vee b) = ca \vee cb$, and $ac\downarrow, bc\downarrow$ implies $(a \vee b)c = ac \vee bc$.

We may now consider a transformation Φ on $\mathcal{T}(A)^{(-)}$ which sends every downwards closed subset of A to its closure under pushouts. Since application preserves pushouts, this is clearly order-preserving; it is trivially idempotent, and it preserves finite meets: suppose S and T are closed under pushouts. Their meet in $\mathcal{T}(A)^1$ is $S \wedge T = \downarrow\{pst \mid s \in S, t \in T\}$. If pst and $ps't'$ are elements of $S \wedge T$ which have a common lower bound c, then $p_0 c$ is a lower bound for $p_0(pst) = s$ and $p_0(ps't') = s'$ so $s \vee s' \in S$ and similarly $t \vee t' \in T$; hence $p(s \vee s')(t \vee t')$ is in $S \wedge T$ and is an upper bound of pst and $ps't'$, so $pst \vee ps't' \in S \wedge T$ since it is downward closed. So $S \wedge T$ is closed under pushouts. We conclude that Φ is a closure transformation on $\mathcal{T}(A)^{(-)}$, which therefore determines a subtripos.

An example somewhat similar to this is discussed in Hyland's paper [73]: suppose D is a domain model of the λ-calculus, which is a complete lattice. One can show that the realizability tripos on D has a subtripos given by maps into the collection of subsets of D which are closed under joins $\bigvee$. In this case, the map left adjoint to the inclusion is *not* given by pointwise closure under joins.

2.6.6   Extensional realizability

Our next example is Pitts' topos for *extensional realizability*([123]). Let Σ be the set of pairs $(A, \sim)$ where A is a subset of $\mathbb{N}$ and $\sim$ is an equivalence relation on A. For $\phi, \psi \in \Sigma^X$ define $\phi \leq \psi$ if there is an $e \in \mathbb{N}$ such that for all x and for all $a \sim a'$ in $\phi(x)$, $ea\downarrow$, $ea'\downarrow$ and $ea \sim ea'$ in $\psi(x)$.

We can show right away that this defines a tripos, by exhibiting $\Sigma^{(-)}$ as the image of a closure transformation on the tripos $T(T(\mathcal{K}_1))$. Here $\mathcal{K}_1$ is a discrete order-pca, so $T(\mathcal{K}_1)$ consists of the nonempty subsets of $\mathbb{N}$, with the inclusion order. For any downwards closed subset S of $T(\mathcal{K}_1)$ we form an equivalence relation on $A = \bigcup S$: it is the least equivalence relation $\sim$ such that $x \sim y$ whenever there is an $\alpha \in S$ such that $x, y \in \alpha$. Define $\Phi(S)$ as $\{\alpha \subseteq A \mid \forall xy \in \alpha(x \sim y)\}$. Clearly, $S \subseteq \Phi(S)$. A moment's reflection will convince you that $S = \Phi(S)$ if and only if S satisfies the following property: whenever $\alpha, \beta \in S$ and $\alpha \cap \beta \neq \emptyset$, then $\alpha \cup \beta \in S$. That is, the set S is *closed under pushouts* in the order $T(\mathcal{K}_1)$. And $\Phi(S)$ is the closure of S under pushouts. So we see that this is an application of the construction given in the previous item.

The extensional realizability interpretation was studied and applied in [16],[17],[129] and [36]; a further study of the topos, and similar toposes, is in [171].

Extensional realizability is treated in more detail in section 4.1 below.

2.6.7   Modified realizability

Another important example is *modified realizability*. First we consider a variation on the realizability tripos on $\mathcal{K}_1$: let Σ_2 be the set of *inclusions* of subsets of $\mathbb{N}$: $\Sigma_2 = \{(A, B) \mid A \subseteq B \subseteq \mathbb{N}\}$. We shall write $A = (A_0, A_1)$ for elements of Σ_2. For $\phi, \psi \in \Sigma_2^X$ we say $\phi \leq \psi$ if and only if there is an $e \in \mathbb{N}$ such thet for all $x \in X$, if $n \in \phi(x)_0$ then $en \in \psi(x)_0$ and if $n \in \phi(x)_1$ then $en \in \psi(x)_1$. It is not hard to work out that this defines a tripos on Set.

We define a closure transformation Φ on $\Sigma_2^{(-)}$ as follows. By the recursion theorem, there is a number a such that for all n, $an = a$. There are elements q, q_0, q_1 such that for all n, m, $q_0(qnm) = n$, $q_1(qnm) = m$, $q(q_0n, q_1n) = n$ and moreover $qaa = a$. Clearly, in Σ_2^1, $(A_0, A_1) \wedge (B_0, B_1)$ is isomorphic to $(\{qab \mid a \in A_0, b \in B_0\}, \{qab \mid a \in A_1, b \in B_1\})$. It follows that the subset $\{(A_0, A_1) \in \Sigma_2 \mid a \in A_1\}$ is closed under finite meets in Σ_2^1. Let $F_a : \mathbb{N} \to \mathbb{N}$ be the function such that $F_a(n) = n$ if $n < a$, and $n+1$ if $n \geq a$. Define $\Phi : \Sigma_2 \to \Sigma_2$ by $\Phi(A_0, A_1) = (F_a[A_0], F_a[A_1] \cup \{a\})$. I leave it to you to check that Φ is a closure transformation. And the image of Φ is equivalent to the pseudofunctor induced by the set

$$\{(A_0, A_1) \in \Sigma_2 \mid a \in A_1\}$$

Modified realizability was originally defined by Kreisel ([93]) for a system of arithmetic of all finite types. A collapse of this interpretation to an interpretation of first-order arithmetic (by means of the so-called HRO-interpretation) was given by Troelstra in [161], and this is the notion that is generalized by the sketched tripos above. This tripos is due to Hyland and Grayson and was first defined in [62]. Further work on modified realizability toposes was done in [75, 172, 25].

Modified realizabiity is treated in more detail in section 4.2 below.

2.6.8 Lifschitz realizability

Our next example is *Lifschitz realizability* after an ingenious definition by Vladimir Lifschitz ([98]). Let us write $nm\uparrow$ for: the applicaton nm is undefined. Lifschitz devised the following coding of finite subsets of $\mathcal{K}_1$: let V_e denote the set of numbers $\{x \leq p_1 e \mid p_0 ex\uparrow\}$. This coding has the following properties:

Lemma 2.6.3 *There is no partial recursive function δ such that for all e, if V_e is nonempty then $\delta(e)$ is defined and is an element of V_e.*

Proof. Otherwise, let $F(x)$ be total recursive with the property that for $i = 0, 1$, $F(x)i{\downarrow} \Leftrightarrow xx = i$. Let $G(x) = p(F(x))1$. Then $V_{G(x)} \neq \emptyset$ for all x, so if δ existed, the set $A = \{x \,|\, \delta(G(x)) = 0\}$ would be a recursive separation of the sets $\{x \,|\, xx = 0\}$ and $\{x \,|\, xx = 1\}$. But it is a result of elementary recursion theory that this is impossible. ∎

Lemma 2.6.4 *There is a partial recursive function ζ with the property that if $fx{\downarrow}$ for all $x \in V_e$, then $\zeta(f, e){\downarrow}$ and $V_{\zeta(f,e)} = \{fx \,|\, x \in V_e\}$.*

Proof. Let $T(a, b, c)$ be Kleene's predicate, meaning: c codes a computation on Turing machine a with input b. Let U be the result extracting function, so that if $T(a, b, c)$ holds, then $\varphi_a(b) = U(c)$.

Let γ be total recursive such that for f, e, x, $\gamma(f, e)x$ is the outcome of the least computation which witnesses that $fx{\downarrow}$ or $p_0ex{\downarrow}$. Let Γ be partial recursive such that for all f, e, x,

$$\Gamma(f, e)x \simeq \max\{\gamma(f, e)x \,|\, x \leq p_1e\}$$

Note: if $fx{\downarrow}$ for all $x \in V_e$, then $\gamma(f, e)x{\downarrow}$ for all $x \leq p_1e$, hence $\Gamma(f, e)x{\downarrow}$; moreover in that case $fx \leq \Gamma(f, e)x$ for all $x \in V_e$.

Now a number y is an element of $\{fx \,|\, x \in V_e\}$ if and only if there is an $x \leq p_1e$ such that for all w the statement

$$\neg T(p_0e, x, w) \wedge (T(f, x, w) \to U(w) = y)$$

holds. Equivalently, for all sequences σ of length $p_1e + 1$, there is a number $i \leq p_1e + 1$ such that

$$(*) \quad \neg T(p_0e, i, (\sigma)_i) \wedge (T(f, i, (\sigma)_i) \to U((\sigma)_i) = y)$$

Now let B be total recursive such that for all f, e, y, $B(f, e)y$ is the least sequence σ of length $p_1e + 1$ for which there is *no* $i \leq p_1e + 1$ satisfying $(*)$.

Clearly then, $y \in \{fx \,|\, x \in V_e\}$ if and only if $B(f, e)y{\uparrow}$. So define ζ by $\zeta(f, e) = p(B(f, e))(\Gamma(f, e))$. ∎

Lemma 2.6.5 *There is a total recursive function γ such that for all e,*

$$V_{\zeta(e)} = \bigcup\{V_x \,|\, x \in V_e\}$$

Proof. If $y \in \bigcup\{V_x \mid x \in V_e\}$, then $y \leq \max\{p_1 x \mid x \leq p_1 e\}$ and also, for every sequence σ of length $p_1 e + 1$ there is an $i \leq p_1 e$ such that $y \leq p_1 i$, $\neg T(p_0 e, i, p_0((\sigma)_i))$ and $\neg T(p_0 i, y, p_1((\sigma)_i))$ hold (by similar reasoning as in the previous proof). This last statement can be written as $\forall \sigma P(\sigma)$ with $P(\sigma)$ primitive recursive. So if $B(e) = \max\{p_1 x \mid x \leq p_1 e\}$ and $C(e)y \simeq$ the least σ such that $\neg P(\sigma)$ holds, then $\zeta(e) = p(C(e))(B(e))$ satisfies the lemma. ∎

Lemma 2.6.6 *There is a total recursive function β such that for all x,*
$$V_{\beta(x)} = \{x\}.$$

Proof. Easy. ∎

We can now define a tripos on Set, the *Lifschitz tripos* as follows. First let J be the set of those numbers e such that V_e is nonempty; then, let Σ consist of those subsets H of J that satisfy the following conditions:

i)   For $e, f \in J$, if $e \in H$ and $V_f \subseteq V_e$ then $e \in H$;

ii)   For $e, f \in H$, if $V_g = V_e \cup V_f$ then $g \in H$.

For $\phi, \psi \in \Sigma^X$ we put $\phi \leq \psi$ if there is a number n such that for all $x \in X$ and all $e \in \phi(x)$, $ne\downarrow$ and $ne \in \psi(x)$. This clearly gives a pseudofunctor $\mathsf{P}_L : \mathsf{Set} \to \mathsf{Preord}$; P_L is a subfunctor of the effective tripos $\mathsf{P}_{\mathrm{eff}}$.

On Σ, define the operation $\times$ by

$$H_1 \times H_2 = \{e \in J \mid \forall x \in V_e (p_0 x \in H_1 \wedge p_1 x \in H_2)\}$$

Then if $\phi, \psi \in \mathsf{P}(X)$, the function $x \mapsto \phi(x) \times \psi(x)$ is a meet $\phi \wedge \psi$ for ϕ and ψ. For, suppose $\chi \leq \phi$ and $\chi \leq \psi$ via n and m respectively. Then for all x, if $e \in \chi(x)$ then $\beta(p(ne)(me)) \in (\phi \wedge \psi)(x)$, if β is from lemma 2.6.6; so $\chi \leq \phi \wedge \psi$.

To show that $\phi \wedge \psi \leq \phi$, suppose $e \in (\phi \wedge \psi)(x)$. If ζ is as in Lemma 2.6.4 then $\zeta(p_0, e)$ is defined and $V_{\zeta(p_0, e)} = \{p_0 x \mid x \in V_e\} \subseteq \phi(x)$. Then if γ is as in Lemma 2.6.5,

$$V_{\gamma(\zeta(p_0, e))} = \bigcup\{V_{p_0 x} \mid x \in V_e\}$$

Hence $\gamma(\zeta(p_0, e)) \in \phi(x)$, by condition ii) in the definition of the set Σ. In a similar way one proves $\phi \wedge \psi \leq \psi$.

Define $K : \mathcal{P}(\mathbb{N}) \to \Sigma$ by $K(A) = \{e \,|\, V_e \subseteq A\}$. Then K induces a transformation $\Phi : \mathsf{P}_{\mathrm{eff}} \to \mathsf{P}_L$, for if $\phi \leq \psi$ in $\mathsf{P}_{\mathrm{eff}}(X)$ via f, then any index for the function $e \mapsto \zeta(f, e)$ realizes $\Phi(\phi) \leq \Phi(\psi)$. Moreover, from the ideas in the proof that P has finite meets one easily works out that Φ preserves finite meets, and is left adjoint to the embedding $\mathsf{P}_L \to \mathsf{P}_{\mathrm{eff}}$.

And, to conclude, lemma 2.6.3 can be used to show that this inclusion is *proper*.

Lifschitz realizability was further studied in [165, 167, 170].

More on Lifschitz realizability in section 4.4 below.

2.6.9   Relative realizability

We consider the situation that A is a pca and $A_\sharp$ is an *elementary sub-pca* of A. By this we mean: $A_\sharp$ is a subset of A, closed under the application of A (so if $a, b \in A_\sharp$ and $ab\downarrow$ in A, then $ab \in A_\sharp$) and such that elements witnessing the combinatory completeness of A (see Definition 1.1.2) can be found in $A_\sharp$ (equivalently, elements k and s as in 1.1.3 can be found in $A_\sharp$).

Define a new preorder $\leq_\sharp$ on $\mathcal{P}(A)^X$ by: $\phi \leq_\sharp \psi$ if there is an $a \in A_\sharp$ such that for all $x \in X$ and all $b \in \phi(x)$, $ab\downarrow$ and $ab \in \psi(x)$.

It is not hard to verify that $(\mathcal{P}(A)^{(-)}, \leq_\sharp)$ is a tripos on Set. Since the definition of elementary sub-pca implies that $A_\sharp$ is itself a pca, we can compare this tripos to the ordinary realizability tripos on $A_\sharp$. We claim that there is a geometric inclusion from $\mathcal{P}(A_\sharp)^{(-)}$ into $(\mathcal{P}(A)^{(-)}, \leq_\sharp)$.

Indeed, for $\alpha \subseteq A_\sharp$ define

$$\Phi_*(\alpha) \;=\; \{pab \,|\, \text{if } a \in A_\sharp \text{ then } ba\downarrow \text{ and } ba \in \alpha\}$$

where p is, a combinator for pairing which is, by elementariness of $A_\sharp \subset A$, chosen in $A_\sharp$.

Then if $a' \in A_\sharp$ is such that for all $a'' \in \alpha$, $a'a'' \in \beta$ (that is, a' realizes the inequality $\alpha \leq \beta$ in $\mathcal{P}(A_\sharp)^1$), then the element

$$\langle x \rangle p(p_0 x)(\langle y \rangle a'(by))$$

realizes $\Phi_*(\alpha) \leq_\sharp \Phi_*(\beta)$. So Φ_* induces a transformation of triposes from $\mathcal{P}(A_\sharp)$ to $(\mathcal{P}(A), \leq_\sharp)$. It is not hard to see that Φ_* has a left adjoint, which is induced by the map from $\mathcal{P}(A)$ to $\mathcal{P}(A_\sharp)$ given by intersection with $A_\sharp$. Using elementariness, one also shows that this map preserves finite meets.

Examples of elementary sub-pcas are $\mathcal{K}_2^{\mathrm{rec}} \subset \mathcal{K}_2$ and $\mathcal{P}(\omega)^{\mathrm{re}} \subset \mathcal{P}(\omega)$. In particular the first example has been studied thoroughly: it is Kleene and Vesley's realizability for analysis ([90]). The geometric inclusion given here was discussed in [9]. Further information can be found in [25].

Unlike with realizability triposes over pcas, the Heyting pre-algebra $(\mathcal{P}(A)^1, \leq_\sharp)$ has a very interesting structure: it is dual to the *Medvedev lattice*, introduced in [107]. See section 4.5 below for a definition of this lattice, as well as for more on relative realizability.

More on relative reealizability in section 4.5 below.

2.6.10 Definable subtriposes

It is easy to check that for any C-tripos P, there is a closure transformation Φ on P defined by $\Phi_X(\phi) = \neg\neg\phi$ (in the Heyting prealgebra $\mathsf{P}(X)$. There is an associated subtripos $\mathsf{P}_{\neg\neg}$: $\mathsf{P}_{\neg\neg}(X)$ is the subset of $\mathsf{P}(X)$ consisting of the $\neg\neg$-*stable* elements of $\mathsf{P}(X)$, i.e. those elements ϕ for which $\phi \simeq \neg\neg\phi$.

Let $\mathsf{C[P]}_{\neg\neg}$ be the subtopos of $\mathsf{C[P]}$ of the $\neg\neg$-sheaves, and $L : \mathsf{C[P]} \to \mathsf{C[P]}_{\neg\neg}$ the sheafification functor. Then subobjects of $L(\nabla_{\mathsf{P}}(X))$ in $\mathsf{C[P]}_{\neg\neg}$ are in 1-1 correspondence with $\neg\neg$-stable subobjects of $\nabla_{\mathsf{P}}(X)$ in $\mathsf{C[P]}$, and hence, via proposition 2.4.2, with $\neg\neg$-stable elements of $\mathsf{P}(X)$. It now follows from section 2.7 below, that the toposes $\mathsf{C[P]}_{\neg\neg}$ and $\mathsf{C[P}_{\neg\neg}]$ are equivalent.

As an example, let us look at $\mathsf{P}_{\neg\neg}$ when P is the realizability tripos on a pca A. Since in $\mathsf{P}(X)$, $\neg\phi(x) = \{a \in A \mid \phi(x) = \emptyset\}$, we see that every $\neg\neg$-stable element of $\mathsf{P}(X)$ is isomorphic to an element ϕ with the property that for every $x \in X$, $\phi(x)$ is either A or $\emptyset$. That is, $\mathsf{P}_{\neg\neg}$ is equivalent with the tripos $2^{(-)}$, where 2 is the two element Boolean algebra; and $\mathsf{RT}(A)_{\neg\neg} \simeq \mathsf{Set}$.

At this point we can make a remark about *equivalence of realizability toposes*. When are two realizability toposes $\mathsf{RT}(A)$ and $\mathsf{RT}(B)$ equivalent? If that is the case, then certainly such an equivalence preserves subobjects of $\neg\neg$-sheaves, and hence restricts to an equivalence between the categories of assemblies $\mathrm{Ass}(A)$ and $\mathrm{Ass}(B)$. By theorem 1.6.2, this leads to an equivalence in the 2-category PCA between A and B. In some cases, we can identify properties of pca's which are stable under equivalence; for example, it is fairly easy to prove that *decidability* is such a property. The pca $\mathcal{K}_1$ is decidable; on the other hand, from proposition 1.3.4 it follows easily that a total pca is never decidable. Therefore $\mathsf{RT}(\mathcal{K}_1)$, which we shall later call the *effective topos*, can not be equivalent to a topos $\mathsf{RT}(A)$ if A is a pca which is equivalent to a total pca. This was first shown in [84], but this easy proof was noted by Longley ([99]).

Other definable subtriposes are so-called *open* and *closed* subtriposes. If $\mathcal{E}$ is a topos with subobject classifier Ω and U a subobject of 1 in $\mathcal{E}$, there are maps $j_U, j^U : \Omega \to \Omega$, defined internally by $j_U(x) = (u \Rightarrow x)$ and $j^U(x) = u \vee x$, where u is the global section of Ω that names U. The maps j_U and j^U are local operators; the sheaf subtoposes of $\mathcal{E}$ corresponding to j_U and j^U are called the *open* and *closed* subtopos, respectively. This terminology stems from the fact that if $\mathcal{E}$ is the topos of sheaves on a topological space X, so U is an open subset of X, the sheaf subtopos corresponding to j_U is equivalent to the topos of sheaves on U, and the one corresponding to j^U is equivalent to the topos of sheaves on $X - U$.

These constructions also exist on the level of triposes: if $u \in \mathsf{P}(1)$ then $u \Rightarrow (-)$ and $u \vee (-)$ define closure transformations on P, hence subtriposes which we shall also call open and closed.

For examples of this among realizability toposes, look at example 2.6.7. If P is the Set-tripos induced by the set Σ_2 defined there, and u is the element $(\emptyset, \mathbb{N})$, then the open subtripos of $\Sigma_2^{(-)}$ corresponding to u is equivalent to the effective tripos, and the closed one is equivalent to the modified realizability tripos (this fact was first noted in [172]).

2.7 Iteration

In this short section we study the situation tha P is a tripos on C and Q is a tripos on C[P]. How can we describe the topos (C[P])[Q]? Is it C[R] for some tripos R on C? The answer is yes.

Let P be a pseudofunctor $C^{op} \to$ Heytpre satisfying part i) of definition 2.1.2. By the remark at the end of section 2.2, we can form the category C[P] and prove the "first order part" of the properties discussed in that section and the ones following. In particular, proposition 2.4.2, which establishes an equivalence of pseudofunctors between P and $Sub_{C[P]}(\nabla_P(-))$, still holds. Also, corollary 2.4.5 remains valid.

Now, consider the situation of a finite limit-preserving functor $\nabla :$ $C \to \mathcal{E}$, where $\mathcal{E}$ is a topos. Let P be the pseudofunctor $Sub_{\mathcal{E}}(\nabla(-)) :$ $C \to$ Heytpre. Then P certainly satisfies part i) of definition 2.1.2; we compare $\mathcal{E}$ to C[P].

An object of $Ass_C(P)$ is a subobject in C[P] of an object $\nabla_P(X)$, but these subobjects correspond (by proposition 2.4.2) to elements of $P(X)$, i.e. to subobjects of $\nabla(X)$ in $\mathcal{E}$. Moreover, if $F \in P(X \times Y)$ is a functional relation from $(X, \sim_\phi)$ to $(Y, \sim_\psi)$, then if ϕ and ψ correspond to subobjects $U \rightarrowtail X$ and $V \rightarrowtail Y$ respectively, then $F \rightarrowtail \nabla(X) \times \nabla(Y)$ is such that

$$\mathcal{E} \models \forall x(x \in U \to \exists ! y F(x, y))$$

So in $\mathcal{E}$, F determines a morphism $U \to V$. We see that we have a functor $\bar{\nabla} : Ass_C(P) \to \mathcal{E}$ extending ∇. $\bar{\nabla}$ preserves finite limits, is full and faithful and surjective on subobjects.

Since C[P] is $Ass_C(P)_{ex/reg}$, there is an essentially unique regular functor $\kappa : C[P] \to \mathcal{E}$ which extends $\bar{\nabla}$. From the properties of $\bar{\nabla}$ and the fact that, in C[P], every object is a quotient of an object of $Ass_C(P)$, it follows that κ is also full and faithful.

Hence, if in $\mathcal{E}$ every object is a quotient of some $\bar{\nabla}(X)$ for a P-assembly X, or equivalently: every object of $\mathcal{E}$ is a quotient of a subobject of (a *subquotient* of) some $\nabla(X)$, then κ is an equivalence of categories.

We now have the ingredients for proving a weak version of Pitts' *Iteration Theorem*

Theorem 2.7.1 (Pitts Iteration Theorem) *Suppose* P *is a tripos on a category* C, *and* Q *is a tripos on* C[P] *such that the functor* $\nabla_Q : C[P] \rightarrow$ C[P][Q] *preserves epimorphisms.*

Let R : $C^{op} \rightarrow$ Heytpre *be the functor* $Q \circ \nabla_P^{op}$. *Then there is an equivalence of categories between* C[R] *and* C[P][Q] *which commutes with the functors* ∇_R *and* $\nabla_Q \circ \nabla_P$.

Proof. Certainly R satisfies part i) of definition 2.1.2. We look at the functor $\nabla_Q \circ \nabla_P : C \rightarrow C[P][Q]$. For every object A of C[P][Q] there is a diagram

$$
\begin{array}{ccc}
B & \longrightarrow & \nabla_Q(V) \\
\downarrow & & \\
A & &
\end{array}
$$

with the horizontal arrow monic and the vertical one epic. For the object V of C[P] there is a similar diagram

$$
\begin{array}{ccc}
U & \longrightarrow & \nabla_P(X) \\
\downarrow & & \\
V & &
\end{array}
$$

Using the assumption that ∇_Q preserves epimorphisms and the fact that epimorphisms are stable under pullback, we get a diagram

$$
\begin{array}{ccccc}
W & \longrightarrow & \nabla_Q(U) & \longrightarrow & \nabla_Q\nabla_P(X) \\
\downarrow & & \downarrow & & \\
B & \longrightarrow & \nabla_Q(V) & & \\
\downarrow & & & & \\
A & & & &
\end{array}
$$

in which the upper left hand square is a pullback, all horizontal arrow monic and all vertical ones epic. This establishes A as a subquotient of $\nabla_Q\nabla_P(X)$.

As we have seen, it follows that the composite $\nabla_Q \circ \nabla_P : C \to C[P][Q]$ is equivalent over C to ∇_S where $S : C \to \mathsf{Heytpre}$ is the functor

$$\mathrm{Sub}_{C[P][Q]}(\nabla_Q(\nabla_P(-)))$$

But S is isomorphic to $Q(\nabla_P(-))$, which is R. So we are done. ∎

The stronger theorem that Pitts proved (6.2 in [123]) asserts that in the situation of theorem 2.7.1, R is actually a tripos. We skip that part of the theorem; although not hard, it is somewhat lengthy, and in our examples a quick inspection suffices to see that we are dealing with triposes.

2.8 Glueing of triposes

In this last section of this chapter we deal with the tripos-theoretic analogue of a well-known construction om toposes: glueing.

Suppose $\mathcal{E}$ and $\mathcal{F}$ are toposes and $F : \mathcal{E} \to \mathcal{F}$ a functor which preserves finite limits. Consider the comma category $\mathcal{F}{\downarrow}F$: its objects are triples (X, A, ϕ) where X is object of $\mathcal{F}$, A is object of $\mathcal{E}$ and $\phi : X \to F(A)$ is an arrow in $\mathcal{F}$. An arrow $(X, A, \phi) \to (Y, B, \psi)$ is a pair (f, α) with $f : X \to Y$ in $\mathcal{F}$ and $\alpha : A \to B$ in $\mathcal{E}$, such that the square

$$\begin{array}{ccc} X & \xrightarrow{\ f\ } & Y \\ {\scriptstyle\phi}\downarrow & & \downarrow{\scriptstyle\psi} \\ F(A) & \xrightarrow[F(\alpha)]{} & F(B) \end{array}$$

commutes. Composition of arrows is componentwise.

Clearly, $\mathcal{F}{\downarrow}F$ is a category, but the theorem (by Grothendieck for the case of Grothendieck toposes, by Tierney for the elementary case) is that it is a topos. One says that it is obtained by "glueing $\mathcal{E}$ to $\mathcal{F}$ along F". An elegant proof of this fact is given in [178], where it is observed that $\mathcal{F}{\downarrow}F$ is the category of coalgebras for the comonad $(A, X) \mapsto (A, F(A) \times X)$ on the topos $\mathcal{E} \times \mathcal{F}$.

$\mathcal{F} \downarrow F$ comes equipped with two projection functors $\pi_1 : \mathcal{F} \downarrow F \to \mathcal{F}$ and $\pi_2 : \mathcal{F} \downarrow F \to \mathcal{E}$. Both these functors have a full and faithful right adjoint: we have $q_1 : \mathcal{F} \to \mathcal{F} \downarrow F$ sending X to $(X, 1, !)$ and $q_2 : \mathcal{E} \to \mathcal{F} \downarrow F$ sending A to $(F(A), A, \mathrm{id}_{F(A)})$. Moreover, the functor π_2 is logical, since it exhibits $\mathcal{E}$ as (equivalent to) the slice category $(\mathcal{F} \downarrow F)/(0, 1, !)$.

A similar construction is available for triposes. Suppose P and Q are C-triposes and Φ is a transformation $\mathsf{P} \to \mathsf{Q}$ which preserves finite meets. We form a pseudofunctor $\mathsf{Q} \downarrow \Phi : \mathsf{C} \to \mathsf{Preord}$ by defining

$$(\mathsf{Q} \downarrow \Phi)(X) = \{\phi, \psi) \mid \phi \in \mathsf{P}(X), \psi \in \mathsf{Q}(X), \psi \leq \Phi_X(\phi)\}$$

with pointwise order. For $f : Y \to X$ and $(\phi, \psi) \in (\mathsf{Q} \downarrow \Phi)(X)$ we set

$$(\mathsf{Q} \downarrow \Phi)(f)(\phi, \psi) = (\mathsf{P}(f)(\phi), \mathsf{Q}(f)(\psi))$$

It is easily seen that $(\mathsf{Q} \downarrow \Phi)(X)$ has finite joins and meets which are computed pointwise. As to Heyting implication, we put

$$(\phi_1, \psi_1) \Rightarrow (\phi_2, \psi_2) = (\phi_1 \Rightarrow \phi_2, (\psi_1 \Rightarrow \psi_2) \wedge \Phi_X(\phi_1 \Rightarrow \phi_2))$$

where, in the right hand side, we use the Heyting operations in $\mathsf{P}(X)$ and $\mathsf{Q}(X)$. Again it is easily verified that this defines a Heyting implication.

Existential quantification is also computed pointwise; if $f : Y \to X$, $(\phi, \psi) \in (\mathsf{Q} \downarrow \Phi)(Y)$ and $\exists^{\mathsf{P}}_f \dashv \mathsf{P}(f)$, $\exists^{\mathsf{Q}}_f \dashv \mathsf{Q}(f)$, we can put

$$\exists_f(\phi, \psi) = (\exists^{\mathsf{P}}_f(\phi), \exists^{\mathsf{Q}}_f(\psi))$$

using that we always have the inequality $\exists^{\mathsf{Q}}_f(\psi) \leq \exists^{\mathsf{Q}}_f(\Phi_Y(\phi)) \leq \Phi_X(\exists^{\mathsf{P}}_f(\phi))$.

For the right adjoint to $(\mathsf{Q} \downarrow \Phi)(f)$ we put

$$\forall_f(\phi, \psi) = (\forall^{\mathsf{P}}_f(\phi), \forall^{\mathsf{Q}}_f(\psi) \wedge \Phi_X(\forall^{\mathsf{P}}_f(\phi)))$$

We show that $\mathsf{Q} \downarrow \Phi$ is a tripos in the case that C is cartesian closed, so we only have to check condition ii)$'$ of Remark 3 in 2.1.2. Suppose $\sigma \in \mathsf{P}(\Sigma)$ and $\tau \in \mathsf{Q}(T)$ are generic elements for P and Q respectively, so for $(\phi, \psi) \in (\mathsf{Q} \downarrow \Phi)(X)$ we have $[\phi] : X \to \Sigma$ and $[\psi] : X \to T$ such that $\mathsf{P}([\phi])(\sigma) \simeq \phi$ and $\mathsf{Q}([\psi])(\tau) \simeq \psi$.

Then the element $(\varepsilon, \delta) \in (Q{\downarrow}\Phi)(\Sigma \times T)$ given by

$$(\varepsilon, \delta) \ = \ (P(\pi_1)(\sigma), Q(\pi_2)(\tau) \wedge \Phi_{\Sigma \times T}(P(\pi_1)(\sigma)))$$

is a generic element for $Q{\downarrow}\Phi$: for any $(\phi, \psi) \in (Q{\downarrow}\Phi)(X)$ we have

$$(\phi, \psi) \ \simeq \ (Q{\downarrow}\Phi)(\langle [\phi], [\psi] \rangle)(\varepsilon, \delta)$$

Let us now assume that the transformation $\Phi : P \to Q$ commutes with existential quantification (meaning that $\Phi_Y(\exists_f^P(\phi)) \simeq \exists_f^Q(\Phi_X(\phi)))$, so that Φ induces a regular functor $\bar{\Phi} : \mathrm{Ass}_C(P) \to \mathrm{Ass}_C(Q)$ and hence, by 2.4.5, a regular extension, also denoted $\bar{\Phi}$, from $C[P]$ to $C[Q]$. We have a commutative diagram

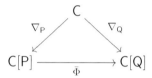

Now, an object of $C[Q{\downarrow}\Phi]$ is a triple $(X, \sim_P, \sim_Q)$ where $\sim_P \in P(X \times X)$ and $\sim_Q \in Q(X \times X)$ are equality predicates, such that $\sim_Q \le \Phi_{X \times X}(\sim_P)$. But this means that we have an arrow in $C[Q]$ from $(X, \sim_Q)$ to $(X, \Phi_{X \times X}(\sim_P))$, which is $\bar{\Phi}(X, \sim_P)$. This arrow is represented by the predicate

$$[x \sim_Q x \wedge \Phi(\sim_P)(x, x')]$$

An arrow $(X, \sim_P, \sim_Q) \to (Y, \sim_P, \sim_Q)$ is represented by functional relations $F_P \in P(X \times Y)$ and $F_Q \in Q(X \times Y)$ from $(X, \sim_P)$ to $(Y, \sim_P)$ and $(X, \sim_Q)$ to $(Y, \sim_Q)$ respectively, such that $F_Q \le \Phi_{X \times Y}(F_P)$. But this means, that if $f : (X, \sim_P) \to (Y, \sim_P)$ is the arrow in $C[Q]$ represented by F_P, and $g : (X, \sim_Q) \to (Y, \sim_Q)$ is the arrow in $C[Q]$ represented by F_Q, we have a commuting diagram

$$
\begin{array}{ccc}
(X, \sim_Q) & \xrightarrow{\;g\;} & (Y, \sim_Q) \\
\downarrow & & \downarrow \\
\bar{\Phi}(X, \sim_P) & \xrightarrow[\bar{\Phi}(f)]{} & \bar{\Phi}(Y, \sim_P)
\end{array}
$$

That is, we have a functor from $\mathsf{C}[\mathsf{Q}{\downarrow}\Phi]$ to $\mathsf{C}[\mathsf{Q}]{\downarrow}\bar{\Phi}$. I leave it to you to convince yourself, that this functor is full and faithful. In some cases, it is an equivalence; but not in general.

However, we have always a logical functor from $\mathsf{C}[\mathsf{Q}{\downarrow}\Phi]$ to $\mathsf{C}[\mathsf{P}]$. In order to see this, note that we have a transformation $\pi_1 : \mathsf{Q}{\downarrow}\Phi \to \mathsf{P}$. From the explicit constructions given, it is immediate that this transformation preserves the Heyting prealgebra structure for each X, and that it commutes with the quantifiers $\exists_f$ and $\forall_f$. So it commutes with the tripos structure except maybe the generic element. However, observe that if $\sigma \in \mathsf{P}(\Sigma)$ is a generic element of some tripos P and T is a weak terminal object in C (meaning that from any object there is at least one map to T), and $\pi_1 : \Sigma \times T \to \Sigma$ is the projection, then $\mathsf{P}(\pi_1)(\sigma) \in \mathsf{P}(\Sigma \times T)$ is also a generic element for P. And if T is the carrier object for a generic element of some tripos on C, then T is weakly terminal.

Hence, $\pi_1 : \mathsf{Q}{\downarrow}\Phi \to \mathsf{P}$ preserves all the tripos structure. By the tripos-to-topos construction, it follows that π_1 induces a logical functor $\mathsf{C}[\mathsf{Q}{\downarrow}\Phi] \to \mathsf{C}[\mathsf{P}]$.

We will apply this glueing construction in section 4.6.1 below.

Chapter 3

The Effective Topos

Definition 3.0.1 The *effective topos* is the topos $\mathsf{RT}(\mathcal{K}_1)$. It arises out of the effective tripos on Set.

We denote the effective topos by $\mathcal{E}\!f\!f$.

This chapter intends to investigate toposes of the form $\mathsf{RT}(A)$ in detail; but for definiteness, we focus on the effective topos. Virtually everything we meet in this chapter, carries over to the more general situation, with appropriate changes.

3.1 Recapitulation and arithmetic in $\mathcal{E}\!f\!f$

First, we recapitulate what we know from chapter 2 about $\mathsf{RT}(\mathcal{K}_1)$. This will also provide us with an opportunity to see the abstract theory 'at work'.

Objects of $\mathcal{E}\!f\!f$ are pairs $(X, =)$; X is a set, and for every $x, y \in X$ a subset $[x = y]$ of $\mathbb{N}$ is given, and this system satisfies the requirement that for suitable elements s and t of $\mathbb{N}$ we have

$$\mathsf{s} \in [x = y] \Rightarrow [y = x] \quad \text{for all } x, y \in X$$
$$\mathsf{t} \in ([x = y] \wedge [y = z]) \Rightarrow [x = z] \quad \text{for all } x, y, z \in X$$

Here $\Rightarrow$ and $\wedge$ are as in the definition of the effective tripos. So, if $n \in [x = y]$ then $\mathsf{s}n{\downarrow}$ and $\mathsf{s}n \in [y = x]$; if $n \in [x = y]$ and $m \in [y = z]$ then $\mathsf{t}(pnm){\downarrow}$ and $\mathsf{t}(pnm) \in [x = z]$.

Note furthermore: if $n \in [x = y]$ then $\mathsf{t}(pn(\mathsf{s}n)) \in [x = x]$.

An arrow $f : (X, =) \rightarrow (Y, =)$ is represented by a function $F : X \times Y \rightarrow \mathcal{P}(\mathbb{N})$ such that for suitable elements st, rl, sv and tl of $\mathbb{N}$ we have

$$
\begin{aligned}
\mathsf{st} &\in F(x, y) \Rightarrow ([x = x] \wedge [y = y]) &&\text{for all } x \in X, y \in Y \\
\mathsf{rl} &\in ([x' = x] \wedge F(x, y) \wedge [y = y']) \Rightarrow F(x', y') &&\text{for all } x, x' \in X, y, y' \in Y \\
\mathsf{sv} &\in (F(x, y) \wedge F(x, y')) \Rightarrow [y = y'] &&\text{for all } x \in X, y, y' \in Y \\
\mathsf{tl} &\in [x = x] \Rightarrow \bigcup_{y \in Y} F(x, y) &&\text{forall } x \in X
\end{aligned}
$$

Two such functions F, F' represent the same arrow in $\mathcal{E}ff$ if and only if $F \simeq F'$ in $\mathsf{P}(X \times Y)$ for the effective tripos P.

In many cases, an arrow $f : (X, =) \rightarrow (Y, =)$ is actually determined by a *function* $\varphi : X \rightarrow Y$, such that f is then represented by the element

$(*)$ $[x = x] \wedge [\varphi(x) = y]$

of $\mathcal{P}(\mathbb{N})^{X \times Y}$. This element is always strict, relational and single-valued; for it to be total there should be a number e such that for all $x \in X$, $e \in [x = x] \Rightarrow [\varphi(x) = \varphi(x)]$.

Cases where every $f : (X, =) \rightarrow (Y, =)$ is always given by such a function, include (we assume in the following cases, that $[x = x]$ is nonempty for every $x \in X$):

1. if $[x = x]$ is a singleton for every $x \in X$. For, the conditions on F imply that there is an a such that for all $x \in X$ and all $n \in [x = x]$ there is a $y \in Y$ with $an \in F(x, y)$. So if $[x = x]$ is always a singleton, one can use the axiom of choice to find a function φ such that for the unique $n \in [x = x]$, $an \in F(x, \varphi(x))$. It is then easily seen that f is represented by the relation $(*)$.

   Examples of such objects $(X, =)$ are objects in the image of ∇, for $\nabla(X)$ is isomorphic to $(X, =)$ with $[x = y] = \{0 \mid x = y\}$.

2. if $(Y, =)$ is Ω, the subobject classifier, or more generally a power object. This actually holds for any topos $\mathsf{C}[\mathsf{P}]$: suppose $f : (X, =) \rightarrow (\Sigma, \Leftrightarrow)$ is represented by $F \in \mathsf{P}(X \times \Sigma)$. Let $\top : 1 \rightarrow \Sigma$ be an arrow such that $\top^*(\sigma)$ is a top element in the Heyting prealgebra

P(1). For a variable a of type Σ we then have $\mathsf{P} \models a \leftrightarrow (a \Leftrightarrow \top)$. Using this and the single-valuedness of F we see that

$$\mathsf{P} \models F(x, a) \rightarrow (a \Leftrightarrow F(x, \top))$$

So if $\varphi : X \rightarrow \Sigma$ is an arrow such that $\varphi^*(\sigma)$ is the relation $F(x, F(x, \top))$ then f is represented by $[x = x \wedge (a \Leftrightarrow \varphi(x)]$.

3. if $(Y, =)$ has the property that $[y = y'] = \emptyset$ if $y \neq y'$. Work this out for yourself!

Let us look at the category $\mathrm{Ass}_{\mathsf{Set}}(\mathsf{P})$ for the effective tripos P. Objects are of the form $(X, \sim_\phi)$ for some $\phi \in \mathsf{P}(X)$; $\sim_\phi$ is $\exists_\delta(\phi)$. This means that $[x \sim_\phi y] = \phi(x)$ if $x = y$, and $\emptyset$ otherwise. So these objects fall under the situation discussed above, and we arrive at the following presentation of $\mathrm{Ass}_{\mathsf{Set}}(\mathsf{P})$: objects (now just called *assemblies* in the context of $\mathcal{E}ff$) are pairs (X, E) where $E(x)$ is a nonempty subset of $\mathbb{N}$; arrows $(X, E) \rightarrow (Y, E')$ are functions $f : X \rightarrow Y$ such that for some $e \in \mathbb{N}$ it holds that for every $x \in X$ and every $n \in E(x)$, $en{\downarrow}$ and $en \in E'(f(x))$. In other words, this is the category $\mathrm{Ass}(\mathcal{K}_1)$ from definition 1.5.1.

The assembly (X, E) corresponds to the object $(X, =)$ of $\mathcal{E}ff$ where $[x = y] = \emptyset$ if $x \neq y$, and $[x = x] = E(x)$.

From sections 2.6.3 and 2.6.10 we know that $\nabla : \mathsf{Set} \rightarrow \mathcal{E}ff$ is full and faithful and has a left adjoint Γ, and this geometric morphism is the embedding of the category of $\neg\neg$-sheaves in $\mathcal{E}ff$. The assemblies, being the subobjects of the $\neg\neg$-sheaves, are the $\neg\neg$-*separated* objects in $\mathcal{E}ff$: the objects for which the equality relation is $\neg\neg$-stable. By section 2.3, the objects $(X, =)$ for which $\mathsf{P} \models \forall xy(x = x \wedge y = y \wedge \neg\neg(x = y) \rightarrow x = y)$. You can also verify this directly.

I recall corollary 2.4.5, which states that $\mathcal{E}ff$ is the ex/reg completion of the category of assemblies.

An important assembly is $N = (\mathbb{N}, E)$ with $E(n) = \{n\}$. Recall that a *natural numbers object* or *NNO* in a topos is an object N together with maps $1 \xrightarrow{0} N$ and $N \xrightarrow{S} N$, such that for any other such diagram

$1 \xrightarrow{a} A \xrightarrow{f} A$ there is a unique arrow $g : N \to A$ such that the diagram

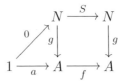

commutes.

Proposition 3.1.1 *With the obvious maps* $1 \xrightarrow{0} N \xrightarrow{S} N$, N *is a natural numbers object in* $\mathcal{E}ff$.

To prove proposition 3.1.1, it is easy to check that N is an NNO in the category of assemblies; since every NNO in any topos is $\neg\neg$-separated, this would prove the proposition *provided we know that* $\mathcal{E}ff$ *has a natural numbers object*. There are several ways to prove this (including a direct proof that N is an NNO in $\mathcal{E}ff$), but I prefer the following general lemma, which also appears as Corollary D5.1.3 in [83], with a slightly different proof.

Lemma 3.1.2 *Suppose in a topos* $\mathcal{E}$ *there is an object* X *together with maps* $1 \xrightarrow{x_0} X$ *and* $X \xrightarrow{S} X$, *such that* S *is monic and the sentence* $\forall v \in X \neg (S(v) = x_0)$ *is true in* $\mathcal{E}$. *Then* $\mathcal{E}$ *has a natural numbers object.*

Proof. Let $N \subseteq X$ be the least subobject which contains x_0 and is closed under S (that is, N is the intersection of all those subobjects of X). I claim that $1 \xrightarrow{x_0} N \xrightarrow{S} N$ is an NNO in $\mathcal{E}$.

To prove this, let $1 \xrightarrow{a_0} A \xrightarrow{f} A$ be a diagram in $\mathcal{E}$. We have to find a unique $g : N \to A$ such that $g(x_0) = a_0$ and $\forall v \in N(g(S(v)) = f(g(v)))$. This is a nice exercise in higher-order logic.

For any $y \in N$, let N_y be the least subobject M of X such that $y \in M$ and, if $S(v) \in M$ then $v \in M$. N_y has the following properties:

i) $y \in N_y$

ii) $x_0 \in N_y$

iii) $N_{S(y)} = N_y \cup \{S(y)\}$, i.e. $\forall v \in N_{S(y)}(v \in N_y \lor v = S(y))$ holds.

For, the subobject of X consisting of those y for which N_y has these properties, contains x_0 and is closed under S. Note, moreover, that $N_{x_0} = \{x_0\}$.

Now let $K \subseteq N$ consist of those $y \in N$ for which there exists a unique function $g_y : N_y \to A$ such that $g_y(x_0) = a_0$ and if $S(v) \in N_y$ then $g_y(S(v)) = f(g_y(v))$. Then certainly $x_0 \in K$ since $N_{x_0} = \{x_0\}$, and from property iii) of $N_{S(y)}$ it follows at once that if $y \in K$, also $S(y) \in K$. Hence $K = N$.

Define $g : N \to A$ by $g(y) = g_y(y)$. By a now familiar reasoning one shows that the subset of N of those y for which the restriction of g to N_y is equal to g_y, is the whole of N; hence g satisfies $g(x_0) = a_0$ and $g(S(v)) = f(g(v))$.

For uniqueness of g, it is immediate that any g' satisfying the same equations must have the same restrictions to each N_y (by uniqueness of g_y). So $g = g'$, as required. ∎

In every cartesian closed category with natural numbers object N, there is a straightforward interpretation of the primitive recursive (in fact, ε_0-recursive) functions: see [95]. In $\mathcal{E}ff$, morphisms $N^k \to N$ are determined by functions $\mathbb{N}^k \to \mathbb{N}$, so the standard interpretation of a primitive recursive function F in the category of assemblies is itself; when viewed in $\mathcal{E}ff$, it is represented by the functional relation

$$(n, m) \mapsto \{pnm \mid m = F(n)\}$$

The *language of arithmetic* is (in this book) the first-order language with function symbols for each primitive recursive function. For every formula $\varphi(x_1, \ldots, x_n)$ of this language, we have a straightforward interpretation $[\![\varphi]\!]$ in $\mathcal{E}ff$ as subobject of N^n. Subobjects of N^n are given by strict relations on $\mathbb{N}^n$, that is: functions $f : \mathbb{N}^n \to \mathcal{P}(\mathbb{N})$ such that for some $e \in \mathbb{N}$ we have: for all $k_1, \ldots, k_n \in \mathbb{N}$ and all $a \in f(k_1, \ldots, k_n)$,

$$ea = \langle k_1, \ldots, k_n \rangle$$

(here $\langle k_1, \ldots, k_n \rangle$ denotes the code of the n-tuple $k_1, \ldots, k_n$)
According to section 2.3 we have (assuming φ a formula with free vari-

ables $x_1, \ldots, x_n$; I write $\vec{k}$ for the n-tuple $k_1, \ldots, k_n$ of natural numbers):

$$
\begin{aligned}
[\![\, t = s \,]\!](\vec{k}) &= \{\langle k_1, \ldots, k_n \rangle \mid (t = s)(k_1, \ldots, k_n) \text{ is true}\} \\
[\![\, \varphi \wedge \psi \,]\!](\vec{k}) &= \{pab \mid a \in [\![\, \varphi \,]\!](\vec{k}), b \in [\![\, \psi \,]\!](\vec{k})\} \\
[\![\, \varphi \vee \psi \,]\!](\vec{k}) &= \{p0a \mid a \in [\![\, \varphi \,]\!](\vec{k})\} \cup \\
& \quad\, \{p1b \mid b \in [\![\, \psi \,]\!](\vec{k})\} \\
[\![\, \varphi \to \psi \,]\!](\vec{k}) &= \{p\langle k_1, \ldots, k_n \rangle e \mid e \in [\![\, \varphi \,]\!](\vec{k}) \Rightarrow [\![\, \psi \,]\!](\vec{k})\} \\
[\![\, \exists y \varphi \,]\!](\vec{k}) &= \{pab \mid b \in [\![\, \varphi \,]\!](\vec{k}, a)\} \\
[\![\, \forall y \varphi \,]\!](\vec{k}) &= \{p\langle k_1, \ldots, k_n \rangle e \mid \text{for all } m, \\
& \quad\, em{\downarrow} \text{ and } em \in [\![\, \varphi \,]\!](\vec{k}, m)\}
\end{aligned}
$$

This is very similar to Kleene's definition of *realizability* given in [88]. There, he defined a relation between natural numbers and sentences of the language of arithmetic, expressed as "n realizes ϕ". The idea is that if n realizes ϕ, n codes some information which suggests that ϕ is constructively true. The definition is by the following inductive clauses:

1. n realizes an atomic sentence ϕ, if and only if that sentence is true in $\mathbb{N}$;

2. n realizes a conjunction $\phi \wedge \psi$ if and only if n codes a pair (n_0, n_1) such that n_0 realizes ϕ and n_1 realizes ψ;

3. n realizes a disjunction $\phi \vee \psi$ if and only if n codes a pair (n_0, n_1) such that either $n_0 = 0$ and n_1 realizes ϕ, or $n_0 \neq 0$ and n_1 realizes ψ;

4. n realizes $\phi \to \psi$ if and only if for every m realizing ϕ, nm is defined and realizes ψ;

5. n realizes $\exists x \phi(x)$ if and only if n codes a pair (n_0, n_1) such that n_1 realizes $\phi(n_0)$;

6. n realizes $\forall x \phi(x)$ if and only if for every m, nm is defined and realizes $\phi(m)$.

Indeed, we have the following proposition, which justifies the name 're-alizability topos':

Proposition 3.1.3 *For every formula $\varphi(x_1,\dots,x_n)$ there are primitive recursive functions t_φ and s_φ of n arguments, such that for every n-tuple $k_1,\dots,k_n$ and every natural number a the following hold:*

i)   *if a realizes $\varphi(k_1,\dots,k_n)$ then $t_\varphi(k_1,\dots,k_n)a$ is defined and is an element of $[\![\,\varphi\,]\!](k_1,\dots,k_n)$;*

ii)   *if $a \in [\![\,\varphi\,]\!](k_1,\dots,k_n)$ then $s_\varphi(k_1,\dots,k_n)a$ is defined and realizes $\varphi(k_1,\dots,k_n)$.*

Therefore, a sentence ϕ of the language of arithmetic is true in the standard interpretation in εff, if and only if ϕ has a realizer in Kleene's sense.

Proof. This is straightforward and left to you.   ■

Markov's Principle is the axiom scheme:

(MP) $\forall x(\phi(x) \vee \neg\phi(x)) \wedge \neg\neg\exists x\phi(x) \rightarrow \exists x\phi(x)$

and *Extended Church's Thesis* is:

(ECT$_0$) $\forall x(\phi(x) \rightarrow \exists y\psi(x,y)) \rightarrow \exists e\forall x(\phi(x) \rightarrow \exists u\,(T(e,x,u)\wedge\psi(x,U(u))))$

where T and U are, as before, Kleene's computation predicate and result extraction function. Moreover, the formula ϕ is required to be *almost negative*, which means that an existential quantifier only occurs directly before an atomic formula, and a disjunction also only occurs between atomic formulas.

Markov's Principle implies for any term t which is built up from numbers and application, that t denotes whenever the assumption to the contrary leads (with classical logic!) to a contradiction. The principle is almost indispensible if one wishes to develop recursion theory in intuitionistic logic. Extended Church's Thesis is a principle which is a bit different from what is usually understood by 'Church's Thesis': it says that every relation on an almost negatively defined domain, contains a partial recursive function which is defined on that domain. If one would drop the requirement 'almost negatively defined', the principle would be absurd (see [161],3.2.20).

Corollary 3.1.4 *The principles* MP *and* ECT_0 *are true in* $\mathcal{E}\!f\!f$.

Proof. Every instance of one of these principles has a realizer (see also [161]). ∎

Some other principles which are often considered in the context of intuitionistic first-order arithmetic are:

(CT_0) $\forall x \exists y \psi(x,y) \rightarrow \exists e \forall x \exists u (T(e,x,u) \wedge \psi(x,U(u)))$ (Church's Thesis)

(IP) $\forall x(\neg\varphi(x) \rightarrow \exists y \psi(x,y)) \rightarrow \forall x \exists y(\neg\varphi(x) \rightarrow \psi(x,y))$ (Independence of Premiss)

(IP_0) $\forall x(\varphi(x) \vee \neg\varphi(x)) \wedge (\forall x \varphi(x) \rightarrow \exists y \psi(y)) \rightarrow \exists y(\forall x \varphi(x) \rightarrow \psi(y))$

Theorem 3.1.5 (Troelstra)

i) IP+ECT_0 *is inconsistent relative to first-order intuitionistic arithmetic.*

ii) *The principle* CT_0 *is strictly weaker than* ECT_0.

iii) *The principle* IP_0 *is a consequence of* MP $+$ ECT_0.

Proof. i) can be found in [161], 3.4.14.

ii) follows from i), as soon as we know that IP $+$ CT_0 is consistent. This can be shown by modified realizability.

iii) is stated (in a weaker form) in [161], 3.2.26, but the proof there contains an inaccuracy; so I give the argument here. Reason inside first-order intuitionistic arithmetic. Suppose $\forall x(\varphi(x) \vee \neg\varphi(x))$. Then by ECT_0 there is an n such that for all x, $nx{\downarrow}$ and $\forall x(\varphi(x) \leftrightarrow nx = 0)$.

Suppose $\forall x \varphi(x) \rightarrow \exists y \psi(y)$, hence $\forall x(nx = 0) \rightarrow \exists y \psi(y)$. By ECT_0 there is m such that $\forall x(nx = 0) \rightarrow m0{\downarrow} \wedge \psi(m0)$. Let k be an index of a partial recursive function, such that for all a,b:

$$kab \simeq \mu x.(ax \neq 0 \vee T(b,0,x))$$

Since n is total we have $\neg\neg(\exists x(nx \neq 0) \vee \forall x(nx = 0))$, so $\neg\neg(knm{\downarrow})$. By MP, $knm{\downarrow}$. Now we have a case distinction:

- If $n(knm) \neq 0$ then $\neg\forall x\varphi(x)$

- if $T(m, 0, knm)$ then $(\forall x\varphi(x) \to \psi(U(knm)))$

So in both cases, $\forall x\varphi(x) \to \psi(U(knm))$, hence $\exists y(\forall x\varphi(x) \to \psi(y))$ as desired. ∎

Remark. IP_0 is an example of a purely predicate logical scheme which is not provable in intuitionistic predicate calculus, but forced to hold under realizability by theorem 3.1.5iii).

De Jongh's Theorem (proved in a weak form by De Jongh in [35]; the full result was proved by Leivant in [96] and Van Oosten in [168]) states that if $\phi(P_1, \ldots, P_n)$ is a sentence in intuitionistic predicate logic involving relation symbols $P_1, \ldots, P_n$ and for every n-tuple $\psi_1, \ldots, \psi_n$ of formulas in the language of arithmetic such that ψ_i has exactly as many free variables as P_i, the substitution $\phi(\psi_1, \ldots, \psi_n)$ is provable in intuitionistic arithmetic, then $\phi(P_1, \ldots, P_n)$ is provable in the intuitionistic predicate calculus. In other words, the axioms of arithmetic do not force any new *logical* truth on us; in De Jongh's words, intuitionistic logic is *maximal* for first-order arithmetic.

From 3.1.5iii) one sees that intuitionistic logic is *not* maximal for arithmetic with ECT_0 andf MP added. Albert Visser has raised the question whether it is maximal for arithmetic with only ECT_0 added (it can be shown that ECT_0 alone does not imply IP_0; see [161], remark following 3.2.26; a proof which uses another theorem of De Jongh, namely the maximality of propositional logic w.r.t. Σ_1^0-substitutions). As far as I am aware, this question is still open.

Let us look at the space of functions from N to N in $\mathcal{E}ff$: the exponential N^N. In every topos, the subcategory of $\neg\neg$-separated objects is a so-called *exponential ideal*, meaning that if Y is $\neg\neg$-separated, then so is every exponential Y^X. Moreover, this subcategory is also closed under finite products in the topos, and hence is a cartesian closed subcategory. So the exponential N^N can be computed in the category of assemblies; by theorem 1.5.2, it has as underlying set the set Rec of total recursive functions $\mathbb{N} \to \mathbb{N}$, and function $E : \text{Rec} \to \mathcal{P}(\mathbb{N})$ given by $E(f) = \{e \mid e \text{ is an index for } f\}$.

Similarly, the iterated exponential $N^{(N^N)}$ has as underlying set the set of *effective operations*, that is: the set of functions $F : \text{Rec} \to \mathbb{N}$ such that there is a partial recursive function φ with the property that for every total recursive f and every index e of f, we have $\varphi(e) = F(f)$. We then let $E(F)$ be the set of indices for such φ.

We can now consider the following well-known principles from the intuitionistic literature:

(CT) $\forall f \in N^N \exists e \in N \forall x \in N \exists z \in N(T(e,x,z) \wedge U(z) = f(x))$
      (*Church's Thesis*)

(WCN) $\forall f \in N^N \exists x \in N \varphi(f,x) \to \forall f \in N^N \exists xy \in N \forall g \in N^N$
      $(\bar{f}y = \bar{g}y \to \varphi(g,x))$
      where $\bar{f}y = \bar{g}y$ is short for $\forall z < y(f(z) = g(z))$
      (*Weak Continuity for Numbers*)

(BP) $\forall F \in N^{(N^N)} \forall f \in N^N \exists x \in N \forall g \in N^N (\bar{f}x = \bar{g}x \to F(f) = F(g))$
      (*Brouwer's Principle*)

You notice that these names are somewhat nonstandard. Church's Thesis, again, says nothing like you expected it would, but blandly asserts that *every* function from N to N is recursive. Brouwer's Principle says that every function from N^N to N is continuous if we give N the discrete topology and N^N the product topology. *Weak* Continuity for Numbers is much stronger than that and says that every total relation from N^N to N is open (as subset of $N^N \times N$; note that this implies BP).

Proposition 3.1.6 *In $\mathcal{E}ff$, Church's Thesis and Brouwer's Principle are true, but Weak Continuity for Numbers fails.*

Proof. For Church's Thesis, let $f \in \text{Rec}$, and $e \in [f = f]$. Then e is an index for f. So it is easy to find, recursively in e, an element a of $[\![\forall x \in N \exists z \in N(T(e,x,z) \wedge U(z) = f(x))]\!]$. So the element $\langle e \rangle pea$ realizes Church's Thesis.

For Brouwer's Principle, one uses the *Kreisel-Lacombe-Shoenfield theorem* from recursion theory, which says that every effective operation is continuous in the following strog sense: there is a partial recursive function ψ with the property that for any effective operation F and any

$a \in E(F)$, for any total recursive function f and index b for f, whenever a total recursive function g coincides with f on the initial segment $\{0, \ldots, \psi(a, b)\}$, then $F(f) = F(g)$. From this, it is straightforward to calculate a realizer for Brouwer's Principle.

Weak Continuity for Numbers is simply inconsistent with Church's Thesis. Take, in WCN, for $\varphi(f, x)$ the formula $\forall y \in N \exists z \in N(T(x, y, z) \wedge U(z) = f(y))$, expressing that x is an index for f. Then the premiss of WCN is true by Church's Thesis, but the conclusion is absurd. ∎

Corollary 3.1.7 *The axiom of choice fails for the object N^N.*

Proof. Under the axiom of choice for N^N, Brouwer's Principle would imply WCN. ∎

3.1.1 Second-order arithmetic in ℰff

We now turn to second-order arithmetic. First of all, it is convenient to have a good representation of the power object $\mathcal{P}(N)$ in ℰff. Due to the particular equality relation on N, every function $\phi \in \mathcal{P}(N)^N$ is automatically relational: $\phi(x) \wedge x = y \rightarrow \phi(y)$ holds in the effective tripos. Therefore the power-object $\mathcal{P}(N)$ can be given as $(\mathcal{P}(N)^N, \sim)$ with

$$[R \sim S] = [\forall n (R(n) \rightarrow \{n\}) \wedge \forall n (R(n) \leftrightarrow S(n))]$$

We can simplify a bit. Let X be the set of those functions $\phi : \mathbb{N} \to \mathcal{P}(\mathbb{N})$ such that for every $n, x \in \mathbb{N}$, if $x \in \phi(n)$ then $p_1 x = n$. Then it is easily seen that $(\mathcal{P}(\mathbb{N})^{\mathbb{N}}, \sim)$ is isomorphic to $(X, \sim)$. Now there is a bijection between X and $\mathcal{P}(\mathbb{N})$ given by $G(\phi) = \{y \in \mathbb{N} \mid y \in \phi(p_1 y)\}$, with inverse $H(A)(n) = \{x \in A \mid p_1 x = n\}$. We conclude that the power object $\mathcal{P}(N)$ in ℰff is isomorphic to the object $(\mathcal{P}(\mathbb{N}), \approx)$ where

$$[A \approx B] = \bigcap_n H(A)(n) \leftrightarrow H(B)(n)$$

The element relation is represented by

$$[n \in A] = H(A)(n)$$

Recall the definition of uniform objects from the discussion before proposition 2.4.6. By that proposition, interpreted in $\mathcal{E}\!f\!f$ we see that an object is uniform (a quotient of an object $\nabla(X)$) if and only if it is isomorphic to an object $(X, =)$ for which $\bigcap_{x \in X}[x = x]$ is nonempty. We note that $\mathcal{P}(N)$ is uniform, since $pii \in \bigcap_{A \in \mathcal{P}(\mathbb{N})}[A \approx A]$ (recall that i abbreviates $\langle x \rangle x$).

Therefore, in spelling out the logic of $\mathcal{P}(N)$, we see that $[\forall A(A \approx A \to \psi)]$ is isomorphic (in the effective tripos) to $[\forall A \psi]$, for a variable A of type $\mathcal{P}(\mathbb{N})$; and similarly $[\exists A(A \approx A \land \psi]$ is isomorphic to $[\exists A \psi]$. We arrive at the following definition and proposition.

Definition 3.1.8 (Extension to second-order arithmetic) Define for numbers $n \in \mathbb{N}$ and sentences ϕ of second-order arithmetic (with constants for every subset A of $\mathbb{N}$) the relation 'n realizes ϕ', extending Kleene's definition, by:

$$
\begin{array}{ll}
n \text{ realizes } (m \in A) & \text{if } pnm \in A \\
n \text{ realizes } \forall X \psi & \text{if for all } A \subseteq \mathbb{N}, \ n \text{ realizes } \psi(A) \\
n \text{ realizes } \exists X \psi & \text{if for some } A \subseteq \mathbb{N}, \ n \text{ realizes } \psi(A)
\end{array}
$$

Here X is a second-order variable.

This definition is due to Troelstra ([161]). The following proposition was first proved in [166].

Proposition 3.1.9 *For every formula $\phi(x_1, \ldots, x_n, X_1, \ldots, X_m)$ of second-order arithmetic there are primitive recursive functions s_ϕ and t_ϕ of n arguments, such that for every n-tuple $k_1, \ldots, k_n$ of numbers and every m-tuple $A_1, \ldots, A_m$ of subsets of $\mathbb{N}$ we have:*

i)   If a realizes $\phi(k_1, \ldots, k_n, A_1, \ldots, A_m)$ then $t_\phi(k_1, \ldots, k_n)a{\downarrow}$ and

$$t_\phi(k_1, \ldots, k_n)a \in [\![\,\phi\,]\!](k_1, \ldots, k_n, A_1, \ldots, A_m)$$

ii) If $a \in [\![\,\phi\,]\!](k_1, \ldots, k_n, A_1, \ldots, A_m)$ then $s_\phi(k_1, \ldots, k_n)a{\downarrow}$ and

$$s_\phi(k_1, \ldots, k_n)a \text{ realizes } \phi(k_1, \ldots, k_n, A_1, \ldots, A_m)$$

Consequently, a sentence of second-order arithmetic is true in ℰff if and only it has a realizer.

Let us look at $\neg\neg$-stable subsets of N. Since, for any formula φ, the number 0 realizes $\neg\neg\varphi$ if and only if φ has a realizer, we see that for $A \subseteq \mathbb{N}$, a number a realizes $\forall x(\neg\neg(x \in A) \to x \in A)$ if for all n, $an{\downarrow}$ and, if $n \in A$ has a realizer, then $an0{\downarrow}$ and $an0$ realizes $n \in A$. Abbreviate the formula $\forall x(\neg\neg(x \in A) \to x \in A)$ by $\mathrm{Stab}(A)$ ("A is $\neg\neg$-stable").

Examples

a)   Suppose $f : \mathbb{N} \to \mathbb{N}$ is any non-recursive function and

$$A = \{p(f(n))n \mid n \in \mathbb{N}\}$$

Then $\mathrm{Stab}(A)$ has no realizer.

b)   For any $B \subseteq \mathbb{N}$, the set $\tilde{B} = \{p0b \mid b \in B\}$ is such that $\mathrm{Stab}(\tilde{B})$ is realized by $\langle xy \rangle p0x$, and $n \in B$ holds if and only if the sentence $n \in \tilde{B}$ has a realizer.

There is a primitive recursive bijection $\mathbb{N} \times \mathbb{N} \to \mathbb{N}$ with primitive recursive inverse, for example $n, m \mapsto \frac{(n+m)^2+3n+m}{2}$. There is a function symbol for this in the language of arithmetic; let us write $n, m \mapsto (n, m)$. Clearly, there are total recursive functions δ and ζ such that $\delta((n, m)) = pnm$ and $\zeta(pnm) = (n, m)$, so from the point of view of realizability we may assume that in fact, $pnm = (n, m)$.

Now we see from example b) above, that the sentence

(SHP) $\forall X \exists Y (\mathrm{Stab}(Y) \wedge \forall x(x \in X \leftrightarrow \exists y((y, x) \in Y)))$

is realizable. This principle is called *Shanin's Principle* in the literature ([59]): it says that every subset of N (internally) is the projection of a stable subset.

The following extension of the principle ECT_0 to second-order arithmetic is also realizable:

(ECT) $\forall X (\mathrm{Stab}(X) \wedge \forall x \in X \exists y \phi(x, y) \to$
$\exists e \forall x \in X \exists v (T(e, x, v) \wedge \phi(x, U(v))))$

which says that every relation contains, for every stable part of its domain, a partial recursive function defined on that input.

A further principle which holds in $\mathcal{E}\!f\!f$ is the *Uniformity Principle*, which says that every total relation from $\mathcal{P}(N)$ to N contains a constant function:

$$(\text{UP}) \quad \forall X \exists x \phi(X, x) \rightarrow \exists x \forall X \phi(X, x)$$

The principle was discovered and named by Troelstra; the later terminology of 'uniform objects' derives from this.

Digression As a slight digression we remark that, nonclassical as the Uniformity Principle may be, unlike a principle such as ECT_0 it has no non-classical first-order consequences. This can be seen as follows: in every realizability topos $\mathsf{RT}(A)$ it holds. Now there are pca's A for which the first-order arithmetic in $\mathsf{RT}(A)$ is classical true arithmetic ($\mathcal{K}_2$ is an example). So we see that true arithmetic plus the Uniformity Principle, taken as a theory in intuitionistic logic, is consistent.

There is another principle of second-order arithmetic which is true in the effective topos. We shall call it 'double negation shift for stable sets', or $\neg\neg$-Stab:

$$\neg\neg-\text{Stab} \quad \neg\neg\exists X(\text{Stab}(X) \wedge \varphi) \rightarrow \exists X(\text{Stab}(X) \wedge \neg\neg\varphi)$$

For, suppose we have a realizer for the premiss. That just means that for some A, there is a realizer e_0 for $\text{Stab}(A)$ and a realizer e_1 for $\varphi(A)$. Given such A, let

$$\bar{A} = \{p0n \mid \exists x \in A(p_1 x = n)\}$$

We have:

i) There is a *canonical* realizer, namely $\langle x \rangle 0$, for $\text{Stab}(\bar{A})$ (recall the notation $\langle x \rangle t$ from definition 1.1.4);

ii) From e_0 we can find a realizer for $\forall x(x \in A \leftrightarrow x \in \bar{A})$, hence for $\varphi(A) \leftrightarrow \varphi(\bar{A})$.

From the existence of e_0, e_1 we conclude that there exists a realizer for $\varphi(\bar{A})$; hence 0 is a realizer for $\neg\neg\varphi(\bar{A})$. We conclude that $p(\langle x \rangle p0x)0$ is a realizer for the conclusion.

It is worth-while to give another proof of the validity of $\neg\neg$-Stab, which is more general and uses some concepts of categorical logic.

First we remark that the object of stable subsets of N is isomorphic to $\nabla(\mathcal{P}(\mathbb{N}))$, with element relation

$$[n \in A] = \{n \mid n \in A\}$$

This is standard topos theory: $\mathcal{P}_{\neg\neg}(N) = (\Omega_{\neg\neg})^N = \nabla(2)^N \simeq \nabla(2^{\Gamma N}) = \nabla(\mathcal{P}(\mathbb{N}))$. Our second remark is that if $A \rightarrowtail X$ is a subobject in $\mathcal{E}ff$, then the $\neg\neg$-closure of A, or $[\![\, x \in X \mid \neg\neg x \in A \,]\!]$, is given by the pullback square

$$\begin{array}{ccc} \neg\neg A & \longrightarrow & \nabla\Gamma A \\ \downarrow & & \downarrow \\ X & \longrightarrow & \nabla\Gamma X \end{array}$$

Thirdly, the functor $\nabla\Gamma : \mathcal{E}ff \to \mathcal{E}ff$ preserves epi-mono factorizations since both ∇ and Γ do.

Now suppose $\phi \rightarrowtail \nabla X \times Y$ is a subobject in $\mathcal{E}ff$. We consider the formula $\exists \xi \phi$, where ξ is a variable of type ∇X; then

$$[\phi] \to [\exists \xi \phi] \rightarrowtail Y$$

is the epi-mono factorization of the composite $[\phi] \to \nabla X \times Y \to Y$.

Consider now the pullback diagrams

$$\begin{array}{ccc} [\neg\neg\phi] & \longrightarrow & \nabla\Gamma[\phi] \\ \downarrow & & \downarrow \\ \nabla X \times Y & \longrightarrow \nabla X \times \nabla\Gamma Y \simeq \nabla\Gamma(\nabla X \times Y) \\ \downarrow & & \downarrow \\ Y & \longrightarrow & \nabla\Gamma Y \end{array}$$

Then the subobject $[\exists \xi \neg \neg \phi]$ of Y is the mono-part of the left hand composite. Since $\nabla \Gamma$ preserves epi-mono factorizations we see that we have pullbacks:

$$
\begin{array}{ccc}
[\neg \neg \phi] & \longrightarrow & \nabla \Gamma [\phi] \\
\downarrow & & \downarrow \\
[\exists \xi \neg \neg \phi] & \longrightarrow & \nabla \Gamma [\exists \xi \phi] \\
\downarrow & & \downarrow \\
Y & \longrightarrow & \nabla \Gamma Y
\end{array}
$$

In particular, the bottom diagram is a pullback; but this exhibits $[\exists \xi \neg \neg \phi]$ as isomorphic to $[\neg \neg \exists \xi \phi]$, by our second remark.

From the given presentation of the object of stable subsets of N it is immediate that we also have a 'uniformity principle for stable subsets of N':

$$
\mathrm{UP}_{\mathrm{Stab}} \quad \forall X (\mathrm{Stab}(X) \to \exists n \phi) \to \exists n \forall X (\mathrm{Stab}(X) \to \phi)
$$

Note that, in the presence of SHP, UP is a consequence of $\mathrm{UP}_{\mathrm{Stab}}$.

In [169], a precise sense was formulated in which one can say that the principles MP, ECT, $\neg \neg$-Stab, $\mathrm{UP}_{\mathrm{Stab}}$ and SHP 'axiomatize the second-order arithmetic that can be constructively shown to be true under realizability'.

As a last remark about realizability for second-order arithmetic, we observe that the following principle is realizable:

$$
\mathrm{IP}_{\mathcal{P}(N)} \quad (\neg \phi \to \exists X \psi) \to \exists X (\neg \phi \to \psi)
$$

where X runs over $\mathcal{P}(N)$, and ϕ does not contain X. Principles of this form are often called 'Independence of Premiss'.

It seems worthwhile to record that the principles of double negation shift and Independence of Premiss hold more generally for uniform objects:

Proposition 3.1.10 *Let X be a uniform object. Then the principles*

$$
\begin{array}{ll}
\neg \neg \exists & \neg \neg \exists x {:} X \varphi \to \exists x {:} X \neg \neg \varphi \\
IP & (\neg \varphi \to \exists x {:} X \psi) \to \exists x {:} X (\neg \varphi \to \psi) \quad x \text{ not in } \varphi
\end{array}
$$

are true in $\mathcal{E}\!f\!f$.

The last principle to be recorded here which is valid in $\mathcal{E}ff$, follows at once from the given description of $\mathcal{P}_{\neg\neg}(N)$ and the element relation:

Proposition 3.1.11 *The following principe holds in $\mathcal{E}ff$:*

$$\Omega\text{-}cov \quad \forall p{:}\Omega \exists A{:}\mathcal{P}_{\neg\neg}(N)(p \leftrightarrow \exists n{:}N(n \in A))$$

3.1.2 Third-order arithmetic in $\mathcal{E}ff$

If we want to go one level higher, it is good to review proposition 2.4.7 again, and in particular its proof. It says that in a topos $\mathsf{C}[\mathsf{P}]$, if $(X, \sim)$ is uniform, and (as we may assume) $(X, \sim)$ is a quotient of $\nabla_{\mathsf{P}}(X)$, then $\mathcal{P}(X, \sim)$ is a quotient of $\nabla_{\mathsf{P}}(\pi(X))$: $\mathcal{P}(X, \sim)$ is isomorphic to $(\pi(X), \approx')$ where $[R \approx' S]$ is $[\zeta(R) \approx \zeta(S)]$ for an arrow $\zeta : \pi(X) \to \pi(X)$ such that

$$\mathsf{P} \models \forall R \forall x (\exists x'(x \sim x' \wedge x' \in R) \leftrightarrow x \in \zeta(R))$$

and $\approx$ is such that

$$[R \approx S] \;=\; [\forall x x'(x \sim x' \to (x \in R \leftrightarrow x' \in S))]$$

In the effective tripos, $\pi(X)$ is $\mathcal{P}(\mathbb{N})^X$ and $\nabla(\mathcal{P}(\mathbb{N})^X)$ is $\mathcal{P}_{\neg\neg}(N \times \nabla X)$, the object of stable subsets of $N \times \nabla X$, with element relation

$$[(n, x) \in G] \;=\; G(x) \cap \{n\}$$

If one writes out the fact that there is an epi ϕ in $\mathcal{E}ff$ from $\nabla(\mathcal{P}(\mathbb{N})^X)$ to $(\mathcal{P}(\mathbb{N})^X, \approx')$ one arrives at the following *covering axiom* (see also [169]):

$$\forall F : \mathcal{P}(X, \sim) \exists G : \mathcal{P}_{\neg\neg}(N \times \nabla X) \forall x : (X, \sim)\, [x \in F \leftrightarrow$$
$$\exists x'(\phi(x') = x \wedge \exists n(n, x') \in G)]$$

Applying this to the covering of $\mathcal{P}(N)$ by $\nabla(\mathcal{P}(\mathbb{N}))$, which is $\mathcal{P}_{\neg\neg}(N)$, we obtain the following sentence of third-order arithmetic which is true in $\mathcal{E}ff$:

$$\forall \mathcal{X} \exists \mathcal{U} \forall X (X \in \mathcal{X} \leftrightarrow \exists A(\forall x(x \in X \leftrightarrow \exists y(y, x) \in A) \wedge$$
$$\exists n((n, A) \in \mathcal{U})))$$

where $\mathcal{X}$ is of type $\mathcal{PP}(N)$, $\mathcal{U}$ of type $\mathcal{P}_{\neg\neg}(N \times \mathcal{P}(N))$, X of type $\mathcal{P}(N)$ and A of type $\mathcal{P}_{\neg\neg}(N)$.

3.2   Some special objects and arrows in $\mathcal{E}\!ff$

3.2.1   Closed and dense subobjects

As already remarked in section 3.1.1, a subobject $A \rightarrowtail X$ is $\neg\neg$-closed
(or, $\neg\neg$-stable) if and only if the square

$$
\begin{array}{ccc}
A & \longrightarrow & \nabla\Gamma A \\
\downarrow & & \downarrow \\
X & \longrightarrow & \nabla\Gamma X
\end{array}
$$

is a pullback. That means, that if X is $(X, \sim)$, A is isomorphic to $(A, \sim)$
with $A \subseteq X$ a subset which is closed under the equivalence relation
$[x \sim x'] \neq \emptyset$, and $\sim$ on A is the restriction of $\sim$ on X.

For $\neg\neg$-separated objects we have the following useful proposition.

Proposition 3.2.1 *Suppose $m : A \to B$ is a monomorphism between
assemblies. Then m represents a closed subobject in $\mathcal{E}\!ff$ if and only if
m is a regular mono in* Ass.

Proof. If m is a regular mono in Ass, so $m : A \to B$ is the equalizer in
Ass of $f, g : B \to C$, then this is also an equalizer in $\mathcal{E}\!ff$, and in $\mathcal{E}\!ff$ we
have for $x \in B$:

$$
\neg\neg(x \in A) \leftrightarrow \neg\neg(f(x) = g(x)) \leftrightarrow f(x) = g(x) \leftrightarrow x \in A
$$

(since C is $\neg\neg$-separated), so m is closed in $\mathcal{E}\!ff$.

Conversely, if m is closed in $\mathcal{E}\!ff$ then we know that

$$
\begin{array}{ccc}
A & \xrightarrow{\eta_A} & \nabla\Gamma A \\
\downarrow & & \downarrow \\
B & \xrightarrow[\eta_B]{} & \nabla\Gamma B
\end{array}
$$

is a pullback. Combining this with the pullback diagram

$$
\begin{array}{ccc}
\nabla\Gamma A & \longrightarrow & 1 \simeq \nabla 1 \\
\downarrow & & \downarrow{\scriptstyle \nabla t} \\
\nabla\Gamma B & \xrightarrow[\nabla\phi]{} & \nabla 2
\end{array}
$$

(where ϕ is the characteristic function of $\Gamma A \subseteq \Gamma B$ in Set), we get that m is the equalizer of $\nabla \phi \circ \eta_B$ and $\nabla \mathrm{to!} : B \to 1 \to \nabla 2$, so m is regular mono. ∎

I mention the following standard fact without proof.

Proposition 3.2.2 *If $A, B \rightarrowtail X$ are closed subobjects, then so are $A \wedge B$, $A \to B$, $\neg A$ and, for any map $X \xrightarrow{f} Y$, $\forall_f(A)$.*

A subobject $A \rightarrowtail X$ is $\neg\neg$-*dense* if the sentence $\forall x : X \neg\neg(x \in A)$ is true. Equivalently, if $\nabla \Gamma A \to \nabla \Gamma X$ is an isomorphism. It means in $\mathcal{E}ff$ that if $X = (X, \sim)$ and A is given by a strict predicate $A : X \to \mathcal{P}(\mathbb{N})$, then $A(x)$ is nonempty for every $x \in X$.

For example: suppose $A \rightarrowtail N \times N$ is the graph of some non-recursive function, then the first projection $\pi_1 : A \rightarrowtail N$ is a dense mono which is not an isomorphism.

3.2.2 Infinite coproducts and products

In chapter 2 we have seen how to compute finite limits and colimits in toposes of the form $\mathsf{C}[P]$. It is worth remarking that in $\mathcal{E}ff$, in contrast to the case for Grothendieck toposes, the natural numbers object N is *not* the countable coproduct of copies of 1 (since the arrows $N \to N$ in $\mathcal{E}ff$ are just the total recursive functions); in fact, we have the following proposition:

Proposition 3.2.3 *In $\mathcal{E}ff$, the countable coproduct of copies of 1 does not exist. For any object $(X, \sim)$ there exist at most countably many arrows to N.*

Proof. If such a coproduct existed, then there would be $2^{\aleph_0}$ arrows in $\mathcal{E}ff$ from this coproduct to N: for any function $f : \mathbb{N} \to \mathbb{N}$ in Set we would have an arrow in $\mathcal{E}ff$ sending the i-th summand to $f(i)$ in N. So it suffices to prove the second statement.

For any arrow $(X, \sim) \to N$, represented by $F : X \times \mathbb{N} \to \mathcal{P}(\mathbb{N})$, we have seen that there is a function $\phi : \{x \in X \mid [x \sim x] \neq \emptyset\} \to \mathbb{N}$ and a partial recursive function $g : \bigcup_{x \in X}[x \sim x] \to \mathbb{N}$ such that for each x and each $n \in [x \sim x]$, $g(n) = \phi(x)$ and $F(x, n) \neq \emptyset$. And the arrow is completely determined by the function g. So there can be at most countably many arrows $(X, \sim) \to N$ in $\mathcal{E}ff$. ∎

Corollary 3.2.4 *The functor* $\Gamma : \mathcal{E}ff \to \mathrm{Set}$ *does not have a left adjoint.*

Proof. Suppose $L \dashv \Gamma$. Then since Γ is the global sections functor, for any object $(X, \sim)$ of $\mathcal{E}ff$ we would have naturally in $(X, \sim)$:

$$\mathcal{E}ff(1, (X, \sim)) \simeq \Gamma(X, \sim) \simeq \mathrm{Set}(1, \Gamma(X, \sim)) \simeq \mathcal{E}ff(L(1), (X, \sim))$$

so that by the Yoneda Lemma, $L(1) \simeq 1$. But then, since L preserves coproducts, the countable coproduct of copies of 1 would exist in $\mathcal{E}ff$; contradiction with 3.2.3. ∎

Corollary 3.2.5 *In* $\mathcal{E}ff$, *the countable product of copies of* Ω *does not exist.*

Proof. The Monadicity Theorem in topos theory (see [83], A2.2) says that for every topos $\mathcal{E}$, the category of algebras for the double-powerset monad $\mathcal{P}^2$ is equivalent to $\mathcal{E}^{\mathrm{op}}$, the equivalence being given by a functor $\mathcal{E}^{\mathrm{op}} \to \mathcal{P}^2 - \mathrm{Alg}$ which sends an object X to an algebra with underlying object $\mathcal{P}(X)$. Since the forgetful functor from $\mathcal{P}^2 - \mathrm{Alg}$ to $\mathcal{E}$ creates limits, this means that if I is a diagram in $\mathcal{E}^{\mathrm{op}}$ such that its $\mathcal{P}$-image has a limit in $\mathcal{E}$, then I has a limit in $\mathcal{E}^{\mathrm{op}}$. Applying this to the constant functor with value 1 from the discrete category $\mathbb{N}$, we see that a countable product of copies of Ω in $\mathcal{E}ff$ would give us a countable coproduct of copies of 1 in $\mathcal{E}ff$, which contradicts proposition 3.2.3. ∎

3.2.3 Projective and internally projective objects, and choice principles

In $\mathcal{E}ff$, every object is a quotient of a $\neg\neg$-separated object (since these are the assemblies). More special coverings are available: given $(X, \sim)$, let $P(X, \sim)$ be the object $(X', \approx)$, where

$$
\begin{aligned}
X' &= \{(x, n) \mid n \in [x \sim x]\} \\
[(x, n) \approx (x', n')] &= \{n \mid x = x' \text{ and } n = n'\}
\end{aligned}
$$

Then there is an arrow $\pi : (X', \approx) \to (X, \sim)$ represented by

$$\Pi((x, n), x') = \{n\} \wedge [x \sim x']$$

This is an epimorphism. Note that the object $P(X, \sim)$ has the properties that $[\xi \approx \eta] = \emptyset$ if $\xi \neq \eta$ (so, $P(X, \sim)$ is an assembly), and $[\xi \approx \xi]$ is always a singleton. Objects with these properties we shall call *partitioned assemblies*. So we see that every object is covered by a partitioned assembly. Let us note a consequence of this fact:

Proposition 3.2.6 *In $\mathcal{E}ff$, every power object is uniform.*

Proof. If $(X, \sim)$ is covered by the partitioned assembly $(X', \approx)$ as above, then $\mathcal{P}(X, \sim)$ is covered by $\mathcal{P}(X', \approx)$ by the map which takes the image of a subobject under the original covering. So it suffices to show that $\mathcal{P}(X', \approx)$ is uniform. Now every element of $\mathcal{P}(\mathbb{N})^{X'}$ is automatically relational, and if ϕ is such an element, then the map $(x, n) \mapsto \{n\} \wedge \phi(x, n)$ is strict. So we see that $\mathcal{P}(X', \approx)$ is a quotient of $\nabla(\mathcal{P}(\mathbb{N})^{X'})$. ∎

Recall that in a regular category, an object P is called *projective* if for any regular epimorphism $f : A \to B$, any arrow from P to B factors through f. Equivalently: every regular epi with codomain P is split. The axiom of choice for Set is equivalent to the statement that every object of Set is projective.

The following proposition relies on the axiom of choice in Set.

Proposition 3.2.7 *In $\mathcal{E}ff$, an object is projective if and only if it is isomorphic to a partitioned assembly. Every object is covered by a projective object. The full subcategory of $\mathcal{E}ff$ on the projective objects is closed under finite limits in $\mathcal{E}ff$.*

Proof. The second claim follows from the first, by the remarks we just made about every object being covered by a partitioned assembly. The third claim is also straightforward, as it is easy to see that the partitioned assemblies are closed under finite limits in $\mathcal{E}ff$.

So let $(X, \sim)$ be a partitioned assembly and $(Y, \sim) \to (X, \sim)$ be an epimorphism represented by F. From a realizer for the statement that

F represents an epi, we get a partial recursive function g such that for every $x \in X$ there is a $y \in Y$ such that $g(n) \in F(y, x)$, where n is the unique element in $[x \sim x]$. Using Choice in Set, let $\phi : X \to Y$ be such that $g(n) \in F(\phi(x), x)$. The the relation $[x \sim x] \wedge [y \sim \phi(x)]$ defines a section for the epi represented by F. So $(X, \sim)$ is projective.

Conversely, suppose $(X, \sim)$ is projective. Then $(X, \sim)$ is $\neg\neg$-separated; for $(X, \sim)$ is covered by a separated object, and this cover has a section, so $(X, \sim)$ is a subobject of a separated object. So we may assume that $(X, \sim)$ is an assembly. Now $(X, \sim)$ is also covered by a partitioned assembly $P(X, \sim)$ as above. Then the section $(X, \sim) \to P(X, \sim)$ is a regular mono in Ass, hence by 3.2.1 a closed mono in $\mathcal{E}ff$. But this presents $(X, \sim)$ as a partitioned assembly itself.   ∎

Proposition 3.2.7 allows $\mathcal{E}ff$ to be seen as a universal construction, see subsection 3.2.4 below.

An object P in a topos $\mathcal{E}$ is called *internally projective* if the functor $(-)^P : \mathcal{E} \to \mathcal{E}$ preserves epimorphisms. Logically this means that the axiom of choice holds for P in the following form: for every arrow $f : Y \to P$ the sentence

$$\forall x : P \exists y : Y (f(y) = x) \to \exists g : Y^P \forall x : P(f(g(x)) = x)$$

is true in $\mathcal{E}$. It is easy to see that if 1 is projective in $\mathcal{E}$ then every internally projective object is projective: suppose P is internally projective and $Y \xrightarrow{f} P$ an epimorphism. Then $f^P : Y^P \to P^P$ is epi since P is internally projective. Let $1 \to P^P$ be the arrow corresponding to the identity on P; then as 1 was assumed projective, this arrow factors through an arrow $1 \to Y^P$. This gives an arrow $P \to Y$ which is a section for f.

In $\mathcal{E}ff$, 1 is projective, so every internally projective object is isomorphic to a partitioned assembly. But the converse holds too (assuming choice for Sets). To show this we construct, for a partitioned assembly $(P, \sim)$ and an object $(A, \sim)$ the exponential $(A, \sim)^{(P, \sim)}$ as follows: define $\approx$ on the set of functions A^P by

$$[f \approx g] = [\forall p \in P((p \sim p) \to (f(p) \sim g(p)))]$$

Then we can show that $(A, \sim)^{(P,\sim)}$ is isomorphic to the object $(A^P, \approx)$: the exponential is of the form $(\mathcal{P}(\mathbb{N})^{P \times A}, \sim)$ with

$$[R \sim S] = [\text{“}R \text{ is a functional relation”} \wedge \forall pa(R(p,a) \leftrightarrow S(p,a))]$$

One now defines a map $G : \mathcal{P}(\mathbb{N})^{P \times A} \times A^P \to \mathcal{P}(\mathbb{N})$ by

$$G(R, f) = [\text{“}R \text{ is a functional relation”} \wedge \forall p : P(R(p, f(p)))]$$

Then G is strict, relational and single-valued; using choice it is total. So G represents a morphism: $(A, \sim)^{(P,\sim)} \to (A^P, \approx)$. It is easy to see that this is in fact an isomorphism in $\mathcal{E}ff$. Now using this representation for the exponential and choice in Set, one readily deduces that $(-)^{(P,\sim)}$ preserves epimorphisms. So we have proved the following proposition.

Proposition 3.2.8 *In $\mathcal{E}ff$, the classes of the projective objects and the internally projective objects coincide.*

For reference, I single out a particular instance of this fact as a corollary.

Corollary 3.2.9 *In $\mathcal{E}ff$, the principle of countable choice is valid:*

$$\forall x{:}N \exists y{:}X \psi(x, y) \to \exists f{:}X^N \forall x{:}N \psi(x, f(x))$$

for any object X of $\mathcal{E}ff$.

We can get a little bit beyond that, using the representation of exponentials for partitioned assemblies given above. First, a definition.

Definition 3.2.10 *Let $\mathcal{E}$ be a topos, and X an object of $\mathcal{E}$. We say that $\mathcal{E}$ satisfies* dependent choices *for X, or $DC(X)$, if for every relation $A \rightarrowtail X \times X$ the sentence*

$$\forall x : X \exists y : X \, A(x, y) \to \forall x : X \exists f : X^N \, (f(0) = x \wedge \forall n : N \, A(f(n), f(n+1)))$$

is true in $\mathcal{E}$.

Proposition 3.2.11 *In $\mathcal{E}ff$, the principle of dependent choices holds for every object.*

3.2.4 $\mathcal{E}\!f\!f$ as a universal construction

In [32], a construction is given (it is due to A. Joyal) for the so-called *ex/lex completion* of a category $\mathcal{C}$ with finite limits ('lex', or 'left exact', is old terminology for having finite limits). Let FL denote the category of categories with finite limits and finite limit-preserving functors. The ex/lex completion of $\mathcal{C}$, which results in a finite limit-preserving functor $\eta : \mathcal{C} \to \mathcal{C}_{\mathrm{ex/lex}}$, is determined up to equivalence of categories by the requirement that $\mathcal{C}_{\mathrm{ex/lex}}$ is exact and composition with η induces, for every exact category $\mathcal{D}$, an equivalence of categories

$$FL(\mathcal{C},\mathcal{D}) \simeq REG(\mathcal{C}_{\mathrm{ex/lex}},\mathcal{D})$$

In *l.c.*, the following facts are shown (the precise construction does not matter here):

1)   Every object of $\mathcal{C}$ becomes (via η) a projective object in $\mathcal{C}_{\mathrm{ex/lex}}$ and every projective object of $\mathcal{C}_{\mathrm{ex/lex}}$ is isomorphic to one in the image of η.

2) η is full and faithful.

3)   An exact category is an ex/lex completion (necessarily, by 1 and 2, of its full subcategory of projective objects), if and only if every object is covered by a projective object, and the full subcategory on the projective objects is closed under finite limits in the category.

After these definitions and facts, the following corollary, first recorded in [134], follows directly from proposition 3.2.7:

Corollary 3.2.12 $\mathcal{E}\!f\!f$ *is the* ex/lex *completion of its full subcategory on the projective objects.*

I should reiterate, however, that corollary 3.2.12, like its father proposition 3.2.7, relies on the axiom of choice in Set (and is in fact equivalent to it). Therefore, despite its obvious appeal to category theorists (the effective topos is a universal construction!), applications of this fact have been limited. Realizability toposes constructed over other toposes than Set, which do not satisfy the axiom of choice, are not exact completions.

However, the only obstacle is that the partitioned assemblies are not necessarily projective, and one feels that there might be a more general formulation of the ex/lex completion result.

In fact, a more subtle approach is possible. Suppose the effective tripos is defined over a topos $\mathcal{E}$, so elements of $\mathsf{P}_{\mathrm{eff}}(C)$, for $C \in \mathcal{E}$, are maps in $\mathcal{E}$ from C to $\mathcal{P}(N)$, N being the natural numbers object in $\mathcal{E}$. For two such maps ϕ and ψ then, one defines $\phi \leq \psi$ if and only if

$$\mathcal{E} \models \exists a : N \forall x : C \forall n : N(n \in \phi(x) \rightarrow \exists z : N(T(a,n,z) \wedge U(z) \in \psi(x)))$$

One can easily prove that this gives a tripos.

One has the category of *partitioned assemblies* over $\mathcal{E}$: objects are maps $X \rightarrow N$, and arrows are functions which are (internally in $\mathcal{E}$, as in the definition of the tripos) tracked by a partial recursive function.

There is the regular 'constant objects' functor $\nabla : \mathcal{E} \rightarrow \mathcal{E}[\mathsf{P}_{\mathrm{eff}}]$, which factors through the category of partitioned assemblies over $\mathcal{E}$. Now such a partitioned assembly $X \rightarrow N$ is 'as projective in $\mathcal{E}[\mathsf{P}_{\mathrm{eff}}]$, as X is projective in $\mathcal{E}$'. So in what sense can $\mathcal{E}[\mathsf{P}_{\mathrm{eff}}]$ be seen as an 'exact completion' of the partitioned assemblies?

The answer, as explained in detail in [67], is that instead of looking at the categories FL and REG, one looks at the 'co-slices' $\mathcal{E}/FL$ and $\mathcal{E}/REG$. Objects of $\mathcal{E}/FL$ are finite limit-preserving functors $\mathcal{E} \rightarrow \mathcal{C}$, with $\mathcal{C}$ a category with finite limits; morphisms are commutative triangles

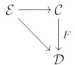

where, again, F preserves finite limits. The category $\mathcal{E}/REG$ is defined likewise, now we have regular functors into a regular category, and commutative triangles of regular functors. Of course, both $\mathcal{E}/FL$ and $\mathcal{E}/REG$ are 2-categories just as FL and REG.

The 'exact completion relative to $\mathcal{E}$' constructs, for an object $\mathcal{E} \rightarrow \mathcal{C}$ of $\mathcal{E}/FL$, an object $\mathcal{E} \rightarrow \mathcal{C}_{\mathrm{ex}/\mathcal{E}}$ of $\mathcal{E}/REG$ such that $\mathcal{C}_{\mathrm{ex}/\mathcal{E}}$ is exact, and an arrow

$$\eta/\mathcal{E} : (\mathcal{E} \rightarrow \mathcal{C}) \rightarrow (\mathcal{E} \rightarrow \mathcal{C}_{\mathrm{ex}/\mathcal{E}})$$

in $\mathcal{E}/FL$, such that for any object $\mathcal{E} \to \mathcal{D}$ of $\mathcal{E}/REG$ with $\mathcal{D}$ exact, composition with $\eta/\mathcal{E}$ induces an equivalence of categories

$$\mathcal{E}/FL(\mathcal{E} \to \mathcal{C}, \mathcal{E} \to \mathcal{D}) \;\simeq\; \mathcal{E}/REG(\mathcal{E} \to \mathcal{C}_{\mathrm{ex}/\mathcal{E}}, \mathcal{E} \to \mathcal{D})$$

One can now prove:

Theorem 3.2.13 (Hofstra) *Let* $\mathsf{P}_{\mathrm{eff}}$ *be the effective tripos on a topos* $\mathcal{E}$, *and let* $\mathrm{PAss}_{\mathcal{E}}$ *be the category of partitioned assemblies over* $\mathcal{E}$. *Then* $\mathcal{E}[\mathsf{P}_{\mathrm{eff}}]$ *is the exact completion relative to* $\mathcal{E}$ *of the functor* $\mathcal{E} \to \mathrm{PAss}_{\mathcal{E}}$.

There is a similar story about the relationship between partitioned assemblies and assemblies. Carboni and Rosolini (see [30]) have given a general construction for the 'regular completion' of a category with finite limits (or, reg/lex completion), and proved that Ass is the reg/lex completion of the category of partitioned assemblies.

Again, this result depends on choice in Set; however, again a relative version, due to Hofstra (l.c.) also holds.

3.2.5   Real numbers in $\mathcal{E}ff$

The principle of countable choice (3.2.9) is useful for the calculation of the real numbers in $\mathcal{E}ff$. Let Q be the object of rational numbers. Q is easily constructed: fix a bijection $\shortmid\shortmid : \mathbb{N} \to \mathbb{Q}$ such that the basic operations $+, \cdot$ and the order on $\mathbb{Q}$ are given primitive-recursively in codes. Then Q is the partitioned assembly $(\mathbb{Q}, E)$ with $E(r) = \mathbf{q}^{-1}(r)$.

In constructive mathematics, some care is needed in defining the real numbers as equivalence classes of Cauchy sequences. The usual treatment (e.g. in [163], section 5.2) defines a Cauchy sequence as a pair $((r_n)_n, \beta)$ where $(r_n)_n$ is a sequence of rational numbers and $\beta : N \to N$ is its *modulus of convergence*, that is: the pair satisfies

$$\forall knm(|r_{\beta(k)+n} - r_{\beta(k)+m}| < 2^{-k})$$

Two such pairs $((r_n)_n, \beta)$ and $((s_n)_n, \gamma)$ define the same real number, if

$$\forall k \exists n \forall m(|r_{n+m} - s_{n+m}| < 2^{-k})$$

Equivalently, given that β and γ are moduli of convergence,

$$\forall km(|r_{\delta(k)+m} - s_{\delta(k)+m}| < 2^{-k})$$

where $\delta(k) = \max\{\beta(k+2), \gamma(k+2)\}$. Although the moduli of convergence are not part of the definition of the equivalence relation which gives the real numbers, the explicit information they provide is usually necessary for establishing basic properties about the real line.

In $\mathcal{Eff}$, thanks to countable choice, we can always find a modulus of convergence for $(r_n)_n$ provided $\forall k \exists n \forall mm'(|r_{n+m} - r_{n+m'}| < 2^{-k})$. And given a modulus β for $(r_n)_n$, we can find a sequence $(r'_n)_n$ which defines the same real number, and which satisfies

$$\forall k(|r'_k - r'_{k+1}| < 2^{-(k+1)})$$

Note, that the identity function is a modulus of convergence for $(r'_n)_n$.

We define therefore, in $\mathcal{Eff}$, the object of Cauchy sequences as a subobject of Q^N, defined by:

(C1) $C = \{(r_n)_n \in Q^N \,|\, \forall k(|r_k - r_{k+1}| < 2^{-(k+1)})\}$

C is obviously a closed subobject of Q^N: it is the assembly $(\mathbb{C}, E)$ where $\mathbb{C}$ is the set of recursive sequences satisfying (C1), and $E(f)$ is the set of indices for f.

The object R_c of *Cauchy reals* in $\mathcal{Eff}$ is the quotient of C by the equivalence relation

$$(r_n)_n \sim (s_n)_n \equiv \forall k \exists n \forall m |r_{n+m} - s_{n+m}| < 2^{-k}$$

Proposition 3.2.14 $\sim$ *is a closed equivalence relation.*

Proof. In order to see this, define for $(r_n)_n, (s_n)_n$:

$$(r_n)_n \sharp (s_n)_n \equiv \exists kn \forall m |s_{n+m} - r_{n+m}| > 2^{-k}$$

Then clearly, $(r_n)_n \sim (s_n)_n$ implies $\neg((r_n)_n \sharp (s_n)_n)$, but also the converse holds: suppose $\neg((r_n)_n \sharp (s_n)_n)$. Then

(1) $\forall kn \neg \forall m |s_{n+m} - r_{n+m}| > 2^{-k}$

(2) $\forall knm |s_{k+n} - s_{k+m}| < 2^{-k}$

(3) $\forall knm |r_{k+n} - r_{k+m}| < 2^{-k}$

(since the identity is a modulus for r and s). Combining these and taking $k + 2$ for k and n in (2) we get

(4) $\forall k \neg \forall m |s_{k+m+2} - s_{k+m+2}| > 2^{-(k+2)}$

Now suppose that for some m we have $|r_{k+m+2} - s_{k+m+2}| > 2^{-k}$. Then for all m' we have

$$
\begin{aligned}
|r_{k+m'+2} - s_{k+m'+2}| &\geq |s_{k+m+2} - r_{k+m+2}| - |s_{k+m'+2} - s_{k+m+2}| - \\
& \qquad |r_{k+m'+2} - r_{k+m+2}| \\
&> 2^{-k} - 2^{-(k+2)} - 2^{-(k+2)} \\
&= 2^{-(k+1)} \\
&> 2^{-(k+2)}
\end{aligned}
$$

But this contradicts (4). Hence $|r_{k+m+2} - s_{k+m+2}| \leq 2^{-k}$ for all m; it follows that $(r_n)_n \sim (s_n)_n$. ∎

We arrive at the following characterization:

Proposition 3.2.15 (Hyland) *The object R_c of Cauchy reals in $\mathcal{E}ff$ is isomorphic to the assembly $(\mathbb{R}_{rec}, E)$, where $\mathbb{R}_{rec}$ is the set of recursive real numbers (i.e. the set of real numbers represented by a recursive Cauchy sequence), and $E(r)$ is the set of indices a such that a defines a Cauchy sequence of rationals converging to r, and $\forall n(|an - a(n+1)| < 2^{-(n+1)})$ holds.*

In general, there is more than one notion of 'real number', in constructive logic. The *Dedekind reals* are given by Dedekind cuts: a Dedekind cut is a pair (L, R) of subsets of Q such that L is downward closed and open, R is upward closed and open, $L \cap R = \emptyset$, both L and R are inhabited, and the pair is *located*, that is: for every pair $q, r \in Q$ we have $q < r \to q \in L \vee r \in R$. Given a Dedekind cut (L, R), it is easy to show that $\forall n \exists qr \in Q(q \in L \wedge r \in R \wedge |r - q| < \frac{1}{2^n})$, so using Choice for numbers one finds a Cauchy sequence $(r_n)_n$ which represents the same real as the cut (L, R). Therefore, the following proposition holds.

Proposition 3.2.16 *In $\mathcal{E}ff$, the objects of Dedekind reals and Cauchy reals are isomorphic.*

In view of this proposition we shall just write R for "the" object of reals in $\mathcal{E}ff$. For further information about R, see section 3.3 below.

3.2.6   Discrete and modest objects

Considerable attention has been devoted to the class of objects that we shall discuss now, the *discrete objects*.

Definition 3.2.17 A *discrete object* is a quotient of a subobject of N.

Let us notice at once that in $\mathcal{E}ff$ every subobject of N is covered by a *closed* subobject of N. This can be seen as a consequence of Shanin's principle (combined with the fact that 1 is projective); concretely, if $A : \mathbb{N} \to \mathcal{P}(\mathbb{N})$ is a strict predicate for N, hence giving a subobject of N, this subobject is covered by the closed subobject of N determined by the subset $\{pnx \mid x \in A(n)\}$ of $\mathbb{N}$. Therefore, discrete objects can also be defined as quotients of closed subobjects of N. A discrete object is therefore isomorphic to one of the form $(A, \sim)$ with $A \subseteq N$ and $\sim$ an equality predicate such that the functions $\lambda n.[n \sim n]$ and $\lambda n.\{n\}$ are isomorphic in $\mathsf{P}(A)$ (where P is the effective tripos).
   The following proposition gives another characterization of the discrete objects.

Proposition 3.2.18 *An object is discrete if and only if it is isomorphic to an object $(X, \sim)$ which satisfies the condition that $[x \sim x] \cap [y \sim y] = \emptyset$ whenever $x \neq y$.*

Proof. If $(A, \sim)$ is discrete, with $A \subseteq N$ and $\sim$ such that $[n \sim n] \simeq \{n\}$, then clearly it is of the form in the proposition.
   Conversely, suppose $(X, \sim)$ satisfies the condition in the proposition. Let $A = \bigcup_{x \in X}[x \sim x]$. Then by assumption on $(X, \sim)$ there is a function $f : A \to X$ such that for all $n \in A$, $n \in [f(n) \sim f(n)]$. Define an equivalence relation on A:

$$R(n, m) \;=\; \{n\} \wedge \{m\} \wedge [f(n) \sim f(m)]$$

Then clearly $R(n,n) \simeq \{n\}$ in $\mathsf{P}(A)$, so the object (A, R) is discrete. Moreover, if $F : A \times X \to \mathcal{P}(\mathbb{N})$ is defined by

$$F(n, x) \;=\; \{n\} \wedge [f(n) \sim x]$$

then it is easily verified that F represents an isomorphism $(A, R) \to (X, \sim)$. ∎

Proposition 3.2.19

i) *The discrete objects are closed under finite products, quotients and subobjects.*

ii) *The discrete objects form an exponential ideal in $\mathcal{E}ff$.*

iii) *The full subcategory of $\mathcal{E}ff$ on the discrete objects is* reflective, *that is: the inclusion functor into $\mathcal{E}ff$ has a left adjoint.*

Proof. i) For products, it is easiest to use the representation given in proposition 3.2.18. Clearly the objects of the form in that proposition are closed under finite products. Closure under quotients follows at once from the definition. For subobjects one considers a pullback diagram:

$$
\begin{array}{ccc}
B & \longrightarrow & A \\
\downarrow & & \downarrow{\scriptstyle r} \\
Y & \longrightarrow & X
\end{array}
$$

If r presents X as a quotient of the subobject A of N and $Y \to X$ is monic, then since epis are stable, Y is a quotient of the subobject B of N.

ii) We need to prove that for $(X, \sim)$ discrete and $(Y, \sim)$ arbitrary, $(X, \sim)^{(Y, \sim)}$ is discrete. To this end, let P be a partitioned assembly which covers $(Y, \sim)$. Since the partitioned assemblies are internally projective in $\mathcal{E}ff$ and $(X, \sim)$ is covered by a closed subobject A of N, we have a diagram

$$A^P \xrightarrow{\;e\;} (X, \sim)^P \xleftarrow{\;m\;} (X, \sim)^{(Y, \sim)}$$

with e epi and m mono. By part i) therefore, it suffices to prove that A^P is discrete. The exponential A^P can be computed in the category of assemblies; clearly it is a quotient of the closed subobject of N determined by the set of indices of partial recursive functions which track an arrow $P \to A$.

iii) We define, for every object $(X, \sim)$ of $\mathcal{Eff}$, a discrete object $(A_X, \sim_X)$ and an arrow $\eta : (X, \sim) \to (A_X, \sim_X)$ such that every arrow from $(X, \sim)$ to a discrete object factors uniquely through η.

Let $A_X = \bigcup_{x \in X}[x \sim x]$. For $n, m \in A_X$, define $[n \sim_X m]$ as the set of all codes σ of sequences $\langle n_0, a_0, n_1, a_1, \dots, n_{k-1}, a_{k-1}, n_k \rangle$ which satisfy:

1) $k \geq 1$

2) $n_0 = n$ and $n_k = m$

3) For every $i < k$ there are $x, y \in X$ such that $n_i \in [x \sim x]$, $n_{i+1} \in [y \sim y]$ and $a_i \in [x \sim y]$

Then $\sim_X$ is a good equality relation on A_X: if $\sigma \in [n \sim_X m]$ and $\sigma = \langle n_0, a_0, n_1, a_1, \dots, n_{k-1}, a_{k-1}, n_k \rangle$, then

$$\sigma^* = \langle n_k, \mathsf{s}(a_{k-1}), n_{k-1}, \dots, n_1, \mathsf{s}(a_1), n_0 \rangle$$

is an element of $[m \sim_X n]$, where s is a realizer for the symmetry of $\sim$ on X. And if $\sigma \in [n \sim_X m]$ and $\tau \in [m \sim_X k]$ then $\sigma * \langle m \rangle * \tau$ is an element of $[n \sim_X k]$, where $*$ stands for the operation of codes of sequences which mirrors concatenation.

Notice that for each $n \in A_X$, $\langle n, n, n \rangle$ is an element of $[n \sim_X n]$, so we have a discrete object.

Next, we define a functional relation G from $(X, \sim)$ to $(A_X, \sim_X)$: let $G(x, n)$ consist of those sequences σ such that for some $n_0 \in [x \sim x]$, $\sigma \in [n_0 \sim_X n]$. It is straightforward to check that G is indeed a functional relation, and that it represents an epimorphism $(X, \sim) \to (A_X, \sim_X)$. This is our promised map η.

We have to prove the universal property of η. Suppose $f : (X, \sim) \to (A, R)$ is a map from $(X, \sim)$ to a discrete object. We assume without loss of generality that $A \subseteq \mathbb{N}$, and R an equality relation satisfying $R(n, n) \simeq \{n\}$ in $\mathsf{P}(A)$. We show that f factors through η; the factorization is unique since η is epi.

Suppose f is represented by $F \in \mathsf{P}(X \times A)$. Using totality of F and the assumed property of R, we see that there are partial recursive functions φ and ψ such that for every $x \in X$ and every $n \in [x \sim x]$:

$$\psi(n) \in F(x, \psi(n))$$

Now if $\langle n_0, a_0, n_1 \rangle$ is such that for some $x, y \in X$, $n_0 \in [x \sim x]$, $a_0 \in [x \sim y]$ and $n_1 \in [y \sim y]$, then we have $\psi(n_0) \in F(x, \varphi(n_0))$ and $\psi(n_1) \in F(y, \varphi(n_1))$. If r realizes that F is relational for $(X, \sim)$ then $\mathsf{r}(\psi(n_0), a_0) \in F(y, \varphi(n_0))$. So if sv realizes the single-valuedness of F we have $\mathsf{sv}(\mathsf{r}(\psi(n_0), a_0)) \in R(\varphi(n_0), \varphi(n_1))$. It is now easy to define by recursion on σ a partial recursive function $\chi(\sigma)$ such that for all n, m and $\sigma \in [n \sim_X m]$:

$$\chi(\sigma) \in R(\varphi(n), \varphi(m))$$

Define $H \in \mathsf{P}(A_X \times A)$ by putting

$$H(n, k) \;=\; [n \sim_X n] \wedge R(\varphi(n), k)$$

H is clearly strict and single-valued. That it is relational and total follows from the existence of χ above, so H represents a map $h : (A_X, \sim_X) \to (A, R)$. The verification that the diagram

$$
\begin{array}{ccc}
(X, \sim) & & \\
\eta \downarrow & \searrow^{f} & \\
(A_X, \sim_X) & \xrightarrow[h]{} & (A, R)
\end{array}
$$

commutes, is left to you.   ∎

The following corollary will be useful when we consider *families* of discrete objects, in section 3.4.

Corollary 3.2.20 *Suppose* $(X, \sim)$ *is an object of* $\mathcal{E}ff$ *such that the set*

$$\bigcap_{x, x' \in X} (E(x) \cap E(x') \to [x \sim x'])$$

is nonempty. Then $(X, \sim)$ is discrete.

Proof. It is easy to see that any element of the given set gives a realizer for the statement that the map $\eta : (X, \sim) \rightarrow (A_X, \sim_X)$, constructed in the proof of proposition 3.2.19iii), is monic, hence an isomorphism. ∎

The discrete objects give rise to the following generalization of the Uniformity Principle, which is an easy exercise:

Proposition 3.2.21 *Suppose X is discrete and Y uniform. Then the statement*

$$\forall \phi \in \mathcal{P}(X \times Y)[\forall y \in Y \exists x \in X \phi(x, y) \rightarrow \exists x \in X \forall y \in Y \phi(x, y)]$$

is true in Eff. In particular, the map $x \mapsto \lambda y.x : X \rightarrow X^Y$ is an isomorphism.

The converse holds too.

Proposition 3.2.22 *Suppose $(X, \sim)$ is an object of Eff with the property that the diagonal map*

$$(X, \sim) \rightarrow (X, \sim)^{\nabla(2)}$$

is an epimorphism. Then $(X, \sim)$ is discrete.

Proof. By the description of exponentials of the form $(X, \sim)^P$ with P a partitioned assembly, in 3.2.3, we can write $(X, \sim)^{\nabla(2)}$ as the object $(X^2, \sim)$ with

$$[(x_0, x_1) \sim (y_0, y_1)] = [x_0 \sim y_0] \cap [x_1 \sim y_1]$$

Hence $E((x_0, x_1)) = E(x_0) \cap E(x_1)$. The diagonal embedding is represented by

$$(x, (x_0, x_1)) \mapsto [x \sim x_0] \cap [x \sim x_1]$$

The requirement that this represents a surjection forces that there is an element e such that for all x_0, x_1 and all $n \in E(x_0) \cap E(x_1)$, $en\downarrow$ and $en \in [x_0 \sim x_1]$. By corollary 3.2.20, $(X, \sim)$ is discrete. ∎

Definition 3.2.23 A *modest set* or *modest object* is a separated discrete object.

The modest sets were introduced by Hyland in [70] under the name "effective objects" (however, as a category, outside the context of $\mathcal{E}ff$, they had already been studied by Kreisel: see [93]. See also the model HEO of "hereditarily effective operations" in Troelstra's [161]). The terminology "modest sets" was coined by Scott ([146]).

Clearly, an object is modest if and only if it is a quotient of a closed subobject of N by a *closed* equivalence relation. Proposition 3.2.19 also holds for modest objects, provided one replaces 'closed under quotients' in i) by 'closed under quotients by closed equivalence relations'. This follows easily from the corresponding properties of the separated objects.

Examples. Examples of modest objects are N, N^N and R. More on discrete objects, in particular on *families* of discrete objects, in section 3.4 below.

3.2.7   Decidable and semidecidable subobjects

In $\mathcal{E}ff$, the coproduct $2 = 1 + 1$, which classifies decidable subobjects, is (up to isomorphism) the modest object $(\{0,1\}, E)$ with $E(0) = \{0\}$ and $E(1) = \{1\}$. For any object X there is a natural 1-1 correspondence between decidable subobjects of X (subobjects A such that $\forall x{:}X(x \in A \vee \neg(x \in A))$ holds), and arrows $X \to 2$; and the object of decidable subobjects of X is the exponential 2^X.

'Cantor space' is the object 2^N, the assembly (R, E) where R is the set of recursive functions $\mathbb{N} \to \{0,1\}$, and $E(f)$ is the set of indices of f.

A valuable tool for studying 2^N is the so-called *Kleene tree*.

Definition 3.2.24 The *Kleene tree* T is the set of those 01-sequences

$$(a_0, \ldots a_{n-1})$$

which satisfy the following condition: for all $i, k < n$, if $T(i, i, k) \wedge U(k) \leq 1$ holds then $a_i = U(k)$.

In $\mathcal{E}ff$, T can be seen as a decidable subobject of the free monoid on 2, i.e. the assembly 2^* which has the set of finite 01-sequences as underlying set, and $E(\sigma)$ consists only of the code for σ.

For a subtree U of 2^* we shall say that every branch is finite, if

$$\forall f : N \to 2 \exists n((f(0), \dots, f(n-1)) \notin U)$$

holds. Recall that the *Fan Theorem* (Brouwer) asserts that every decidable subtree U of 2^* in which every branch is finite, has a branch of maximal length. In $\mathcal{E}ff$, the Fan Theorem *fails*, as the following proposition shows.

Theorem 3.2.25 *In $\mathcal{E}ff$, the following statements hold for the Kleene tree T:*

i)   *T contains arbitrarily long branches*

ii)   *For all $f : N \to T$ there is an n such that $(f(0), \dots, f(n)) \notin T$.*

Proof. i) is obvious: to construct an element of T of length n, just go through all $i, k < n$.

For ii), suppose $f : N \to 2$ is such that $(f(0), \dots, f(n-1)) \in T$ for all n. Then it holds that for all i, if $ii\!\downarrow$ and $ii \leq 1$, then $f(i) = ii$. Let $g : N \to 2$ be defined by $g(i) = 1 - f(i)$. By Church's Thesis, g has an index a. But now we have:

$$g(a) = 0 \to f(a) = 1 \to aa = 1$$
$$g(a) = 1 \to f(a) = 0 \to aa = 0$$

contradicting that a is an index for g. This contradiction shows that in $\mathcal{E}ff$,

$$\forall f : N \to 2 \neg\forall n((f(0), \dots, f(n-1)) \in T)$$

hence by decidability of T and Markov's principle we get

$$\forall f : N \to 2 \exists n((f(0), \dots, f(n-1)) \notin T)$$

as claimed.   ∎

Proposition 3.2.26 *In $\mathcal{E}ff$, the objects 2^N and N^N are isomorphic.*

Proof. Let U be the subset of 2^* given by

$$U = \{\sigma = (a_0, \ldots, a_n) \mid n > 0, \sigma \notin T, (a_0, \ldots, a_{n-1}) \in T\}$$

Then U is a decidable subobject of 2^*. Hence, since T has arbitrarily long branches, there is an isomorphism $\zeta : N \to U$.

Define an arrow $F : 2^N \to N \times 2^N$ by:

$$F(\alpha) = (\zeta^{-1}((\alpha(0), \ldots, \alpha(n))), \lambda k.\alpha(n + 1 + k))$$

where n is the unique number such that $(\alpha(0), \ldots, \alpha(n)) \in U$, which exists by theorem 3.2.26ii). Write:

$$F(\alpha) = (F_1(\alpha), F_2(\alpha))$$

Now define $G : 2^N \to N^N$ by $G(\alpha)(n) = F_1(F_2^n(\alpha))$. It is easily checked that G is an isomorphism.   ∎

Semidecidable or *r.e.* subobjects are classified by another subobject of Ω. The *r.e. subobject classifier* Σ is defined by:

$$\Sigma = \{p \in \Omega \mid \exists f{:}N^N (p \leftrightarrow \exists n(f(n) = 0))\}$$

By Markov's Principle, we see that $\Sigma \subseteq \{p \in \Omega \mid \neg\neg p \to p\}$, so Σ is separated.

Let K be the standard set from recursion theory: $K = \{n \mid nn{\downarrow}\}$, and let $\bar{K}$ its complement.

Proposition 3.2.27 Σ *is isomorphic to the assembly* $(\{\bot, \top\}, E_\Sigma)$ *where*

$$
\begin{aligned}
E_\Sigma(\top) &= K \\
E_\Sigma(\bot) &= \bar{K}
\end{aligned}
$$

Proof. According to standard realizability semantics, Σ is the object $(\mathcal{P}(\mathbb{N}), \sim)$ where $\sim$ is defined as follows. Let for $A \subseteq \mathbb{N}$, $E(A)$ be defined as the set of coded triples $\langle e, a, b \rangle$ where e is an index of a total recursive function, and a and b satisfy: if $x \in A$ then $ax{\downarrow}$ and $e(ax) = 0$, and if

$ex = 0$ then $bx{\downarrow}$ and $bx \in A$. Let $A \leftrightarrow B$ be the standard equality on Ω; then

$$A \sim B \;\equiv\; E(A) \wedge (A \leftrightarrow B)$$

Let F be partial recursive such that for every index e of a total recursive function, $F(e){\downarrow}$ and

$$F(e) \in K \Leftrightarrow \exists n(en = 0)$$

Define $\Phi : \mathcal{P}(\mathbb{N}) \times \{\bot, \top\} \to \mathcal{P}(\mathbb{N})$ by:

$$\Phi(A, i) \;=\; \begin{aligned} &\{\langle e, a, b, c\rangle \mid \langle e, a, b\rangle \in E(A), c \in E_\Sigma(i) \\ &\qquad \text{and } i = \top \Leftrightarrow \exists n(en = 0)\} \end{aligned}$$

Φ is strict and relational (check), and clearly single-valued; by construction of F it is total. So Φ represents an arrow $(\mathcal{P}(\mathbb{N}), \sim) \to (\{\bot, \top\}, E_\Sigma)$ which is easily seen to be an epimorphism. Given elements $\langle e, a, b\rangle$ of $E(A)$, $\langle e', a', b'\rangle$ of $E(A')$ and elements in $\Phi(A, i)$ and $\Phi(A', i)$ for $i \in \{\bot, \top\}$, one easily finds an element of $A \leftrightarrow A'$, so the map represented by Φ is also monic. ∎

The name 'r.e. subobject classifier' is justified by the following proposition, whose proof is straightforward.

Proposition 3.2.28

  i)   *Let (X, E) be an assembly. There is a 1-1 correspondence between arrows $(X, E) \to \Sigma$ and subsets $X' \subseteq X$ such that for some r.e. set $A \subseteq \mathbb{N}$, the following hold:*

$$x \in X' \Rightarrow E(x) \subseteq A$$
$$x \notin X' \Rightarrow E(x) \cap A = \emptyset$$

  ii)   *The exponential Σ^N is isomorphic to the assembly (RE, W) where RE is the set of r.e. subsets of $\mathbb{N}$ and $W(R) = \{e \mid R = W_e\}$.*

Uniform objects do not have nontrivial decidable subobjects, because 2 is modest; every map $\nabla(A) \to 2$ is constant. But there are many more objects which don't have nontrivial decidable subobjects: later we shall see that this also holds for the real numbers R, for example. Proposition 3.2.28 gives us another example.

Proposition 3.2.29 *The object Σ^N has no nontrivial decidable subobjects; in fact, the exponential $2^{(\Sigma^N)}$ is isomorphic to 2.*

Proof. Note that this is just Rice's Theorem in Recursion theory.   ∎

Since Σ is a subobject of Ω, we have for every object X an element relation as a subobject of $X \times \Sigma^X$, and an inclusion order on Σ^X. We can now express also part of the Rice-Shapiro theorem in Recursion theory in $\mathcal{E}ff$ in the following way:

Proposition 3.2.30 *For the object $\Sigma^{(\Sigma^N)}$ the following statements are true in $\mathcal{E}ff$:*

i) $\;\; \forall \mathcal{R}{:}\Sigma^{(\Sigma^N)} \forall R, S{:}\Sigma^N (R \in \mathcal{R} \wedge R \subseteq S \to S \in \mathcal{R})$

ii) $\;\; \forall \mathcal{R}{:}\Sigma^{(\Sigma^N)} \forall R{:}\Sigma^N (R \in \mathcal{R} \to \exists n{:}N (R \cap \{0, \ldots, n\} \in \mathcal{R}))$

Another way of stating the Rice-Shapiro theorem is as follows. RE, the set of r.e. subsets of $\mathbb{N}$, is a subset of $2^{\mathbb{N}}$, which we can topologize by giving 2 the Sierpinski topology (one open point), and $2^{\mathbb{N}}$ the product topology. RE gets the subspace topology. Then the Rice-Shapiro theorem says that every r.e. subset of RE is *open* in the topology on RE.

One might think that a similar result might hold for the function space N^N, if we see this as a subspace of Baire space $\mathbb{N}^{\mathbb{N}}$. However, this is not true.

Proposition 3.2.31 *There is a semidecidable subobject of N^N which does not determine an open set in the space of total recursive functions (seen as subspace of $\mathbb{N}^{\mathbb{N}}$).*

Proof. This follows by an old result of Friedberg (see [135], theorem 15-XXXI). Consider the set

$$X \;=\; \{e \,|\, \forall y \le e(ey = 0) \vee$$
$$\exists z[ez > 0 \wedge \forall y < z(ey = 0) \wedge \exists e' < z \forall u \le z(e'u = eu)]\}$$

Then X is an r.e. set which is extensional for indices of total recursive functions (if e and e' are indices of the same total recursive function then $e \in X$ if and only if $e' \in X$), so X determines a semidecidable subobject of N^N. However this does not correspond to an open subset of the space of total recursive functions. ∎

I close this section with a propsition about decidable objects. An object X in a topos is *decidable* if the diagonal embedding $X \rightarrowtail X \times X$ is a decidable subobject; in other words, if the sentence

$$\forall x^X y^X (x = y \vee \neg(x = y))$$

holds in the topos.

Clearly, every decidable object is $\neg\neg$-separated. Suppose (X, E) is a decidable assembly; then there is a partial recursive φ such that for all $x, y \in X$, $n \in E(x)$ and $m \in E(y)$, $\varphi(n, m)$ is defined and satisfies: $\varphi(n, m) = 0 \Leftrightarrow x = y$. It follows at once that (X, E) is modest.

This was noted in [82], where the question was asked: is maybe in $\mathcal{E}ff$ every decidable object a subobject of N? This can be equivalently formulated as a purely recursion-theoretic question: suppose we are given a subset A of $\mathbb{N}$ and a recursive equivalence relation on A, that is: there is a partial recursive function F, defined on $A \times A$, such that $F(x, y) = 0$ precisely when x is equivalent to y. Does there always exist a partial recursive function G, defined on A, such that for $x, y \in A$ we have $G(x) = G(y)$ if and only if $F(x, y) = 0$? The answer to this is *no* as the following proposition shows.

Proposition 3.2.32 *There exist decidable modest sets which are not subobjects of N.*

Proof. This proof was communicated to me by Bas Terwijn. Let R be the least reflexive and symmetric relation on $\mathbb{N}$ which relates, for every $e \in \mathbb{N}$, the elements $3e, 3e + 1$ and the elements $3e, 3e + 2$. Then clearly R is recursive; there is a recursive function F such that $F(x, y) = 0$ if and only if $(x, y) \in R$. R is not an equivalence relation, but it suffices to take away one element from each triple $3e, 3e + 1, 3e + 2$ to obtain a set A on which R is an equivalence relation. This allows us to diagonalize away from every candidate partial recursive G as above. We define A as $\bigcup_e A_e$ where A_e is defined as follows:

> If the partial recursive function φ_e is undefined at some element $3e + i$ ($0 \le i \le 2$), pick such i and let $A_e = \{3e + i\}$;

If φ_e is total on $\{3e, 3e+1, 3e+2\}$ and $\varphi_e(3e) \neq \varphi_e(3e+1)$, let $A_e = \{3e, 3e+1\}$;

If φ_e is total on $\{3e, 3e+1, 3e+2\}$, $\varphi_e(3e) = \varphi_e(3e+1)$ and $\varphi_e(3e) \neq \varphi_e(3e+2)$, let $A_e = \{3e, 3e+2\}$;

If φ_e is total on $\{3e, 3e+1, 3e+2\}$ and $\varphi_e(3e) = \varphi_e(3e+1) = \varphi_e(3e+2)$, let $A_e = \{3e+1, 3e+2\}$.

An inspection of the cases now suffices to see that no φ_e can be total on A and satisfy: $\varphi_e(x) = \varphi_e(y)$ if and only if $R(x,y)$.

For the lovers of arithmetic complexity: the set A constructed, is recursive in the Halting problem and therefore Δ_2^0. It is not hard to show that a counterexample cannot be constructed with A recursively enumerable.

∎

3.3   Some analysis in $\mathcal{E}ff$

In this short section I present some facts about real analysis in $\mathcal{E}ff$. Most of these results have been developed by the Russian school of 'Constructive Recursive Mathematics', pioneered by Markov. Other important names are Shanin, Zaslavskii, Ceitin, Kushner. Very often the results follow (in higher order intuitionistic type theory, or topos logic) axiomatically from a few basic principles that we have seen to be true in $\mathcal{E}ff$, such as ECT_0 and MP.

   Another stream of thought is so-called 'recursive analysis', which studies mathematical objects which are endowed with some recursive structure, such as the recursive real numbers, but using classical reasoning. A good introduction to this field is the book [127]. Finally, there is considerable literature on 'computable analysis', which understands mathematical structures as assemblies on $\mathcal{K}_1$ or $\mathcal{K}_2$; see [177]. For an analysis of the relation between Weihrauch's approach and realizability, see [97].

   For a more detailed introduction into various flavours of constructive analysis, see [163]. In fact, the few sample theorems treated here are all in that book (apart from a new proof of theorem 3.3.8). The reason to give them here is to give you a taste of how the internal logic of $\mathcal{E}ff$ works in this area.

Furthermore I should like to stress emphatically Hyland's point from [70]: that recursive analysis 'finds its natural home' in $\mathcal{E}ff$. Indeed, it is only in a model of full higher-order type theory that the notions of real-valued functions, functionals of any type, subsets of the reals etc. are totally unproblematic. It is good to contrast this with the treatment in [127], where after lengthy cogitations about what a 'computable real-valued function' should be, at last a definition is presented in which continuity is required. Instead, for us the notion of a map $R \to R$ exists without further ado, and the fact that such maps are (internally in $\mathcal{E}ff$) continuous is a *theorem* (see 3.3.8 below).

3.3.1 General facts about R

We start by reviewing some general facts about the Cauchy reals in a constructive setting, and which have nothing to do with $\mathcal{E}ff$ (although, occasionally, there will be invoking of countable choice).

The order on Cauchy reals is defined as follows: if ξ, η are represented by Cauchy sequences $(x_n)_n, (y_n)_n$ respectively, we put $\xi < \eta$ iff

$$\exists kn \forall m (y_{n+m} - x_{n+m} > 2^{-k})$$

This is independent of the choice of representatives.

For $q \in Q$ we let q^* be the constant sequence with value q. The map which sends $q \in Q$ to the real represented by q^* is an order-preserving embedding, and we regard Q as a subobject of R.

The order $\leq$ is defined by negation: $x \leq y$ iff $\neg(y < x)$. The relation $\sharp$ from the proof of proposition 3.2.14 respects the equivalence $\sim$ between Cauchy sequences, and gives therefore rise to a relation $\sharp$ between real numbers, which is called the *apartness* relation. It is easy to see that $\xi \sharp \eta$ is equivalent to $\xi < \eta \lor \eta < \xi$, and in 3.2.14 we have seen that $\xi = \eta$ is equivalent to $\neg(\xi \sharp \eta)$. The relation $\leq$ is therefore antisymmetric: $\xi \leq \eta \land \eta \leq \xi$ implies $\xi = \eta$. It is a partial order which is, in general, not linear (see also 3.3.6 below): $\xi \leq \eta \lor \eta \leq \xi$ need not hold.

Addition, multiplication, subtraction are easily defined on R such that they extend the corresponding operations on Q; also we have the absolute value $|\xi|$: if ξ is represnted by $(x_n)_n$ then $|\xi|$ by $(|x_n|)_n$. We have therefore the usual metric $|\xi - \eta|$, satisfying the well-known laws. Note, that for our representation with Cauchy sequences satisfying the condition

(C1) $\forall n(|x_n - x_{n+1}| < 2^{-(n+1)})$

we have that if $(x_n)_n$ represents ξ, then

$$\forall n(|x_n - \xi| < 2^{-n})$$

Although $\leq$ is in general not a linear order, we can nevertheless define the maximum and minimum of two reals: if ξ, η are represented by $(x_n)_n, (y_n)_n$ then $\max(\xi, \eta)$ is represented by $(\max(x_n, y_n))_n$. Note that this sequence satisfies (C1) if x_n and y_n do. Note also, that $\xi \leq \eta$ is equivalent to $\max(\xi, \eta) = \eta$.

An important property relating R and Q is given as proposition 5.3.6 in [163]:

Proposition 3.3.1 *Let $\varphi(x_1, \ldots, x_n) = 0$ be any algebraic equation involving $+, \cdot, |\cdot|, \max, \min$ which holds in Q. Then it also holds in R.*

So we can conclude that R is an ordered commutative ring, for example.

A *Cauchy sequence of reals* with *modulus of convergence* α, is a function $(\xi_n)_n : N \to R$ such that

$$\forall k m m'(|\xi_{\alpha(k)+m} - \xi_{\alpha(k)+m'}| < 2^{-k})$$

In our situation, where countable choice holds, we may define a Cauchy sequence of reals $(\xi_n)_n$ simply as satisfying

$$\forall k \exists n \forall m m'(|\xi_{n+m} - \xi_{n+m'}| < 2^{-k})$$

It is straightforward to define what it means that a Cauchy sequence converges to a limit ξ, and we have:

Theorem 3.3.2 *Every Cauchy sequence converges to a limit in R.*

A simple consequence of this is:

Corollary 3.3.3 R *is connected in the metric topology.*

Less straightforward, but essentially also a corollary of 3.3.2, is the result that R is a real closed field. This is best formulated as the statement: whenever a polynomial with real coefficients takes on values both < 0 and > 0, it has a root.

3.3.2 Specker sequences and singular coverings

As a first peculiarity of R in $\mathcal{E}ff$ we note the existence of a so-called *Specker sequence*. This refutes the Bolzano-Weierstrass property for R.

Definition 3.3.4 A *Specker sequence* is a bounded monotone sequence of rational numbers which has no limit in R.

Proposition 3.3.5 *A Specker sequence exists.*

Proof. Let $f : N \to N$ be an injective function whose range is un-decidable (e.g., f enumerates the standard set K without repetition). Let

$$r_k \;=\; \sum_{i=0}^{k} 2^{-f(i)}$$

Then clearly $(r_n)_n$ is a bounded, monotone sequence of rationals. Suppose it has a limit ξ. Then for all k there is an n such that

$$\forall m \left(|r_{n+m} - \xi| < 2^{-(k+1)} \right)$$

By countable choice, we have then a (recursive) function g such that

$$\forall m \left(|r_{g(k)+m} - \xi| < 2^{-(k+1)} \right)$$

But now one sees that $k \in \mathrm{im}(f)$ if and only if $\exists i \leq g(k)\,(f(i) = k)$; and this contradicts the non-decidability of $\mathrm{im}(f)$. ∎

Proposition 3.3.6

   i)   In $\mathcal{E}ff$, $\neg \forall x{:}R(x \leq 0 \vee 0 \leq x)$ *holds.*

ii) In $\mathcal{E}ff$, the intermediate value theorem fails.

Proof. i) is easily proved, for example using the recursion theorem. Statement ii) follows from i) by a standard argument (see [163], section 6.1). ∎

Theorem 3.3.7 *In $\mathcal{E}ff$, for every $\varepsilon > 0$ there exists a sequence $(I_n)_n$ of intervals with rational endpoints, with the properties:*

i) *For every n, $\sum_{i=0}^{n} |I_i| < \varepsilon$ (here $|I_i|$ denotes the length of the interval I_i).*

ii) *For every sequence of intervals $(J_n)_n$ with the property that*

$$\lim_{n \to \infty} |J_n| = 0$$

there exist n and m such that $I_n = J_m$.

In particular, the sequence $(I_n)_n$ covers R.

Proof. Let $\psi(m,n)$ be a function of two arguments such that for each m, the function $n \mapsto \psi(m,n)$ enumerates all rational intervals of length $< 2^{-m}$. Let γ enumerate the standard set K without repetition. Choose n_0 such that $2^{-n_0} < \varepsilon$. Define:

$$I_m = \psi(n_0 + \gamma(m) + 1, \gamma(m)\gamma(m))$$

(Note: $\gamma(m)\gamma(m)$ is partial recursive application, *not* multiplication!) Then

$$\sum_{n=0}^{k} |I_m| \leq \sum_{n=0}^{k} 2^{-(n_0 + \gamma(m)+1)} \leq \sum_{m=0}^{k} 2^{-(n_0+m+1)} < 2^{-n_0} < \varepsilon$$

For the second inequality, let $\{\gamma(0), \ldots, \gamma(k)\} = \{m_0 < m_1 < \cdots < m_k\}$. Then $p \leq m_p$ for $0 \leq p \leq k$, so $2^{-(n_0+m_p+1)} \leq 2^{-(n_0+p+1)}$. This proves property i).

For property ii), suppose $(J_n)_n$ is a sequence of rational intervals as in ii). Let δ be such that $|J_{\delta(n)}| < 2^{-n}$, and let $J'_n = J_{\delta(n)}$. Then by the property of ψ, $\forall n \exists m (J'_n = \psi(n,m))$; say δ' is such that $\forall n (J'_n = \psi(n, \delta'(n)))$. Then

$$J'_{n_0+n+1} = \psi(n_0 + n + 1, \delta'(n_0 + n + 1))$$

Let k be an index such that for all n, $kn = \delta'(n_0 + n + 1)$. Then $kk\downarrow$, so $k \in K$, and $k = \gamma(m)$ for some m. We find, since $kk = \delta'(n_0 + k + 1) = \delta'(n_0 + \gamma(m) + 1)$,

$$
\begin{aligned}
J'_{n_0+\gamma(m)+1} &= \psi(n_0 + \gamma(m) + 1, \delta'(n_0 + \gamma(m) + 1)) \\
&= \psi(n_0 + \gamma(m) + 1, \gamma(m)\gamma(m)) \\
&= I_m
\end{aligned}
$$

which proves ii).   ∎

One cannot immediately conclude from theorem 3.3.7 that R 'has measure zero' (whichever way one defines this), for one can prove that whenever $(I_n)_n$ is a sequence as in that theorem, the sequence

$$r_n = \sum_{k+0}^{n} |I_k|$$

is a Specker sequence, and has therefore no limit.

3.3.3   Real-valued functions

Since R is an assembly, an arrow $R \to R$ is a function $\mathbb{R}_{\mathrm{rec}} \xrightarrow{F} \mathbb{R}_{\mathrm{rec}}$ for which there is a tracking: a partial recursive function f such that, if $x \in E(\xi)$ (that is, x is an index of a recursive Cauchy sequence which satisfies (C1) and represents ξ), then $fx \in E(F(\xi))$.

Such a function is (in $\mathcal{E}ff$) continuous if the statement

$C(F)$ $\forall \xi{:}R\forall k{:}N\exists \delta{:}R\forall \eta{:}R\,(|\xi - \eta| < \delta \Rightarrow |F(\xi) - F(\eta)| < 2^{-k})$

is true in $\mathcal{E}ff$. That means, if we, for any $x \in E(\xi)$ and every $k \in \mathbb{N}$ can find, recursively in x, k, an element of some $E(\delta)$ such that

$$\forall \eta \in \mathbb{R}_{\mathrm{rec}}(|\xi - \eta| < \delta \Rightarrow |F(\xi) - F(\eta)| < 2^{-k})$$

is true in Set. Of course, it is clearly enough if the last statement holds for all $\eta \in Q$, since Q is dense in R.

Theorem 3.3.8 ("Brouwer's Theorem" in $\mathcal{E}\!f\!f$) *In $\mathcal{E}\!f\!f$, the statement that 'every function from R to R is continuous' holds. That is:*

$$\mathcal{E}\!f\!f \models \forall F{:}R^R\, C(F)$$

Proof. Rather than copying the proof given in [163] (6.4.12), which avoids the recursion theorem, or invoking 'Hyland's formula' ("the reader will have to do this himself",[70], p.201), I have preferred to give a proof based on the recursion theorem, which is very similar to the proof of the Kreisel-Lacombe-Shoenfield-Ceitin theorem as in [135], theorem XXXII.

Let F be a function $R \to R$ in $\mathcal{E}\!f\!f$, and let f track F. Let $\xi \in \mathbb{R}_{\mathrm{rec}}$ and $y \in E(\xi)$. Let $k \in \mathbb{N}$. By the recursion theorem it is possible to find an index z, primitive-recursively in f, y, k, such that the partial recursive function coded by z is given by the following instructions:

1. $zn \simeq yn$ if there is no $i < n$ which testifies

    (1) $|fz(k+3) - fy(k+3)| \le 2^{-(k+2)}$

2. If W is minimal such that W testifies (1), search for an $r \in \mathbb{Q}$ such that $|yW - r| < 2^{-W}$ and

    (2) $|fy(k+3) - fr^*(k+3)| > 2^{-(k+1)}$

    Here r^* is a standard index for the sequence which is constant r. If such r is not found, zn is undefined for all $n > W$. If r is found, put $zn = r - 2^{-(n-W)}\!\cdot\!(r - yW)$ for all $n > W$.

Then, first I claim that $fz{\downarrow}$ and there is a W testifying (1). For otherwise, $zn = yn$ always; hence fz and fy represent the same real $F(\xi)$ (if $y \in E(\xi)$), hence

$$
\begin{aligned}
|fz(k+3) - fy(k+3)| &\le |fz(k+3) - F(\xi)| + |F(\xi) - fy(k+3)| \\
&< 2^{-(k+3)} + 2^{-(k+3)} \\
&= 2^{-(k+2)}
\end{aligned}
$$

so that (1) holds after all. Applying Markov's Principle we see that this is then computed by some W.

Next, I claim that there is *no* $r \in Q$ such that $|yW - r| < 2^{-W}$ and (2) hold. For suppose otherwise; then for the first such r found, we would have $zn = r - 2^{-(n-W)} \cdot (r - yW)$ for all $n > W$, which means that z represents the same real as r^*, which is $F(r)$. We obtain:

$$
\begin{aligned}
|fz(k+3) - fr^*(k+3)| &\leq |F(r) - fz(k+3)| + |F(r) - fr^*(k+3)| \\
&< 2^{-(k+3)} + 2^{-(k+3)} \\
&= 2^{-(k+2)}
\end{aligned}
$$

Hence,

$$
\begin{aligned}
|fz(k+3) - fy(k+3)| &> |fr^*(k+3) - fy(k+3)| - \\
& \quad |fz(k+3) - fr^*(k+3)| \\
\text{by (2)} \quad &> 2^{-(k+1)} - 2^{-(k+2)} \\
&= 2^{-(k+2)}
\end{aligned}
$$

which contradicts (1).

We conclude, that if $|yW - r| < 2^{-W}$, then $|fy(k+3) - fr^*(k+3)| \leq 2^{-(k+1)}$, so that if y represents the real ξ,

$$
\begin{aligned}
|F(\xi) - F(r)| &\leq |F(\xi) - fy(k+3)| + |fy(k+3) - fr^*(k+3)| \\
& \quad + |F(r) - fr^*(k+3)| \\
&< 2^{-(k+1)} + 2 \cdot 2^{-(k+2)} \\
&= 2^{-k}
\end{aligned}
$$

To finish the argument: let $\delta = 2^{-W} - |\xi - yW|$ (for ξ the real represented by y; this is a positive number since y satisfies (C1)). Then for $|\xi - r| < \delta$, $|yW - r| < 2^{-W}$, so $|F(\xi) - F(r)| < 2^{-k}$, as desired. It is left to you to convince yourself that an element of $E(\delta)$ can be found recursively in y, k, f. ∎

Corollary 3.3.9 *R has no nontrivial decidable subobjects.*

Proof. Since $2 = 1 + 1$ is clearly embedded in R, as $\{0, 1\}$ say, any map $F : R \to 2$ can be considered as a map $R \to R$ which is continuous by 3.3.8; so $F^{-1}(0)$ and $F^{-1}(1)$ are open, disjoint subsets of R which together cover R. But this contradicts the connectedness of R (3.3.3). ∎

The following theorem is 6.4.4 in [163].

Theorem 3.3.10

i)   There is a uniformly continuous function defined on $[0,1]$ such that for all $x \in [0,1]$ $f(x) > 0$, yet $\inf_{x \in [0,1]} f(x) = 0$.

ii) There is a continuous function f on $[0,1]$ which is unbounded, and therefore not uniformly continuous.

Proof. (i) Let $(I_n)_n$ be a covering of $[0,1]$ by open intervals (r_n, s_n) which has the property of the covering in theorem 3.3.7, that for every n, $\sum_{k=0}^{n}(s_k - r_k) < \frac{1}{2}$ say. For every n let f_n be defined by

$$f_n(x) = \max\{0, \frac{1}{2}(s_n - r_n) - |x - \frac{1}{2}(r_n + s_n)|\}$$

Define f by $f(x) = \sum_{n=0}^{\infty} 2^{-n} f_n(x)$.

Then f is defined everywhere, and is uniformly continuous: if $|x - y| < \delta$ then $|f_n(x) - f_n(y)| < \delta$ for all n, so $|f(x) - f(y)| < 2\delta$. Furthermore, for every $x \in I_n$, $f_n(x) > 0$ so since $(I_n)_n$ covers, $f(x) > 0$ everywhere. But by the property of this cover, it follows that no finite part of it covers $[0,1]$; if $x \notin I_0 \cup \cdots \cup I_n$, then $f(x) \leq 2^{-n}$. This means that $\inf_{x \in [0,1]} f(x) = 0$, as claimed.

(ii) Take the function f from i), and define g by $g(x) = f(x)^{-1}$.   ∎

For material on differential equations in $\mathcal{E}ff$, see [141].

3.4   Discrete families and Uniform maps

Proposition 3.2.21 relates discrete and uniform objects in $\mathcal{E}ff$ in a way which is studied in category theory under the name 'orthogonality'.

In any category, for two arrows $f : A \to B$ and $g : C \to D$ one says that f is *orthogonal* to g, and writes $f \perp g$, if for any commutative diagram

$$
\begin{array}{ccc}
A & \xrightarrow{\ f\ } & B \\
{\scriptstyle u}\downarrow & & \downarrow{\scriptstyle v} \\
C & \xrightarrow[\ g\ ]{} & D
\end{array}
$$

there is a unique arrow $w : B \to C$ such that $u = wf$ and $gw = v$.

For example, in a regular category one has $e \perp m$ whenever e is regular epi and m is mono.

Proposition 3.2.21 implies that every arrow from a uniform object to a discrete object is constant (factors through 1); this means that if U is uniform and D discrete, then $!_U : U \to 1$ is orthogonal to $!_D : D \to 1$.

Proposition 3.4.1 *Let $\mathcal{D}$ be the full subcategory of $\mathcal{E}ff$ on the discrete objects and $r : \mathcal{E}ff \to \mathcal{D}$ the reflection (which exists by 3.2.19iii)). If Σ is the class of all arrows f such that $r(f)$ is an isomorphism, then an object X of $\mathcal{E}ff$ is discrete, if and only if for all $g \in \Sigma$, g is orthogonal to $!_X : X \to 1$.*

Proof. This is general category theory, see e.g. [28], I.5.4.4. ∎

We now wish to see to what extent the reflectivity of discrete objects extends to *slices* of $\mathcal{E}ff$. To this end we need to say what a 'discrete map' into an object $(X, \sim)$ is (or, a 'family of discrete objects indexed by $(X, \sim)$'), and what a 'uniform map' is.

Definition 3.4.2

i) A map $f : (Y, \sim) \to (X, \sim)$ is *discrete* iff f is, in the topos $\mathcal{E}ff/(X, \sim)$, a subquotient of the natural numbers object.

ii) A map $f : (Y, \sim) \to (X, \sim)$ is *uniform* iff f is, in the topos $\mathcal{E}ff/(X, \sim)$, a quotient of a $\neg\neg$-sheaf.

First, I recall from topos theory that the $\neg\neg$-sheafification functor on the slice $\mathcal{E}ff/(X, \sim)$ is given as follows: given $(Y, \sim) \xrightarrow{f} (X, \sim)$ its sheafification is the left hand side vertical map in the pullback square

$$
\begin{array}{ccc}
L(f) & \longrightarrow & \nabla\Gamma(Y, \sim) \\
\downarrow & & \downarrow {\scriptstyle \nabla\Gamma(f)} \\
(X, \sim) & \xrightarrow[\eta_{(X,\sim)}]{} & \nabla\Gamma(X, \sim)
\end{array}
$$

I also recall that the functor $(X, \sim)^* : \mathcal{E}ff \to \mathcal{E}ff/(X, \sim)$ which sends $(Y, \sim)$ to the projection $(Y, \sim) \times (X, \sim) \to (X, \sim)$, is logical. Therefore the natural numbers object of $\mathcal{E}ff/(X, \sim)$ is $N \times (X, \sim) \to (X, \sim)$.

The fact that every subobject of N is covered by a $\neg\neg$-closed subobject of N holds also in every slice $\mathcal{E}ff/(X,\sim)$. This is so because Shanin's Principle is true in $\mathcal{E}ff$ with arbitrary parameters. Therefore, we might as well have formulated the notion of a discrete map as: quotient of a $\neg\neg$-closed subobject of N in definition 3.4.2. Now it is easy to see that if $A \to N \times (X,\sim)$ is a monomorphism, then the commutative triangle

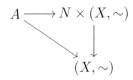

is a $\neg\neg$-closed mono in $\mathcal{E}ff/(X,\sim)$ if and only if $A \to N \times (X,\sim)$ is $\neg\neg$-closed in $\mathcal{E}ff$. The following proposition is then immediate:

Proposition 3.4.3

i)   A map $A \xrightarrow{f} (X,\sim)$ is a $\neg\neg$-closed subobject of N in $\mathcal{E}ff/(X,\sim)$ if and only if there is a map $P : \Gamma(X,\sim) \to \mathcal{P}(\mathbb{N})$ such that A is isomorphic to the object $(A',\sim)$ defined as follows:

$$A' = \{(n,x) \,|\, n \in P([x])\}$$
$$[(n,x) \sim (n',x')] = [n \sim_N n'] \wedge [x \sim x']$$

and f is, relative to this isomorphism, the projection $(A',\sim) \to (X,\sim)$ (i.e., by the functional relation $((n,x),x') \mapsto \{n\} \wedge [x \sim x']$).

ii) A map f into $(X,\sim)$ is discrete if and only if its domain is isomorphic to an object (A',R) where A' is as in i) and R is an equality relation on A' such that the formulas

$$R((m,x),(n,x')) \to x \sim x'$$
$$R((n,x),(n,x)) \leftrightarrow \{n\} \wedge [x \sim x]$$
$$\{n\} \wedge [x \sim x'] \to R((n,x),(n,x'))$$

hold in the effective tripos; and the map f is, relative to this isomorphism, represented by the functional relation

$$((m,x),x') \mapsto \{m\} \wedge [x \sim x']$$

It is tempting to try to achieve a characterization of the discrete maps into $(X, \sim)$ in the spirit of proposition 3.2.18 and corollary 3.2.20. It is clear that if $F : Y \times X \to \mathcal{P}(\mathbb{N})$ represents a discrete map, then the formula

$$F(y, x) \wedge F(y', x) \wedge (E(y) \cap E(y')) \to y \sim y'$$

holds in the effective tripos. The converse, however, does not seem to hold in general. But it does work when the object $(X, \sim)$ is $\neg\neg$-separated:

Proposition 3.4.4 *Suppose F represents a map $f : (Y, \sim) \to (X, \sim)$ into a $\neg\neg$-separated object $(X, \sim)$, and the set*

$$\bigcap_{y,x} [F(y, x) \wedge F(y', x) \wedge (E(y) \cap E(y')) \to [y \sim y']]$$

contains an element ϵ. Then f is discrete.

Proof. Consider the object $(A, \sim)$, where

$$A = \{(x, n) \mid \exists y(F(y, x) \neq \emptyset \wedge n \in E(y))\}$$

and $\sim$ is given by

$$[(x, n) \sim (x', n')] = \begin{cases} [x \sim x'] \wedge \{n\} & \text{if } n = n' \\ \emptyset & \text{else} \end{cases}$$

This is a good equality predicate. Note, that if $(x, n) \in A$ and $[x \sim x'] \neq \emptyset$ then $(x', n) \in A$. So $(A, \sim)$ is a $\neg\neg$-closed subobject of $(X, \sim) \times N$.

First I show that there is a partial recursive α such that if $(x, n) \in A$, $pan \in E(x, n)$, $F(y, x) \neq \emptyset$ and $n \in E(y)$, then $\alpha(a, n) \in F(y, x)$. Let rl, st and tl realize the relevant instances of relationalness, strictness and totality of F, and b be such that when $m \in E(x), n \in E(x')$ and $[x \sim x'] \neq \emptyset$, $b(m, n) \in [x \sim x']$; b exists because $(X, \sim)$ is $\neg\neg$-separated. For some x' we have $\mathsf{tl}(n) \in F(y, x')$ and hence $\mathsf{st}(\mathsf{tl}(n)) \in E(x')$. Since $F(y, x) \neq \emptyset$ we have (by single-valuedness of F) $[x \sim x'] \neq \emptyset$, so $b(a, \mathsf{st}(\mathsf{tl}(n))) \in [x \sim x']$. Hence

$$\alpha(a, n) = \mathsf{rl}(\mathsf{tl}(n), b(a, \mathsf{st}(\mathsf{tl}(n)))) \in F(y, x)$$

as claimed.

Define a functional relation $G : A \times Y \to \mathcal{P}(\mathbb{N})$ by

$$G((x,n),y) = E(x,n) \wedge \bigcup_{F(z,x)\neq\emptyset,n\in E(z)} [z \sim y]$$

It is easily verified that G is strict, relational and total. In order to verify the single-valuedness, suppose $p(pan)m \in G((x,n),y)$ and $p(pa'n)m' \in G((x,n),y')$. Then there are z, z' such that

$$\begin{array}{cccc} n \in E(z) & F(z,x) \neq \emptyset & m \in [z \sim y] \\ n \in E(z') & F(z',x) \neq \emptyset & m' \in [z' \sim y'] \end{array}$$

Then $\alpha(a,n) \in F(z,x)$, $\alpha(a',n) \in F(z',x)$, $n \in E(z) \cap E(z')$, so

$$\epsilon(\alpha(a,n),\alpha(a',n),n) \in [z \sim z']$$

where ϵ is as in the proposition. With the transitivity for $\sim$ we easily find a realizer for $y \sim y'$.

So, G represents an arrow $g : (A,\sim) \to (Y,\sim)$ and the triangle

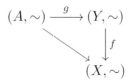

is easily seen to commute.

Finally, it is trivial to check that g is an epimorphism. So f is discrete. ∎

In fact, an easier representation of discrete maps into $\neg\neg$-separated objects is available if we assume that the codomain is an assembly (X,E). Then, a morphism $(Y,\sim) \to (X,E)$ is the same thing as a function $Y \xrightarrow{f} X$ (assuming that $E(y) \neq \emptyset$ for all $y \in Y$) which has the following properties:

a) f is tracked: there is an element in the set $\bigcap_{y\in Y}(E(y) \to E(f(y)))$

b)   whenever $[y \sim y'] \neq \emptyset$, $f(y) = f(y')$

We then have the functional relation

$$F(y,x) \equiv E(y) \wedge \{n \mid n \in E(x) \text{ and } x = f(y)\}$$

Proposition 3.4.5 *A map into an assembly* (X, E) *is discrete if and only if it is isomorphic (in the slice* $\mathcal{E}ff/(X, E)$*) to a map* $f : (Y, \sim) \to (X, E)$ *for which it holds that whenever* $f(y) = f(y')$ *and* $E(y) \cap E(y') \neq \emptyset$*, then* $y = y'$.

Proof. A $\neg\neg$-closed subobject of N in $\mathcal{E}ff/(X, E)$ is given by an assembly (A, E_A) where $A \subseteq N \times X$, and $E_A(n, x) = \{n\} \wedge E(x)$. A quotient of such an object is a map $(A, R) \to (X, E)$ where R is an equivalence relation on (A, E) such that $R((n, x), (n', x')) \neq \emptyset$ implies $x = x'$, and the map $A \to X$ is simply the projection. Since R is an equivalence relation for (A, E_A) we have

$$R((n, x), (n, x)) \leftrightarrow E(n, x)$$

so clearly the map $(A.R) \to (X, E)$ is of the form in the proposition.

Conversely, suppose $f : Y \to X$ determines a map $(Y, \sim) \to (X, E)$ which is of that form, so if $f(y) = f(y')$ and $E(y) \cap E(y') \neq \emptyset$, then $y = y'$. Let $A \subseteq N \times X$ be defined by

$$A = \{(n, x) \mid n \in \bigcup_{f(y)=x} E(y)\}$$

and consider A as a regular ($\neg\neg$-closed) sub-assembly of $N \times (X, E)$. By assumption on f there is then a map $g : A \to Y$ such that for $(n, x) \in A$ we have $n \in E(g(n, x))$ and $f(g(n, x)) = x$. It is easily verified that this is a surjection in $\mathcal{E}ff$; hence the map determined by f is discrete. ∎

We now turn to a characterization of uniform maps. From the definition, a map $(y, \sim) \xrightarrow{f} (X, \sim)$ is uniform if and only if there are commutative diagrams

$$
\begin{array}{ccc}
A & \longrightarrow & \nabla(Z) \\
{\scriptstyle s}\downarrow & & \downarrow{\scriptstyle \alpha} \\
(X, \sim) & \xrightarrow[\eta_{(X,\sim)}]{} & \nabla\Gamma(X, \sim)
\end{array}
\qquad
\begin{array}{ccc}
A & \xrightarrow{r} & (Y, \sim) \\
{\scriptstyle s}\searrow & & \downarrow{\scriptstyle f} \\
& & (X, \sim)
\end{array}
$$

with the left hand square a pullback, and r an epimorphism.

We have the following characterization of uniform maps, analogous to proposition 2.4.6 (note that this means for $\mathcal{E}ff$ that $(X, \sim)$ is uniform if and only if $(X, \sim)$ is isomorphic to an object $(X', \sim)$ for which $\bigcap_{x \in X'} E(x)$ is nonempty).

Proposition 3.4.6 *A map $f : (Y, \sim) \to (X, \sim)$ in $\mathcal{E}ff$ is uniform if and only if for every representing functional relation F of f the following holds: there are numbers a and b such that for all $y \in Y, x \in X, n \in E(x), m \in F(y, x)$, there is a $y' \in Y$ such that $an \in F(y', x)$ and $bnm \in [y' \sim y]$.*

Proof. First suppose f is uniform; consider the diagrams given above. Then the object A in the pullback square is of the form $A, \sim)$ with

$$A = \{(\xi, x) \mid \alpha(\xi) = [x]\}$$
$$[(\xi, x) \sim (\xi', x')] = \begin{cases} [x \sim x'] & \text{if } \xi = \xi' \\ \emptyset & \text{otherwise} \end{cases}$$

The map s is represented by $S((\xi, x), x') = [x \sim x']$.

Let $n \in E(x), m \in F(y, x)$. Suppose c realizes that r is epi, so if R represents r and s realizes the strictness of F, then $c(sm) \in R((\xi, x'), y)$ for some $(\xi, x') \in A$. For this (ξ, x'), $[x \sim x'] \neq \emptyset$ (since $fr = s$), so also $(\xi, x) \in A$, and $n \in [(\xi, x) \sim (\xi, x)]$. By totality and strictness of R there is $y' \in Y$ such that $a_1 n \in R((\xi, x), y')$ and by the commutation $an \in F(y', x)$, for canonical realizers a_1, a. Also, using $c(sm) \in R((\xi, x'), y)$ and $m \in F(y, x)$ we find $b_1 m \in [x \sim x']$ (for a canonical b_1) hence $b_1 m \in [(\xi, x) \sim (\xi, x')]$ which, together with $c(sm) \in R((\xi, x'), y)$ gives $b_2 m \in R((\xi, x), y)$. With $a_1 n \in R((\xi, x), y')$ and single-valuedness of R, we find $bnm \in [y' \sim y]$ as claimed.

For the converse, we look at a projective cover of $(X, \sim)$: let $(P, \sim)$ be given by

$$P = \{(x, n) \mid n \in E(x)\}$$
$$[(x, n) \sim (x', n')] = \{n \mid n = n' \text{ and } x = x'\}$$

There is an epi $\pi : (P, \sim) \to (X, \sim)$ represented by $\Pi((x, n), x) = \{pna \mid a \in [x = x']\}$. Consider the pullback

$$
\begin{array}{ccc}
(Q, \sim) & \longrightarrow & (Y, \sim) \\
\downarrow & & \downarrow f \\
(P, \sim) & \xrightarrow{\pi} & (X, \sim)
\end{array}
$$

Given a and b as in the statement of the proposition, consider the object $(Z, \sim)$ where

$$
Z = \{((x, n), y) \mid n \in E(x), an \in F(y, x)\}
$$

$$
[((x, n), y) \sim ((x', n'), y')] = \begin{cases} [(x, n) \sim (x', n')] & \text{if } y = y' \\ \emptyset & \text{else} \end{cases}
$$

where $[(x, n) \sim (x', n')]$ is the equality of $(P, \sim)$.

We have $w : (Z, \sim) \to (P, \sim)$ represented by

$$
W(((x, n), y), (x', n')) = [(x, n) \sim (x', n')]
$$

and it is easily seen that w is a $\neg\neg$-sheaf in $\mathcal{E}ff/(P, \sim)$.

The object $(Q, \sim)$ can be described by:

$$
Q = \{((x, n), y) \mid n \in E(x), y \in Y, F(y, x) \neq \emptyset\}
$$

$$
[((x, n), y) \sim ((x', n', y')] = [(x, n) \sim (x', n')] \wedge F(y, x) \wedge [y \sim y']
$$

Define $g : (Z, \sim) \to (Q, \sim)$ as represented by G where

$$
G(((x, n), y), ((x', n'), y')) = [((x, n), y) \sim ((x', n'), y')]
$$

Then G is a functional relation, and using the element b from the statement of the proposition, we find that g is an epimorphism.

We have proved: there is a surjection $\pi : (P, \sim) \to (X, \sim)$ such that $\pi^*(f)$ is a quotient of a sheaf in $\mathcal{E}ff/(P, \sim)$. In order to obtain the claimed result, consider the diagram

$$
\begin{array}{ccccc}
(Z, \sim) & \longrightarrow & (P, \sim) & \xrightarrow{\pi} & (X, \sim) \\
\downarrow & & \downarrow{\scriptstyle \eta_P} & & \downarrow{\scriptstyle \eta_X} \\
B & \xrightarrow{a} & \nabla\Gamma(P, \sim) & \xrightarrow{\nabla\Gamma(\pi)} & \nabla\Gamma(X, \sim)
\end{array}
$$

where the left hand square is a pullback and the right hand square a naturality square. The bottom row is a diagram of sets and one sees that for $u, v \in \nabla\Gamma(P, \sim)$ it holds that if $\nabla\Gamma(\pi)(u) = \nabla\Gamma(\pi)(v)$, then $a^{-1}(u) \neq \emptyset \Leftrightarrow a^{-1}(v) \neq \emptyset$. With the axiom of choice this implies that there ia a set C and a function $k : C \to \nabla\Gamma(X, \sim)$, such that for every $u \in \nabla\Gamma(P, \sim)$ we have a surjection from $k^{-1}(\nabla\Gamma(\pi)(u))$ to $a^{-1}(u)$; in other words we have an epi from $(\nabla\Gamma(\pi))^*(k)$ to a in $\mathrm{Set}/\nabla\Gamma(P, \sim)$. If we now pull back k along η_X we get a $\neg\neg$-sheaf in $\mathcal{E}\!f\!f/(X, \sim)$ which covers f, as desired. ∎

Definition 3.4.7 Let $(X, \sim)$ be an object of $\mathcal{E}\!f\!f$. We denote by $\mathcal{D}_{(X,\sim)}$ the full subcategory of the slice $\mathcal{E}\!f\!f/(X, \sim)$ on the discrete maps into $(X, \sim)$.

Proposition 3.4.8 *If $(X, \sim)$ is $\neg\neg$-separated, then the category $\mathcal{D}_{(X,\sim)}$ is a reflective subcategory of $\mathcal{E}\!f\!f/(X, \sim)$.*

Proof. It does no harm to assume $(X, \sim)$ is an assembly (X, E). For a map $(Y, \sim) \to (X, E)$ we may assume it is given by a function $f : Y \to X$ as in the remark before proposition 3.4.5, so $f(y) = f(y')$ whenever $[y \sim y'] \neq \emptyset$, and there is a number $\alpha \in \bigcap_{y \in Y}(E(y) \to E(f(y)))$. The discrete reflection of the map f is constructed in much the same way as in the proof of 3.2.19iii). Let Y_{dis} consist of all pairs (x, n) such that $n \in \bigcup_{f(y)=x} E(y)$. For two such pairs (x, n) and (x', n') let $[(x, n) \sim (x', n')] = \emptyset$ if $x \neq x'$; and $[(x, n) \sim (x, n')]$ consists of all pairs $pa\sigma$ where $a \in E(x)$ and σ is the code of a sequence

$$\sigma = \langle n_0, a_0, n_1, \ldots, n_{k-1}, a_{k-1}, n_k \rangle$$

for $k \geq 1$, such that $n_0 = n$, $n_k = n'$ and for every $i < k$ there are $y_1, y_2 \in f^{-1}(x)$ such that

$$n_i \in E(y_1) \text{ and } a_i \in [y_1 \sim y_2] \text{ and } n_{i+1} \in E(y_2)$$

This is a well-defined equality relation. There is a projection $\pi : Y_{\mathrm{dis}} \to X$ which clearly determines a map $(Y_{\mathrm{dis}}, \sim) \to (X, E)$. It is readily verified (use proposition 3.4.5) that this is a discrete map.

Define a functional relation $G : Y \times Y_{\text{dis}} \to \mathcal{P}(\mathbb{N})$ as follows: $G(y, (x, n)) = \emptyset$ if $f(y) \neq x$, and $G(y, (f(y), n))$ consists of codes σ such that for some $n_0 \in E(y)$ and $a \in E(f(y))$, $pa\sigma$ is an element of $[(f(y), n_0) \sim (f(y), n)]$. This defines a map $\eta_Y : (Y, \sim) \to (Y_{\text{dis}}, \sim)$, and the diagram

$$(Y, \sim) \xrightarrow{\ \eta_Y\ } (Y_{\text{dis}}, \sim)$$
$$f \searrow \qquad \downarrow \pi$$
$$(X, E)$$

commutes. Note, that η_Y is an epimorphism.

To see that η_Y satisfies the universal property, suppose we have another commutative diagram

$$(Y, \sim) \xrightarrow{\ a\ } (Z, \sim)$$
$$f \searrow \qquad \downarrow h$$
$$(X, E)$$

with h a discrete map. We may assume that $(Z, \sim)$ is of the form given in 3.4.5. Suppose A represents a; let tl_A and st_A realize totality and strictness of A, respectively, so for $m \in E(y)$ we have $\mathsf{st}_A(\mathsf{tl}_A(m)) \in E(z)$ for some z with $\mathsf{tl}_A(m) \in A(y, z)$. Then for such z we have that $h(z) = f(y)$, and by the form of $(Z, \sim)$ we see that z is in fact uniquely determined by m and $f(y)$. So we have a function $\tilde{a} : Y_{\text{dis}} \to Z$, which gives a map in $\mathcal{E}\!f\!f$, such that the composite $\tilde{a} \circ \eta_Y$ is equal to a. The factorization is unique since η_Y is epimorphic. ∎

Now, we see a generalization of the Uniformity Principle to slices.

Theorem 3.4.9 *Every uniform epimorphism is orthogonal to every discrete map.*

Proof. Suppose we have a commutative diagram

$$(U, \sim) \xrightarrow{\ g\ } (V, \sim)$$
$$k \downarrow \qquad \qquad \downarrow h$$
$$(Y, \sim) \xrightarrow[\ f\ ]{} (X, \sim)$$

with g surjective (epi) and uniform, and f discrete. Assume every map in the diagram is represented by its upper case functional relation (so, f by F, etc.). We need to find a unique diagonal filler $n : (V, \sim) \to (Y, \sim)$. But let's note at once that uniqueness follows from surjectivity of g (given the required commutations).

Define a relation $N : V \times Y \to \mathcal{P}(\mathbb{N})$ by

$$N(v, y) \equiv \bigcup_{u \in U} (G(u, v) \wedge K(v, y))$$

Then N is clearly relational and strict in v, y; and N is total since g is surjective. So we only have to prove that N is single-valued, for showing that it represents a map $(V, \sim) \to (Y, \sim)$.

Before we do that, let us see that if N does represent a map n, then the two triangles commute, i.e. $ng = k$ and $fn = h$. For, suppose $K(u, y), G(u, v), N(v, y')$; then $N(v, y), N(v, y')$ so by single-valuedness of N, $y \sim y'$. This proves $ng = k$. And this implies $fng = fk = hg$ so $fn = h$ by surjectivity of g.

In order to prove that N is single-valued, suppose $N(v, y), N(v, y')$. We have elements $n \in E(v)$, $m \in G(u, v)$, $l \in K(u, y)$, $m' \in G(u', v)$ and $l' \in K(u', y')$. Let α and β realize the uniformity of the map g in the sense of 3.4.6; so we find elements $u_1, u_2 \in U$, and

$$\alpha n \in G(u_1, v) \quad \beta nm \in [u_1 \sim u]$$
$$\alpha n \in G(u_2, v) \quad \beta nm' \in [u_2 \sim u']$$

From αn we find from the totality and strictness of K, for some $y_1, y_2 \in Y$, elements

$$\gamma n \in K(u_1, y_1) \quad \delta n \in E(y_1)$$
$$\gamma n \in K(u_2, y_2) \quad \delta n \in E(y_2)$$

By totality of H we find $\zeta n \in H(v, x)$ for some $x \in X$. Now using that the square commutes we find, combining these elements of $G(u, v)$, $H(v, x)$, $u_1 \sim u$ and $K(u_1, y_1)$, an element $\kappa_1 nm \in F(y_1, x)$; and combining the eleents of $G(u', v)$, $H(v, x)$, $u_2 \sim u'$ and $K(u_2, y_2)$ we find an element $\kappa_2 nm' \in F(y_2, x)$.

We have found $\delta n \in E(y_1) \cap E(y_2)$, $\kappa_1 nm \in F(y_1, x)$, $\kappa_2 nm' \in F(y_2, x)$. Now we apply the fact that F is discrete (see the remark just preceding proposition 3.4.5), to obtain from these data an element of $[y_1 \sim y_2]$. Now we also had elements of $u_1 \sim u$, $K(u, y)$, $K(u_1, y_1)$ which yield, by relationality and single-valuedness of K, an element of $y \sim y_1$; similarly we find an element of $y' \sim y_2$. Transitivity of $\sim$ now gives us an element of $y \sim y'$, proving the desired single-valuedness of N. ∎

Corollary 3.4.10 *Any map which is both discrete and uniform, is an isomorphism. If a map factors as a uniform surjection followed by a discrete map, then this factorization is unique up to isomorphism.*

Let us look at some easy properties of discrete and uniform maps.

Proposition 3.4.11

i) Uniform and discrete maps are stable under pullback.

ii) Uniform and discrete maps are stable under composition.

iii) If, in a diagram $Z \xrightarrow{g} Y \xrightarrow{f} X$, g is epi and fg is uniform, then f is uniform.

iv) If, in such a diagram, fg is discrete, then so is g.

Proof. i) is straightforward, since sheaves in slices are preserved by pullback functors, as well as closed subobjects of N.

ii) Suppose that in $Z \xrightarrow{g} Y \xrightarrow{f} X$ both maps are uniform. Form a diagram

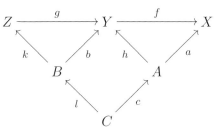

where b is a sheaf in $\mathcal{E}ff/Y$, a a sheaf in $\mathcal{E}ff/X$, k and h epi, and the lower square a pullback. Then l is epi and c is a sheaf in $\mathcal{E}ff/A$. It follows by drawing the obvious pullback diagrams, that ac is a sheaf in $\mathcal{E}ff/X$, which shows that fg is covered by a sheaf, so uniform.

The same diagram can be used for the case that f and g are discrete: now assume in the diagram that a ad b are closed subobjects of N in the respective slices. Then so is c, by stability under pullback; so it suffies to see that this implies that ac is, in $\mathcal{E}ff/X$, a closed subobject of N. We have functions $\bar{A} : \Gamma(X) \to \mathcal{P}(\mathbb{N})$ and $\bar{B} : \Gamma(A) \to \mathcal{P}(\mathbb{N})$ so that $A = \{(n,x) \mid n \in \bar{A}([x])\}$ and $C = \{(m,(n,x)) \mid m \in \bar{B}([(n,x)])\}$ etc. We see that C is isomorphic to $\{(pnm,x) \mid n \in \bar{A}([x]), m \in \bar{B}([(n,x)])\}$.

iii) Suppose G represents g, and F represents f; g epi and fg uniform. In order to prove f uniform we have to find a, b as in 3.4.6 for F. Suppose $n \in E(x)$, $m \in F(y,x)$. By the surjectivity of g we find $sm \in G(z,y)$ for some z, and hence $p(sm)m \in F\circ G(z,x)$. Suppose α, β realize the uniformity of fg; then for some z' we have $\alpha n \in F\circ G(z',x)$ and $\beta n(p(sm)m) \in [z' \sim z]$. By totality of G we have $a'n \in G(z',y')$ for certain y'; then $an \in F(y',x)$ and $bnm \in [y' \sim y]$ as required.

iv) Suppose fg is discrete; then $f^*(fg)$ is a discrete map into Y by i); but g is a subobject of $f^*(fg)$ in $\mathcal{E}ff/Y$ and from the definition of discrete maps it is obvious that they are stable under subobjects. ∎

The fact that discrete maps are stable under pullback means that for any map $X \xrightarrow{f} Y$ in $\mathcal{E}ff$ we have a commutative diagram of categories

$$
\begin{array}{ccc}
\mathcal{D}_Y & \xrightarrow{\ f^\sharp\ } & \mathcal{D}_X \\
{\scriptstyle i_Y}\downarrow & & \downarrow{\scriptstyle i_X} \\
\mathcal{E}ff/Y & \xrightarrow[f^*]{} & \mathcal{E}ff/X
\end{array}
$$

where i_X, i_Y are the inclusion functors and $f^\sharp$ is the restriction of f^* to $\mathcal{D}_Y$. We shall be interested in whether the reflection (if it exists) is *stable*, that is: suppose i_X and i_Y have left adjoints r_X, r_Y; do we have that $f^\sharp \circ r_Y \simeq r_X \circ f^*$?

For this question it is useful to have a look at the right adjoints. I recall that in every topos $\mathcal{E}$ the functors $f^* : \mathcal{E}/Y \to \mathcal{E}/X$ defined by pullback along $f : X \to Y$, have right adjoints $\prod_f : \mathcal{E}/X \to \mathcal{E}/Y$. In set-theoretic terms, if $g : Z \to X$ is an object of $\mathcal{E}/X$, $\Pi_f(g)$ is $W \xrightarrow{h} Y$ with $h^{-1}(y) = \prod_{f(x)=y} g^{-1}(x)$; in other words, $h^{-1}(y)$ consists of partial maps $X \rightharpoonup Z$ with domain $f^{-1}(y)$, which are sections of g.

In $\mathcal{E}ff$, if F represents a map $f : (I, \sim) \to (J, \sim)$ and Φ represents $\phi : (Y, \sim) \to (I, \sim)$, then $\prod_f(\phi)$ can be constructed as an object of pairs (R, j) where $j \in J$ and R is a relation between I and Y; so we have

$$(\mathcal{P}(\mathbb{N})^{I \times Y}, \sim)$$

as a subobject of $\mathcal{P}((I, \sim) \times (Y, \sim)) \times (J, \sim)$ defined by the existence relation $E(R, j)$: $E(R, j)$ is the set of pairs $p\beta n$ with $n \in E(j)$ and β a realizer for

"R is a strict, single-valued relation $\wedge$
$$\forall i (\exists y (R(i, y) \leftrightarrow F(i, j)) \wedge$$
$$\forall i \forall y (R(i, y) \to \Phi(y, i)))$$"

Proposition 3.4.12 *Let $f : (I, \sim) \to (J, \sim)$ be a map with $\neg\neg$-separated codomain. Then if $(Y, \sim) \xrightarrow{\phi} (I, \sim)$ is a discrete map, so is $\prod_f(\phi)$.*

Proof. Referring to the construction of $\prod_f(\phi)$ given above, in order to apply proposition 3.4.4 assume we have an element a of $E(R, j) \cap E(R', j)$. We need to construct from a a realizer for $(R, j) \sim (R', j)$; that is, a realizer for

$$E(j) \wedge \forall i, y (F(i, j) \to (R(i, y) \leftrightarrow R'(i, y)))$$

But a gives, for each realizer for $F(i, j)$, realizers for $R(i, y)$, $R'(i, y')$ and $E(y) \cap E(y')$. Since ϕ is discrete, this gives uniformly a realizer for $y \sim y'$ and this uniformity gives us a realizer for $(R, j) \sim (R', j)$. ∎

Proposition 3.4.12 can *not* be generalized to maps f with arbitrary codomain, as we shall see in a minute.

First, let us conclude that the discrete reflection has nice properties when we restrict ourselves to $\neg\neg$-separated objects.

Proposition 3.4.13 *Suppose $f : X \to Y$ is an arrow such that the functor $\prod_f : \mathcal{E}ff/X \to \mathcal{E}ff/Y$ preserves discrete maps; let $\prod'_f : \mathcal{D}_X \to \mathcal{D}_Y$ be the factorization. Then $\prod'_f$ is right adjoint to $f^\sharp$, and $f^\sharp r_Y \simeq r_X f^*$. Hence for any map between separated objects, the discrete reflection is stable.*

Proof. We have natural isomorphisms

$$
\begin{aligned}
\mathcal{D}_X(f^\sharp r_Y(\phi), \psi) &\simeq \mathcal{E}ff/X(i_X f^\sharp r_Y(\phi), i_X(\psi)) && (i_X \text{ full and faithful}) \\
&\simeq \mathcal{E}ff/X(f^* i_Y r_Y(\phi), i_X(\psi)) && (f^* i_Y \simeq i_X f^\sharp) \\
&\simeq \mathcal{E}ff/Y(i_Y r_Y(\phi), \textstyle\prod_f i_X(\psi)) && (f^* \dashv \textstyle\prod_f) \\
&\simeq \mathcal{E}ff/Y(i_Y r_Y(\phi), i_Y \textstyle\prod_f'(\psi)) && (\textstyle\prod_f i_X \simeq i_Y \textstyle\prod_f') \\
&\simeq \mathcal{D}_Y(r_Y(\phi), \textstyle\prod_f'(\psi)) && (i_Y \text{ full and faithful})
\end{aligned}
$$

so $f^\sharp \dashv \prod_f'$. Using this, we have

$$
\begin{aligned}
\mathcal{D}_X(f^\sharp r_Y(\phi), \psi) &\simeq \mathcal{D}_Y(r_Y(\phi), \textstyle\prod_f'(\psi)) \\
&\simeq \mathcal{E}ff/Y(\phi, i_Y \textstyle\prod_f'(\psi)) \\
&\simeq \mathcal{E}ff/Y(\phi, \textstyle\prod_f i_X(\psi)) \\
&\simeq \mathcal{E}ff/X(f^*(\phi), i_X(\psi)) \\
&\simeq \mathcal{D}_X(r_X f^*(\phi), \psi)
\end{aligned}
$$

whence $f^\sharp r_Y \simeq r_X f^*$ by the Yoneda Lemma.   ∎

Let us now see what can go wrong if the codomain of a map is not necessarily separated.

Proposition 3.4.14

i)   There is an arrow $f : X \to Y$ in $\mathcal{E}ff$ and a discrete map ϕ into X, such that $\prod_f(\phi)$ is not discrete.

ii) There is an epimorphism $z : Z \to Y$ in $\mathcal{E}ff$ and an arrow w into Y, such that $z^*(w)$ is discrete, but w is not.

iii) There is an object Y for which there is no stable discrete reflection $\mathcal{E}ff/Y \to \mathcal{D}_Y$.

Proof. i) This example was given in [77]. Let f be the map 'true': $1 \to \Omega$ and ϕ the map $2 \to 1$. This is certainly a discrete map as 2 is a subobject of N. We consider $\prod_{\text{true}}(2)$ as map into Ω. Now for any $\chi : A \to \Omega$, we have a bijection $\mathcal{E}ff(\text{true}^*(\chi), 2) \simeq \mathcal{E}ff/\Omega(\chi, \prod_{\text{true}}(2)$ and, realizing that maps $A \xrightarrow{\chi} \Omega$ correspond to subobjects of A via $\chi \mapsto \text{true}^*(\chi)$, we see that $\prod_{\text{true}}(2)$ is the map $\mathsf{s} : \tilde{2} \to \Omega$ where $\tilde{2}$ is the partial map classifier of 2 (internally: the object of subsets of 2 having at most one element) and s classifies the subobject 2 of $\tilde{2}$, that is, internally for $\alpha \in \tilde{2}$ we have $s(\alpha) = [\exists x^2 (x \in \alpha)]$. I claim that $\tilde{2} \xrightarrow{s} \Omega$ is not discrete.

To see this note first that $\tilde{2}$ is a retract of $\mathcal{P}(2)$. Indeed, define $R : \mathcal{P}(2) \to \tilde{2}$ by

$$R(U) = \{x \in 2 \mid x \in U \wedge U \in \tilde{2}\}$$

Convince yourself that R is well-defined and is a retraction. Since $\mathcal{P}(2)$ is a uniform object by 3.2.6, $\tilde{2}$ is uniform. If $s : \tilde{2} \to \Omega$ would be discrete, we would have a commutative diagram

$$\begin{array}{ccc} A & \xrightarrow{m} & N \times \Omega \\ \sigma \downarrow & & \downarrow \pi \\ \tilde{2} & \xrightarrow{s} & \Omega \end{array}$$

with m monic, σ epi and π the projection. Then internally the statement

$$\forall \alpha{:}\tilde{2}\exists n{:}N((n, s(\alpha)) \in A \wedge \sigma(n, s(\alpha)) = \alpha)$$

would be true; by uniformity we'd have an n_0 such that $\forall \alpha{:}\tilde{2}(\sigma(n_0, s(\alpha)) = \alpha)$ would hold; which implies $\forall \alpha\beta{:}\tilde{2}(s(\alpha) = s(\beta) \to \alpha = \beta)$. But this is clearly false (take $\alpha = \{0\}$, $\beta = \{1\}$).

ii) Take $f : X \to Y$ and ϕ into X, as in i); so ϕ is discrete but $\prod_f(\phi)$ is not. Let $z : Z \to Y$ be a separated cover of Y, and consider the pullback diagram

$$\begin{array}{ccc} U & \xrightarrow{g} & X \\ h \downarrow & & \downarrow f \\ Z & \xrightarrow{z} & Y \end{array}$$

We have ϕ discrete, so $g^*(\phi)$ discrete by 3.4.11. Since Y is separated, $\prod_h(g^*(\phi))$ is discrete by 3.4.12. Recall from Topos Theory that the Beck-Chevalley condition holds for these pullback squares, that is:

$$\prod_h \circ g^* \simeq z^* \circ \prod_f$$

So if we let $w = \prod_f(\phi)$ then $z^*(w)$ is discrete but w is not.

iii) Consider $Z \xrightarrow{z} Y$ and w into Y satisfying ii). Z is separated so there is a reflection $r_Z : \mathcal{E}ff/Z \to \mathcal{D}_Z$. I claim that there is no reflection $r_Y : \mathcal{E}ff/Y \to \mathcal{D}_Y$ such that $z^\sharp r_Y \simeq r_Z z^*$. For suppose to the contrary that such r_Y exists. Then for the unit $\eta_w : w \to i_Y r_Y(w)$ we have that $z^*(\eta_w) : z^*(w) \to z^*(i_Y r_Y(w)) \simeq i_Z r_Z z^*(w) \simeq z^*(w)$ (since $z^*(w)$ is discrete) is an isomorphism. But since z is epi, $z^* : \mathcal{E}ff/Y \to \mathcal{E}ff/Z$ is a faithful functor between toposes, and such functors reflect isomorphisms. That would mean that η_w is an isomorphism, i.e. w is discrete, quod non.
∎

3.4.1 Weakly complete internal categories in $\mathcal{E}ff$

The importance of discrete maps, to which we have payed considerable attention in this section, lies partly in the fact that they are, internally in $\mathcal{E}ff$, families (indexed by an object of $\mathcal{E}ff$) of objects of an internal category in $\mathcal{E}ff$, a category which is *weakly complete.*

This is remarkable and useful. Remarkable, because (since the category is internal in $\mathcal{E}ff$) from the point of view of $\mathcal{E}ff$ the category is 'small'; yet the category is not a preorder. You recall a little theorem by P. Freyd in Category Theory which says that every small and complete category must be a preorder. In order to see clearly the difference between the world of this classical theorem and $\mathcal{E}ff$ let us review the main argument in the proof: suppose $\mathcal{C}$ is small, with set of arrows $\mathcal{C}_1$, and suppose A, B are two objects of $\mathcal{C}$ with two distinct arrows $f, g : A \to B$. We see then that the existence of a product $\prod_{h \in \mathcal{C}_1} B$ forces an inclusion of sets $2^{\mathcal{C}_1} \rightarrowtail \mathcal{C}_1$, and this runs into a contradiction with Cantor's Theorem in Set Theory.

However, this contradiction evaporates in the context of $\mathcal{E}ff$, where we have already met highly nontrivial objects X for which 2^X embeds into X (let X be, for example, the object R of real numbers (and use a suitable internalization of corollary 3.3.9), or the object Σ^N of r.e. subobjects of N; see 3.2.29).

The result is also useful, because it means that in $\mathcal{E}ff$, a 'set-theoretic' interpretation of the polymorphic λ-calculus of J.-Y. Girard ([56, 57]) is possible; Reynolds ([131]) had shown that such an interpretation cannot exist in Set.

The fact that $\mathcal{E}ff$ contains a weakly complete internal category was discovered by Hyland, who also credits E. Moggi for a first crucial insight, and laid down in [71]. However, the notion of an internal category in a topos which is 'internally full' (that is: relative to the topos, it is really a category of sets and 'all' functions between them) and 'complete', is rather delicate; a minor technical flaw in Hyland's paper was corrected, and an alternative treatment given, in [77].

This last paper, [77], describes the situation in abstract terms and uses the framework of fibrations quite heavily.

In this book I have tried to be as concrete as possible, and the mathematical core of the argument lies already past us. However, for a correct conceptual understanding of what is going on, I think one cannot really avoid a little bit of the theory of fibrations, which we in this book will not use mathematically but only conceptually.

After this, maybe somewhat opaque, introduction, let us get to some specific definitions.

Definition 3.4.15 Let $\mathcal{E}$ be a topos. An *internal category* $\mathcal{C}$ in a topos $\mathcal{E}$ consists of objects C_0, C_1 of $\mathcal{E}$ and arrows:

$$C_1 \underset{d_0}{\overset{d_1}{\rightrightarrows}} C_0 \quad C_0 \xrightarrow{\ i\ } C_1 \quad C_2 \xrightarrow{\ \mu\ } C_1$$

where C_2 is such that

$$\begin{array}{ccc} C_2 & \longrightarrow & C_1 \\ \downarrow & & \downarrow{\scriptstyle d_0} \\ C_1 & \xrightarrow{\ d_1\ } & C_0 \end{array}$$

is a pullback diagram. The object C_0 is the 'object of objects of $\mathcal{C}$', the object C_1 the 'object of arrows of $\mathcal{C}$', d_0 and d_1 are, respectively, the domain and codomain maps so that C_2 is the 'object of composable pairs of arrows of $\mathcal{C}$'; and μ is to be the composition map. Finally the map i assigns the identity arrow to each object. Of course these data must satisfy certain equations (expressed by commutative diagrams), which I trust the reader has no trouble in formulating himself.

If $\mathcal{C}$ and $\mathcal{D}$ are internal categories in $\mathcal{E}$, an *internal functor* $F : \mathcal{C} \to \mathcal{D}$ consists of a pair of arrows $F_0 : C_0 \to D_0$ and $F_1 : C_1 \to D_1$, such that the usual squares commute.

The reader who feels ill at home here, may have a look at the chapter 'Internal Category theory' of [80] for full definitions.

Example. The following example of internal categories will be important to us: given any map $S \xrightarrow{\alpha} T$ in $\mathcal{E}$, construct an internal category $\mathcal{C}_\alpha$ in $\mathcal{E}$ as follows: $(\mathcal{C}_\alpha)_0 = T$, and $(\mathcal{C}_\alpha)_1$ and the pair of maps d_0, d_1 from $(\mathcal{C}_\alpha)_1$ to $(\mathcal{C}_\alpha)_0$ is defined in such a way that the arrow

$$(\mathcal{C}_\alpha)_1 \xrightarrow{(d_0, d_1)} (\mathcal{C}_\alpha)_0$$

is the exponential $\pi_2^*(\alpha)^{\pi_1^*(\alpha)}$ in the slice category $\mathcal{E}/(\mathcal{C}_\alpha)_0 \times (\mathcal{C}_\alpha)_0 = \mathcal{E}/T \times T$.

That means that internally we have a collection of 'sets' $\alpha^{-1}(x)$ for $x \in T$, and functions $f : \alpha^{-1}(x) \to \alpha^{-1}(y)$, which are exactly the arrows in $\mathcal{C}$ from x to y.

A category of this type is called a *full internal subcategory* of $\mathcal{E}$. This terminology is meant to emphasize that in this case $\mathcal{C}$ is a category of 'sets' and 'all' functions between them; be it a bit abusing the language since (at least for now) there is no 'embedding' of $\mathcal{C}$ into $\mathcal{E}$.

The way to achieve such an embedding, is by using the language of fibrations, which I now introduce.

Definition 3.4.16 Suppose $\mathcal{D} \xrightarrow{p} \mathcal{C}$ is a functor between two categories. For an arrow f in $\mathcal{D}$, if $p(f) = g$ we shall say that f *lies over* g. In this case, the arrow $f : U \to V$ is said to be *prone* if whenever $f' : U' \to V$ has the same codomain as f and lies over a composite ga, there is a unique arrow $\alpha : U' \to U$ such that $f\alpha = f'$ and α lies over a:

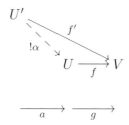

The functor p is called a *fibration* if for every arrow g in $\mathcal{C}$ and for every object V of $\mathcal{D}$ with $p(V) = \mathrm{cod}(g)$, there is a prone arrow f which lies over g and has codomain V.

Suppose $p : \mathcal{D} \to \mathcal{C}$ is a fibration. If X is an object of $\mathcal{C}$, the subcategory of $\mathcal{D}$ consisting of the objects V with $p(V) = X$ and arrows which lie over id_X, is called the *fibre* of p over X, and denoted $\mathcal{D}^X$. A map of $\mathcal{D}$ which lies over an identity is also called *vertical*; prone maps are thought of as 'horizontal', as the word indicates (the word 'prone', invented by Paul Taylor, replaces the meaningless 'cartesian' of the older fibration literature). Note that if p is a fibration, then every arrow of $\mathcal{D}$ factors uniquely as a vertical followed by a prone. Also note that prone maps are stable under composition, and that if, for a composite gf, both gf and g are prone, then f is prone too (compare with the properties of pullback squares).

Given an arrow $g : Y \to X$ in $\mathcal{C}$ we have a functor $g^* : \mathcal{D}^X \to \mathcal{D}^Y$ defined as follows: for any object V of $\mathcal{D}^X$ *choose* a prone arrow f over g with codomain V, and define $g^*(V) = \mathrm{dom}(f)$. If $\alpha : V' \to V$ is an arrow in $\mathcal{D}^X$ and prone f, f' have been have been chosen over g with codomain V, V' respectively, then since $\alpha f'$ lies over g and has codomain V, by proneness of f there is a unique arrow $g^*(\alpha) : \mathrm{dom}(f') \to \mathrm{dom}(f)$ which lies over id_Y and satisfies $f \circ g^*(\alpha) = \alpha f'$. Using the uniqueness of the required factorization in the definition of 'prone', it is straightforward to prove that this gives a functor g^*. Now the functor g^* depends on a choice of prone maps for every object V of $\mathcal{D}^X$; however, if f and f' are both prone maps over g with the same codomain, there is a unique vertical isomorphism between their domains which makes the evident triangle commute, and therefore another choice of prone maps would have resulted in a functor for which there is a unique natural isomorphism with g^*. The functor g^* is usually referred to as the *reindexing functor along g*.

There is a close connection between the notions of fibration and of *indexed category*, which is a 'pseudofunctor $\mathcal{C}^{\mathrm{op}} \to \mathrm{Cat}$', but we shall not pursue this here. Interested readers are referred to the textbook on fibrations [78], or the relevant chapter in [83]. For a readable introduction, see also [157].

Let us see the most important examples. The first example is the *codomain fibration*. For any category $\mathcal{C}$ one can consider the category $\mathcal{C}^{\to}$ which has arrows of $\mathcal{C}$ as objects and commutative squares as arrows. There is an evident functor $\mathrm{cod} : \mathcal{C}^{\to} \to \mathcal{C}$ which assigns to each object of $\mathcal{C}^{\to}$ its codomain in $\mathcal{C}$, and to each commutative square its bottom row. It is easy to see that an arrow in $\mathcal{C}^{\to}$ is prone for cod if and only if it is a pullback square in $\mathcal{C}$, so if the category $\mathcal{C}$ has pullbacks, cod is a fibration. When an older category theorist speaks about 'the canonical fibration', or even 'the category $\mathcal{C}$ canonically fibered over itself', you may wonder why he puts it this way but anyway, what he means is the codomain fibration.

The second example is the *family fibration*. Suppose $\mathcal{C}$ is a category. The category $\mathrm{Fam}(\mathcal{C})$ has as objects pairs $(X, (C_i)_{i \in X})$ where X is a set and $(C_i)_{i \in X}$ is an X-indexed family of objects of $\mathcal{C}$. An arrow $(X, (C_i)_{i \in X}) \to (Y, (D_j)_{j \in Y})$ is a pair $(f, (\phi_i)_{i \in X})$ where $f : X \to Y$ is a function and $(\phi_i)_{i \in X}$ is an X-indexed family of arrows of $\mathcal{C}$ such that for each $i \in X$, $\phi_i : C_i \to D_{f(i)}$. If $(g, (\psi_j)_{j \in Y})$ is an arrow from $(Y, (D_j)_{j \in Y})$ to $(Z, (E_k)_{k \in Z})$, the composition with $(f, (\phi_i)_{i \in X})$ is defined as

$$(gf, (\psi_{f(i)} \phi_i)_{i \in X})$$

and the identity on $(X, (C_i)_{i \in X})$ is $(\mathrm{id}_X, (\mathrm{id}_{C_i})_{i \in X})$. We shall meet the category $\mathrm{Fam}(\mathcal{C})$ again, later on. There is an evident functor $\mathrm{Fam}(\mathcal{C}) \xrightarrow{\pi} \mathrm{Set}$, sending $(X, (C_i)_{i \in X})$ to X and $(f, (\phi_i)_{i \in X})$ to f, and this functor is a fibration: a map $(f, (\phi_i)_{i \in X})$ is prone if and only if every ϕ_i is an isomorphism. Hence, given $f : Y \to X$ and an object $(X, (C_i)_{i \in X})$ over

X, we have a prone map

$$(f, (\mathrm{id}_{C_{f(j)}})_{j \in Y}) : (Y, (C_{f(j)})_{j \in Y}) \to (X, (C_i)_{i \in X})$$

which lies over f.

Suppose $\mathcal{D}_1 \overset{p_1}{\to} \mathcal{C}$ and $\mathcal{D}_2 \overset{p_2}{\to} \mathcal{C}$ are two fibrations over $\mathcal{C}$. A *map of fibrations* from p_1 to p_2 is a functor $\Phi : \mathcal{D}_1 \to \mathcal{D}_2$ such that the diagram

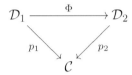

commutes, and which moreover preserves prone maps (if $f : U \to V$ in $\mathcal{D}_1$ w.r.t. p_1, then $\Phi(f)$ is prone in $\mathcal{D}_2$ w.r.t. p_2). If Φ is full and faithful, we call p_2 a *subfibration* of p_1. Note that in this case, the functor Φ not only preserves, but also reflects prone maps. If Φ is full and faithful and essentially surjective on objects, we'll say that Φ is an *equivalence of fibrations*.

Example. Suppose we have a class of maps $\mathcal{D}$ in a topos $\mathcal{E}$ which is stable under pullback. Then we can consider the full subcategory of $\mathcal{E}^{\to}$ on the maps in $\mathcal{D}$, and this forms a subfibration of the codomain fibration. For example, for $\mathcal{D}$ we could take the class of discrete maps in the effective topos.

Let us, for motivation of what is to follow, have another look at the family fibration $\mathrm{Fam}(\mathcal{C})$, where we now assume $\mathcal{C}$ to be small. One of the very first results in category theory ([39]) tells us that $\mathcal{C}$ can be embedded in Set by the assignments $I(C) = \{g \in \mathcal{C}_1 \,|\, \mathrm{cod}(g) = C\}$ and for $f : C \to C'$, $I(f) = f \circ (-) : I(C) \to I(C')$. This embedding can be used to obtain a map of fibrations from the family fibration $\mathrm{Fam}(\mathcal{C})$ to the codomain fibration on Set: define $\Phi : \mathrm{Fam}(\mathcal{C}) \to \mathrm{Set}^{\to}$ by

$$\Phi(X, (C_i)_{i \in X}) = (\{(i, \mu) \,|\, i \in X, \mu \in I(C_i)\} \overset{\pi}{\to} X)$$

(with π the evident projection) and on maps as follows: if $(\alpha, (\phi_i)_{i \in X})$ is a map $(X, (C_i)_{i \in X}) \to (Y, (D_j)_{j \in Y})$ then $\Phi(\alpha, (\phi_i)_{i \in X})$ is the map sending (i, μ) to $(\alpha(i), \phi_i \mu)$. Note that Φ is indeed a map of fibrations: clearly, the required triangle commutes and if $(\alpha, (\phi_i)_{i \in X})$ is prone, that is: all ϕ_i are isomorphisms, then the square

$$
\begin{array}{ccc}
\{(i, \mu) \mid \mathrm{cod}(\mu) = C_i\} & \longrightarrow & \{(j, \nu) \mid \mathrm{cod}(\nu) = D_j\} \\
\downarrow & & \downarrow \\
X & \longrightarrow & Y
\end{array}
$$

where the top horizontal arrow sends (i, μ) to $(j, \phi_i \mu)$, is a pullback diagram, hence a prone arrow for the codomain functor.

Now suppose that the embedding $I : \mathcal{C} \rightarrow \mathrm{Set}$ is actually full, so $\mathcal{C}$ can be identified with a full internal subcategory of Set; which is, a full subcategory of Set on a set $\mathcal{A}$ of sets.

Let $\{\mathcal{C}\}$ be the full subcategory of $\mathrm{Set}^{\rightarrow}$ on objects of the form

$$
\{(i, u) \mid i \in X, u \in A_i\} \xrightarrow{\pi} X
$$

where, again, $(A_i)_{i \in X}$ is an X-indexed family of objects of $\mathcal{C}$, and π is the projection. The restriction of $\mathrm{cod} : \mathrm{Set}^{\rightarrow} \rightarrow \mathrm{Set}$ to $\{\mathcal{C}\}$ is a fibration, and $\{\mathcal{C}\}$ is a subfibration of cod: a map in $\{\mathcal{C}\}$,

$$
\begin{array}{ccc}
\{(i, u) \mid i \in X, u \in A_i\} & \xrightarrow{(\beta_i)_{i \in X}} & \{(j, v) \mid j \in Y, v \in B_j\} \\
\pi \downarrow & & \downarrow \pi \\
X & \xrightarrow{\alpha} & Y
\end{array}
$$

is prone if and only if for every $i \in X$ the map $\beta_i : A_i \rightarrow B_{\alpha(i)}$ is an isomorphism. Since $\mathcal{C}$ is a *full* subcategory of Set, β_i is actually an arrow in $\mathcal{C}$; hence we define a functor $\Psi : \{\mathcal{C}\} \rightarrow \mathrm{Set}^{\rightarrow}$ by putting

$$
\Psi \left(
\begin{array}{c}
\{(i, x) \mid i \in X, u \in A_i\} \\
\downarrow \pi \\
X
\end{array}
\right)
=
\left(
\begin{array}{c}
\{(i, f) \mid \mathrm{cod}(f) = A_i\} \\
\downarrow \pi \\
X
\end{array}
\right)
$$

and $\Psi(\alpha, (\beta_i)_{i \in X}) = (\alpha, (\beta_i \circ (-))_{i \in X})$, and we see that the image of Ψ consists of those objects of $\mathrm{Set}^{\rightarrow}$ which are isomorphic to an object in the image of $\Phi : \mathrm{Fam}(\mathcal{C}) \to \mathrm{Set}^{\to}$. That is, we see that we have an equivalence of fibrations between $\mathrm{Fam}(\mathcal{C})$ and $\{\mathcal{C}\}$.

The fibration $\{\mathcal{C}\}$ has an alternative description as follows. We have a set of objects $\mathcal{A}$ and, 'over $\mathcal{A}$', the 'element relation'

$$\in_{\mathcal{A}} = \{(a, A) \mid A \in \mathcal{A}, a \in A\}$$

with projection $\in_{\mathcal{A}} \overset{\pi_{\mathcal{A}}}{\to} \mathcal{A}$. For every object of $\{\mathcal{C}\}$, say $\{(i, u) \mid i \in X, u \in A_i\} \overset{\pi}{\to} X$, there is an arrow $X \overset{\phi}{\to} \mathcal{A}$ (sending i to A_i) such that there is a pullback diagram

$$
\begin{array}{ccc}
\{(i, u) \mid i \in X, u \in A_i\} & \longrightarrow & \in_{\mathcal{A}} \\
\downarrow & & \downarrow{\scriptstyle \pi_{\mathcal{A}}} \\
X & \underset{\phi}{\longrightarrow} & \mathcal{A}
\end{array}
$$

and conversely, every map $Z \to X$ which is a pullback of $\pi_{\mathcal{A}}$ is isomorphic to an object of $\{\mathcal{C}\}$. So up to equivalence, we might as well have defined $\{\mathcal{C}\}$ as the full subcategory of $\mathrm{Set}^{\to}$ on the objects which are pullbacks of $\pi_{\mathcal{A}}$.

Furthermore let us remark that $\mathcal{C}$ is, of course, isomorphic to the full internal subcategory of Set determined by the map $\in_{\mathcal{A}} \overset{\pi_{\mathcal{A}}}{\to} \mathcal{A}$ in the sense of the Example following definition 3.4.15.

We summarize our findings in the following proposition.

Proposition 3.4.17 *Suppose $\mathcal{C}$ is a full internal subcategory in* Set *determined by a map $S \to T$. Define $\{\mathcal{C}\}$ as the full subcategory of* $\mathrm{Set}^{\to}$ *on those maps $Z \to X$ for which there is a pullback diagram*

$$
\begin{array}{ccc}
Z & \longrightarrow & S \\
\downarrow & & \downarrow \\
X & \longrightarrow & T
\end{array}
$$

Then $\mathrm{cod} : \{\mathcal{C}\} \to \mathrm{Set}$ *is a subfibration of the codomain fibration, and this subfibration is equivalent to the family fibration* $\mathrm{Fam}(\mathcal{C}) \to \mathrm{Set}$.

The point of this whole exercise now is, that the whole procedure can be generalized to (full) internal subcategories in a topos $\mathcal{E}$.

Definition 3.4.18 Suppose $\mathcal{C} = (C_0, C_1, d_0, d_1, i, \mu)$ is an internal category in a topos $\mathcal{E}$. Then there is a fibration $[\mathcal{C}] \xrightarrow{p} \mathcal{E}$, the *externalization* of $\mathcal{C}$, defined as follows: objects of $[\mathcal{C}]$ are maps $X \xrightarrow{f} C_0$ in $\mathcal{E}$. An arrow in $[\mathcal{C}]$ from $(X \xrightarrow{f} C_0)$ to $(Y \xrightarrow{g} C_0)$ is a pair (α, h) where $\alpha : X \to Y$ and $h : X \to C_1$ are maps in $\mathcal{E}$ such that $d_0 h = f$ and $d_1 h = g\alpha$. Given maps

$$(\alpha, h) : (X \xrightarrow{f} C_0) \to (Y \xrightarrow{g} C_0)$$
$$(\beta, k) : (Y \xrightarrow{g} C_0) \to (Z \xrightarrow{m} C_0)$$

we have a factorization of $(h, k\alpha) : X \to C_1 \times C_1$ through a map $\langle h, k\alpha \rangle : X \to C_2$ since $d_0 k\alpha = g\alpha = d_1 h$, and the composition $(\beta, k) \circ (\alpha, h)$ is defined as the pair

$$(\beta\alpha, \mu \circ \langle h, k\alpha \rangle)$$

The functor $p : [\mathcal{C}] \to \mathcal{E}$ sends an object $(X \xrightarrow{f} C_0)$ to X, and an arrow (α, h) to α.

To see that $p : [\mathcal{C}] \to \mathcal{E}$ is indeed a fibration, just note the complete analogy with the family fibration. Just as in that case, an arrow (α, h) is prone if and only if the map $h : X \to C_1$ factors through the object $\mathrm{Iso}(\mathcal{C})$ of internal isomorphisms of $\mathcal{C}$. Given $\alpha : X \to Y$ in $\mathcal{E}$ and an object $Y \xrightarrow{g} C_0$ of $[\mathcal{C}]$, consider the object $X \xrightarrow{g\alpha} C_0$ and the prone map $(\alpha, ig\alpha) : (X \xrightarrow{g\alpha} C_0) \to (Y \xrightarrow{\alpha} C_0)$.

Internalizing the argument leading up to proposition 3.4.17, we obtain:

Proposition 3.4.19 *Suppose $\mathcal{C}$ is a full internal subcategory in a topos $\mathcal{E}$ determined by a map $S \to T$. Define $\{\mathcal{C}\}$ as the full subcategory of $\mathcal{E}^{\to}$ on those maps $Z \to X$ for which there is a pullback diagram*

$$\begin{array}{ccc} Z & \longrightarrow & S \\ \downarrow & & \downarrow \\ X & \longrightarrow & T \end{array}$$

Then $\mathrm{cod} : \{\mathcal{C}\} \to \mathcal{E}$ *is a subfibration of the codomain fibration, and this subfibration is equivalent to the externalization* $[\mathcal{C}] \to \mathcal{E}$ *of* $\mathcal{C}$.

The language of fibrations is used in order to formulate notions of 'completeness' for an internal category. First we formulate the appropriate notions for fibrations. Since we are concerned only with fibrations over toposes, we restrict ourselves to this case (not that it saves much).

Definition 3.4.20 Suppose $\mathcal{D} \to \mathcal{E}$ is a fibration over a topos $\mathcal{E}$. The fibration is *complete* if the following two conditions hold:

a)   every fibre $\mathcal{D}^X$ has finite limits, and every reindexing functor g^* preserves them;

b)   every reindexing functor g^* has a right adjoint $\prod_g$, and the Beck-Chevalley condition holds for this situation: if

$$\begin{array}{ccc} X & \xrightarrow{\ f\ } & Y \\ u \downarrow & & \downarrow v \\ Z & \xrightarrow{\ g\ } & W \end{array}$$

is a pullback diagram in $\mathcal{E}$, then the natural transformation $g^* \circ \prod_v \Rightarrow \prod_u \circ f^*$ which corresponds to $\prod_v(\eta_f) : \prod_v \Rightarrow \prod_v \prod_f f^*$, is an isomorphism.

The fibration is *weakly complete* if, in addition to requirement a) above, the following holds: for every $f : X \to Y$ in $\mathcal{E}$ and every object U in the fibre $\mathcal{D}^X$, there is a pullback diagram

$$\begin{array}{ccc} X' & \xrightarrow{\ g'\ } & X \\ f' \downarrow & & \downarrow f \\ Y' & \xrightarrow{\ g\ } & Y \end{array}$$

such that g is epi, and $\prod_{f'}((g')^*(U))$ exists. Moreover, the Beck-Chevalley condition should hold whenever both $\prod$'s exist.

Examples. 1. Suppose $\mathcal{C}$ has pullbacks. Then the codomain fibration on $\mathcal{C}$ is complete if and only if $\mathcal{C}$ is locally cartesian closed.

2. Suppose $\mathcal{C}$ is an internal category in a topos $\mathcal{E}$. It is easy to express in the internal language that $\mathcal{C}$ 'has a terminal object, binary products and equalizers', and this is equivalent to: the fibration $[\mathcal{C}]$ satisfies requirement a) of definition 3.4.20 above. If $f : X \to Y$ is an arrow in $\mathcal{E}$, we have in $\mathcal{E}$ internal product categories $\mathcal{C}^X$ and $\mathcal{C}^Y$ and an internal projection functor $\mathcal{C}^f : \mathcal{C}^Y \to \mathcal{C}^X$. It seems natural to call $\mathcal{C}$ *complete* if, in addition to finite limits, all such functors $\mathcal{C}^f$ have right adjoints (satisfying Beck-Chevalley conditions), and this is equivalent to requiring that the externalization $[\mathcal{C}]$ is a complete fibration.

3. The subfibration of the codomain fibration on $\mathcal{E}ff$ on the discrete objects is *not* complete as we saw in proposition 3.4.14; however, proposition 3.4.12, together with the fact that every object of $\mathcal{E}ff$ is covered by a $\neg\neg$-separated object, implies that it is weakly complete.

4. An internal category $\mathcal{C}$ in a topos $\mathcal{E}$ is said to be *weakly complete* if its externalization is weakly complete.

Let us now, finally, exhibit a full internal category $\mathcal{Q}$ of $\mathcal{E}ff$ which is weakly complete. In fact, from Example 3. above we see, that it is sufficient to find a full internal category $\mathcal{Q}$ such that the fibration $\{\mathcal{Q}\}$ is equivalent to the fibration of discrete maps. Since a discrete map is a 'family of subquotients of N', the choice of $\mathcal{Q}$ is obvious: we take the full subcategory in $\mathcal{E}ff$ on the set of 'sets of equivalence classes of an equivalence relation on a subset of N'. Accordingly, we define the object of objects $\mathcal{Q}_0$ internally as:

$$\mathcal{Q}_0 = \{F \subset \mathcal{P}(N) \,|\, \forall X{\in}F \exists x{:}N(x \in X) \wedge \forall XY{\in}F\forall x{:}N(x{\in}X \cap Y \to X = Y)\}$$

and we let $S \to \mathcal{Q}_0$ be the restriction of the element relation $\in \mapsto \mathcal{P}(N) \times \mathcal{PP}(N)$ to $\mathcal{Q}_0$ (together with its projection to $\mathcal{Q}_0$), that is:

$$S = \{(A, F) \in \mathcal{P}(N) \times \mathcal{Q}_0 \,|\, A \in F\}$$

Now the category $\{\mathcal{Q}\}$ is the full subcategory of $\mathcal{E}\!f\!f^{\rightarrow}$ on the maps $Z \rightarrow X$ such that there is a pullback diagram

$$
\begin{array}{ccc}
Z & \longrightarrow & S \\
\downarrow & & \downarrow \\
X & \xrightarrow{\phi} & \mathcal{Q}_0
\end{array}
$$

Given such a diagram, we have a subobject A of $N \times X$ defined by $A = \{(n, x) \mid n \in \bigcup \phi(x)\}$ and since for any $(n, x) \in A$ there is a unique $X \in \phi(x)$ with $n \in X$, we have a clear surjection $A \rightarrow Z$ such that the diagram

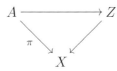

commutes. In other words, $Z \rightarrow X$ is a discrete map.

We see that indeed, $\{\mathcal{Q}\}$ is the subfibration of the codomain fibration on $\mathcal{E}\!f\!f$ on the discrete maps.

Theorem 3.4.21 *The category $\mathcal{Q}$ is weakly complete.*

In [77], another method of proving this result was used: there the authors connect $\{\mathcal{Q}\}$ to the subfibration of cod on the *orthogonal* maps: the maps $Y \rightarrow X$ such that (in $\mathcal{E}\!f\!f/X$) the natural map

$$
(Y \rightarrow X) \rightarrow (Y \rightarrow X)^{X^*(\nabla 2)}
$$

is an isomorphism. It can be rather easily proved that such fibrations of orthogonal maps are always complete. The connection with $\{\mathcal{Q}\}$ is then given as a 'weak equivalence' of fibrations. Some theory (which the authors develop in that paper) is then needed about 'stack completions' and the properties which are preserved by weak equivalences.

Yet another approach, based on the fact that the full subcategory of $\mathcal{E}\!f\!f$ on the discrete objects is the ex/lex completion of the full subcategory of $\mathcal{E}\!f\!f$ on the $\neg\neg$-closed subobjects of N, is presented in [30].

What does 'weakly complete' actually mean? Well, suppose I is an index category (of course, internally in $\mathcal{E}\!f\!f$; we reason 'in $\mathcal{E}\!f\!f$' now); we consider the category $\mathcal{Q}^I$ of functors from I to $\mathcal{Q}$. If F is such a functor, then a limiting cone for F is a constant functor which is universal with the property that there is a natural transformation from it to F. That is: if $\Delta : \mathcal{Q} \to \mathcal{Q}^I$ is the diagonal embedding which assigns to $X \in \mathcal{Q}_0$ the constant functor with value X, then a limiting cone for F has as vertex the value at F of a right adjoint for Δ. Does such a right adjoint exist as a functor $\mathcal{Q}^I \to \mathcal{Q}$? If $\mathcal{Q}$ is complete in the sense of Example 4 following definition 3.4.20, *yes*; intuitionistically as well as classically, limits are produced from products and equalizers so we only need a *choice* for products, but that is exactly what the $\prod$-functors do for us.

However, the weak completeness only gives us that for each index category I, the statement

$$\forall F \text{ functor} : I \to \mathcal{Q}\, \exists \text{ limiting cone for } F$$

is true in $\mathcal{E}\!f\!f$.

Exactly the same reasoning as for $\mathcal{Q}$ can be applied to the subcategory $\mathcal{P}$ of $\mathcal{Q}$ on the $\neg\neg$-separated subquotients of N, the 'internal modest sets'. Like $\mathcal{Q}$, $\mathcal{P}$ is weakly but not strongly complete. It is actually $\mathcal{P}$, rather than $\mathcal{Q}$, which is used for a semantics for the polymorphic λ-calculus (or, 'system F'). Therefore I go a bit into the structure of $\mathcal{P}$ which allows this semantics; a lot of it is surprisingly easy to derive, using the facts of the internal logic of $\mathcal{E}\!f\!f$ we already know.

First, we present $\mathcal{P}$ as follows: $\mathcal{P}_0$ is the object of $\neg\neg$-closed subobjects of $N \times N$ which are, as relations, symmetric and transitive. Given $R \in \mathcal{P}_0$, we write $|R|$ for its field, i.e. $\{n \in N \mid R(n,n)\}$.

The object of $\neg\neg$-closed subobjects of $N \times N$, $\mathcal{P}_{\neg\neg}(N \times N)$ is isomorphic to $\nabla(2^{\mathbb{N}\times\mathbb{N}})$, so it is a sheaf. $\mathcal{P}_0$ is defined from this by the requirements 'symmetric' and 'transitive' which are in the negative fragment (use only the logical symbols $\wedge$, $\to$ and $\forall$), hence $\mathcal{P}_0$ is a closed subobject of a sheaf, and therefore itself a sheaf.

The object of arrows $\mathcal{P}_1$ can be described as the set of triples (R, S, ϕ) where ϕ is a function from the set of R-equivalence classes to the set of S-equivalence classes. We write $\phi : R \to S$.

If we denote the R-class of $n \in |R|$ by $[n]_R$, we have for such a function $\phi : R \to S$:

$$\forall n(n \in |R| \to \exists m(\phi([n]_R) = [m]_S))$$

Applying ECT (since $|R|$ is $\neg\neg$-closed), we find that for ϕ there is a partial recursive index f, such that

$$\forall n(n \in |R| \to fn{\downarrow} \wedge \phi([n]_R) = [fn]_S)$$

We abbreviate this by: 'f tracks ϕ'. This use of the word 'track' is a bit different from earlier use of it; now, 'f tracks ϕ' is a statement in the internal language of $\mathcal{E}ff$. Note that, by Markov's Principle, the statement 'f tracks ϕ' is $\neg\neg$-stable.

It is not hard to convince yourself that the category $\mathcal{P}$ is internally cartesian closed: the total relation $N \times N$ is a terminal object. Given R and S in $\mathcal{P}_0$ we let $R \times S$ be

$$R \times S = \{(pnm, pn'm') \mid R(n, n') \wedge S(m, m')\}$$

(recall that p is our pairing combinator). For the exponent $R \Rightarrow S$ we define

$$|R \Rightarrow S| = \{f \mid \forall n \in |R|(fn{\downarrow} \wedge fn \in |S|) \wedge \\ \forall nm(R(n, m) \to S(fn, fm))\}$$

and

$$(R \Rightarrow S) = \{(f, g) \mid f, g \in |R \Rightarrow S| \wedge \forall n \in |R|\, S(fn, gn)\}$$

For $f \in |R \Rightarrow S|$ we shall use the notation $[f]_{R \Rightarrow S}$ also to denote the unique arrow $R \to S$ which f tracks.

Now, consider an internal functor $F : \mathcal{P} \to \mathcal{P}$. We have $F_0 : \mathcal{P}_0 \to \mathcal{P}_0$ and $F_1 : \mathcal{P}_1 \to \mathcal{P}_1$. For every $R, S \in \mathcal{P}_0$ and $\phi : R \to S$ we have:

$$\forall f(f \text{ tracks } \phi \to \exists g(g \text{ tracks } F_1(\phi)))$$

Rewriting this a bit and applying ECT again, we obtain that there is a number $a_{R,S}$ such that

$(*)$ $\forall f \in |R \Rightarrow S| \, (a_{R,S} f \downarrow \wedge a_{R,S} f$ tracks $F_1([f]_{R \Rightarrow S}))$

So, we have $\forall R, S \in \mathcal{P}_0 \exists a_{R,S} \, (*)$. But $\mathcal{P}_0$ is a sheaf, and therefore satisfies the Uniformity Principle. So,

$$\exists a \forall R, S \forall f \in |R \Rightarrow S| \, (af \downarrow \wedge af \text{ tracks } F_1([f]_{R \Rightarrow S}))$$

which is an important property. In the terminology of [10], one of the fundamental papers in the development of the 'PER' semantics for polymorphism, F is a *realizable functor*.

Suppose F is a functor $\mathcal{P} \rightarrow \mathcal{P}$. We consider cones for F. Such a cone is an object R of $\mathcal{P}$ and a natural transformation from the constant functor with value R to F, which is a $\mathcal{P}_0$-indexed family of arrows $\phi_S : R \rightarrow F(S)$. Applying the Uniformity Principle once again, we see

$$\exists b \forall S \in \mathcal{P}_0 \, (b \text{ tracks } \phi_S)$$

This implies that for $n \in |R|$ we have $bn \in |F(S)|$ for all $S \in \mathcal{P}_0$, and if $R(n,m)$ then $F(S)(bn, bm)$ for all $S \in \mathcal{P}_0$. Moreover, for $n \in |R|$ and $f \in |S \Rightarrow S'|$, since af tracks $[f]_{S \Rightarrow S'}$ and ϕ is a cone, we have $F(S')(bn, af(bn))$. So $R(n,m)$ implies

$$\forall S, S' (F(S)(bn, bm) \wedge \forall f \in |S \Rightarrow S'| \, F(S')(bn, af(bn)))$$

Now if we define a $\neg\neg$-closed binary relation $\lim F$ by

$$\lim F \; = \; \{(n,m) \, | \, \forall S, S' (F(S)(n,m) \wedge \forall f \in |S \Rightarrow S'| \, F(S')(n, afn))\}$$

then it is easily verified that $\lim F$ is symmetric and transitive, there is a cone on F with vertex $\lim F$ (all maps in the cone tracked by the identity), and the cone ϕ factors uniquely through $\lim F$. So $\lim F$ is the vertex of a limiting cone for F.

It is even easier when we just consider products (the kind of limits used in the semantics of type theory): the product $\prod_{R \in \mathcal{P}_0} F(R)$ is just the intersection $\bigcap_{R \in \mathcal{P}_0} F(R)$, as easily follows from the general limit case.

In fact, the situation for the semantics of system F is a little more complicated than sketched here, because the type expressions represent functors of 'mixed variance' (like in $\prod_R (R \Rightarrow R)$) and one has to consider *dinatural transformations*).

The 'PER' models of various type theories are constructed as follows. One works with the category PER which is $\Gamma(\mathcal{P})$ (the functor $\Gamma : \mathcal{E}\!f\!f \to$ Set also maps internal categories to small categories), and functors on (powers of) PER which are also Γ-images of internal functors in $\mathcal{E}\!f\!f$; i.e. realizable functors. One has operations on these functors which are no longer limits, because the reasoning we did about cones, using the Uniformity Principle, no longer applies, but still give sound interpretations for the constructs of type theories. There is by now a vast literature on PER models, of which the following just form a small sample: [1],[6],[10],[20],[34],[38],[45],[76],[139],[130],[140]. Moreover, treatments in textbooks are also available ([111],[7],[78]).

For an analysis of the precise completeness properties of PER, see also [132, 138].

3.5   Set Theory in $\mathcal{E}\!f\!f$

There are at least two interesting models of constructive set theories in $\mathcal{E}\!f\!f$, one of which I present in some detail; the other is indicated (and references are given).

3.5.1   The McCarty model for IZF

Intuitionistic Set Theory IZF is the theory (in intuitionistic logic) in the language with one binary relation symbol ϵ. Its axioms are similar to those of ZF, with the following differences: the axiom of Foundation (every nonempty set has an ϵ-minimal element), which implies Excluded Middle, is replaced by ϵ-Induction:

$$\forall x (\forall y (y \epsilon x \to \phi(y)) \to \phi(x)) \to \forall x \phi(x)$$

and Replacement is 'replaced' by the scheme of Collection:

$$\forall y (y \epsilon x \to \exists w \phi(y, w)) \to \exists z \forall y (y \epsilon x \to \exists w (w \epsilon z \land \phi(y, w)))$$

Recall that Replacement is the scheme like Collection but with an $\exists!w$ in the premiss. Classically, the two schemes are equivalent. The switch from Replacement to Collection is not forced on us; in fact there is also a system IZF_R which has Replacement instead of Collection.

IZF was throroughly studied in the 1970's and 1980's, also using realizability methods, by H. Friedman and A. Scedrov(see e.g. [51, 53, 55, 54, 52, 50, 49]; for an overview, see also [142]), J. Myhill ([118, 117]), W. Powell ([128]), R. Grayson ([60]), M. Beeson ([17]) and others.

One of the obtained results is that IZF and IZF_R are *different*. A theory T of sets is said to have the *set existence property* if whenever $T \vdash \exists x \phi(x)$, there is a formula $\chi(x)$ such that $T \vdash \exists! x \chi(x)$ and $T \vdash \forall x (\chi(x) \to \phi(x))$ (in a language without constants, the formula χ is as close as we can get to a 'term'). Friedman had shown in [51] that IZF_R has the set existence property; [50] proves that IZF hasn't.

The framework I shall use in this section is that of *Algebraic Set Theory*, developed by A. Joyal and I. Moerdijk ([85]). Joyal and Moerdijk formulate axioms for when a class of arrows in a topos $\mathcal{E}$ is called a *class of* IZF-*small maps* (or, 'class of small maps' for short. Their framework is more general than the topos context, but that generality doesn't concern us here). They give the following definition.

Definition 3.5.1 (Joyal-Moerdijk) Let κ be a cardinal number. An arrow $X \xrightarrow{f} Y$ in $\mathcal{E}\!f\!f$ is called κ-*small* if there is a commutative diagram

$$
\begin{array}{ccc}
Q & \longrightarrow & X \\
{\scriptstyle p}\downarrow & & \downarrow{\scriptstyle f} \\
P & \xrightarrow{\pi} & Y
\end{array}
$$

with the following properties:

i) P and Q are projective;

ii) π is an epimorphism;

iii) the canonical arrow from Q to the pullback $P \times_Y X$ is an epimorphism;

iv)   for every $x \in \Gamma(P)$, the fibre $\Gamma(p)^{-1}(x)$ has cardinality $< \kappa$.

An object X is κ-small if the unique map $X \to 1$ is κ-small.

The notion of κ-small is some measure of the 'size' of an object or arrow. The following proposition gives an example: although there are only two 'points' $1 \to \Omega$ in $\mathcal{E}ff$, there are 'many truth-values':

Proposition 3.5.2

i)   If Ω is κ-small, then $\kappa > 2^\omega$;

ii)   There is an object X with $\Gamma(X) \cong 1$, yet if X is κ-small then $\kappa > 2^\omega$.

Proof. For i), it is enough to show that whenever P is projective and P surjects onto Ω, then $|\Gamma(P)| \geq 2^\omega$. We may assume P is a partitioned assembly (P, α) with $\alpha : P \to \mathbb{N}$. Then for every functional relation F from P to Ω there is a function $f : P \to \mathcal{P}(\mathbb{N})$ such that

$$F(x, A) \leftrightarrow \{\alpha(x)\} \wedge [f(x) \leftrightarrow A]$$

holds in the effective tripos; so we assume that F is equal to the expression on the right hand side.

Suppose e realizes that F represents an epimorphism, so for every A and every $n \in E(A)$ there is an x such that $en \in F(x, A)$. For Ω we have that $\bigcap_{A \in \mathcal{P}(\mathbb{N})} E(A) \neq \emptyset$; if I is an element of that set then for all A there is x such that $eI \in F(x, A) = \{\alpha(x)\} \wedge [f(x) \leftrightarrow A]$. We see that if we restrict P to those elements x for which $\alpha(x) = p_0(eI)$, then we have still an epimorphism; in other words we may assume that P is a sheaf, that F is given by $F(x, A) = [f9x) \leftrightarrow A]$, and for all A there is x with $eI \in [f(x) \leftrightarrow A]$. For $x \in P$ define

$$U_x = \{A \in \mathcal{P}(\mathbb{N}) \,|\, eI \in [f(x) \leftrightarrow A]\}$$

Then from eI we find an element J such that for every x,

$$J \in \bigcap_{A, A' \in U_x} (A \to A')$$

Applying this to $A = A' = \{n\}$ for each n we see that J must be an index for the identity function. Hence if $J \in A \to A'$, $A \subseteq A'$ must hold. It follows that every U_x can contain at most one A; there are at least 2^ω x's in P.

For ii), we repeat the story for the object internally defined in $\mathcal{E}\!f\!f$ as

$$T = \{p \in \Omega \,|\, \neg\neg p\}$$

which is given as $(\{A \in \mathcal{P}(\mathbb{N}) \,|\, A \neq \emptyset\}, \leftrightarrow)$. By the same reasonimg as for i) we see that every projective cover of T has cardinality at least 2^ω; and of course $\Gamma(T) \cong 1$. ∎

Recall that a cardinal $\kappa > \omega$ is *strongly inaccessible* if κ is regular and for every $\lambda < \kappa$ it holds that $2^\lambda < \kappa$.

Proposition 3.5.3 (Joyal-Moerdijk) *Suppose κ is a strongly inaccessible cardinal. Then the κ-small maps in $\mathcal{E}\!f\!f$ form a class of IZF-small maps.*

Given a class $\mathcal{S}$ of small maps in a topos $\mathcal{E}$, there is the notion of an $\mathcal{S}$-complete suplattice: suppose $(L, \leq)$ is a partial order in $\mathcal{E}$; then we have a 'pointwise' partial order on the set of arrows $\mathcal{E}(X, L)$ for each object X, and for every $f : Y \to X$ an order-preserving map $\mathcal{E}(f, L) :$ $\mathcal{E}(X, L) \to \mathcal{E}(Y, L)$ by composition with f. We say that $(L, \leq)$ is an $\mathcal{S}$-*complete suplattice* if for each $f \in \mathcal{S}$ the map $\mathcal{E}(f, L)$ has a left adjoint $\bigvee_f$, which system of left adjoints satisfies the Beck-Chevalley condition: if the square

$$
\begin{array}{ccc}
Y' & \xrightarrow{\;g\;} & Y \\
{\scriptstyle f'}\downarrow & & \downarrow{\scriptstyle f} \\
X' & \xrightarrow[\;k\;]{} & X
\end{array}
$$

is a pullback diagram in $\mathcal{E}$ with $f \in \mathcal{S}$, then for any $\phi : Y \to L$ we have $\bigvee_{f'}(\phi g) = (\bigvee_f(\phi))k$ (the axioms for a class of small maps include the requirement that thay are stable under pullback, so in this case also $f' \in \mathcal{S}$).

Of course, we think of the map $\bigvee_f(\phi)$ as the map $x \mapsto \bigvee_{f(y)=x} \phi(y)$.

The axioms for a class of small maps also imply that for every object X of $\mathcal{E}$ we have a 'small power object' : an object $\mathcal{P}_s(X)$ together with a subobject $\in_X \rightarrowtail X \times \mathcal{P}_s(X)$ such that the second projection $\in_X \to \mathcal{P}_s(X)$ is in $\mathcal{S}$ and which has the property that for arbitrary Y and subobject $R \rightarrowtail X \times Y$ such that the composition $R \to X \times Y \to Y$ is in $\mathcal{S}$, there is a unique arrow $\chi_R : Y \to \mathcal{P}_s(X)$ such that we have a pullback diagram

$$
\begin{array}{ccc}
R & \longrightarrow & \in_X \\
\downarrow & & \downarrow \\
X \times Y & \xrightarrow{\ \mathrm{id}_X \times \chi_R\ } & X \times \mathcal{P}_s(X)
\end{array}
$$

This means that we have an 'internal supremum operation' $\bigvee : \mathcal{P}_s(L) \to L$, which is defined as $\bigvee_{\pi_2}(\pi_1)$, where π_1 and π_2 are the projections

$$
\begin{array}{c}
\mathcal{P}_s(L) \\
{\scriptstyle \pi_2}\big\uparrow \\
\in_L \xrightarrow{\ \pi_1\ } L
\end{array}
$$

Obviously, $\mathcal{P}_s(X)$ is a subobject of $\mathcal{P}(X)$.

A *morphism* of $\mathcal{S}$-complete suplattices $L \xrightarrow{\alpha} M$ is an arrow which is order-preserving and such that $\alpha(\bigvee_f \phi) = \bigvee_f(\alpha\phi)$ for each $f : Y \to X$ in $\mathcal{S}$ and each $\phi : Y \to L$.

Definition 3.5.4 (Joyal-Moerdijk) A ZF-*algebra* is an $\mathcal{S}$-complete suplattice $(L, \leq)$ together with a 'successor map' $s : L \to L$.

A *morphism of* ZF-algebras $(L, \leq, s) \to (M, \leq, t)$ is a map $f : L \to M$ which is a morphism of $\mathcal{S}$-complete suplattices and satisfies $fs = tf$.

Theorem 3.5.5 (Joyal-Moerdijk) *Suppose $\mathcal{S}$ is a class of small maps in a topos $\mathcal{E}$. Then the category of ZF-algebras has an initial object, the free ZF-algebra.*

Theorem 3.5.6 (Joyal-Moerdijk) *Let $(L, \leq, s)$ be the free ZF-algebra for a class of small maps in a topos $\mathcal{E}$. Define a relation $\epsilon \rightarrowtail L \times L$ by*

$$ x\epsilon y \leftrightarrow s(x) \leq y $$

Then (L, ϵ) is a model of IZF.

The following lemma is helpful for identifying the free ZF-algebra.

Lemma 3.5.7 ([92]) *Suppose $\mathcal{S}$ is a class of small maps in a topos $\mathcal{E}$ and $(L, \leq, \sigma)$ is a ZF-algebra in $\mathcal{E}$, with induced relation ϵ as in 3.5.6. The $(L, \leq, \sigma)$ is initial if and only if the following conditions hold:*

1. *Extensionality:* $\forall xy(\forall z(z\epsilon x \rightarrow z\epsilon y) \rightarrow x \leq y)$

2. *Strict mono:* $\forall xy(\sigma(x) \leq \sigma(y) \rightarrow x = y)$

3. *Smallness: the map* $\epsilon \rightarrowtail L \times L \xrightarrow{\pi_2} L$ *is in* $\mathcal{S}$

   (equivalently: $\forall x(\{y \in L \mid y\epsilon x\} \in \mathcal{P}_s(L)))$

4. *Irreducibility of successors:*
   $$\forall x \forall E \in \mathcal{P}_s(L)\,[\sigma(x) \leq \bigvee(E) \rightarrow \exists y(y \in_L E \wedge \sigma(x) \leq y)]$$

5. ϵ-*Induction:*
   $$\forall A \in \mathcal{P}(L)\,[\forall x(\forall y(y\epsilon x \rightarrow y \in A) \rightarrow x \in A) \rightarrow A = L]$$

Proof. That the conditions are necessary, is part of the proof of theorem 3.5.6 and can be found in the relevant section of [85]. I sketch the proof that they are sufficient.

We start by noting that conditions 1. and 3. imply that $\forall x \in L\,(x = \bigvee_{y\epsilon x} \sigma(y))$ holds.

Hence, for any homomorphism ϕ of ZF-algebras from L to (M, τ), $\forall x \in L\,(\phi(x) = \bigvee_{y\epsilon x} \tau(\phi(x))$ holds. Conversely, if this last formula is true then ϕ is a homomorphism of ZF-algebras: since $\forall x \in L\,(\forall y \in L\,(y\epsilon\sigma(x) \leftrightarrow y = x))$ holds by 2. and the definition of ϵ, also $\forall x \in L\,(\bigvee_{y\epsilon\sigma(x)} \tau(\phi(y)) = \tau(\phi(x)))$ is true, which means that the map ϕ commutes with the successor operations. Commutation with small sups follows too, because for $E \in \mathcal{P}_s(L)$, $\bigvee_{e\in E} \phi(e) = \bigvee_{e\in E} \bigvee_{y\epsilon e} \tau(\phi(y))$ holds by assumption on ϕ; moreover, the equalities

$$\bigvee_{e\in E} \bigvee_{y\epsilon e} \tau(\phi(y)) = \bigvee_{y\epsilon \bigvee E} \tau(\phi(y)) = \phi(\bigvee E)$$

hold by, respectively, assumption on ϕ, 4. and assumption on ϕ again.

Now suppose that ϕ and ψ are two homomorphisms of ZF-algebras from L to M. Using 5. we can show that $\phi = \psi$ must hold: let $A = \{x \in L \mid \phi(x) = \psi(x)\}$ (and $Z = 1$). From the fact that both ϕ and ψ satisfy the identity just derived it is immediate that A satisfies the hypothesis of the ϵ-Induction scheme, so $A = L$ and $\phi = \psi$.

So, there exists at most one homomorphism of ZF-algebras from L to M. In order to prove that one exists, we first construct a 'transitive closure' operation in L. Let $T = \{x \in L \mid \forall y \epsilon x \forall z \epsilon y \, (z \epsilon x)\}$. Then define

$$A = \{x \in L \mid \exists y \in L \, (y \in T \wedge x \le y \wedge \forall z \in T \, (x \le z \to y \le z))\}$$

We write $TC(x)$ for the unique $y \in L$, if it exists, which witnesses that $x \in A$ (note that $TC(x)$ is indeed uniquely determined). For an application of ϵ-Induction to A, assume $\forall y \epsilon x \, (y \in A)$. By condition 3. and the uniqueness just mentioned we can form $x \vee \bigvee_{z \epsilon x} TC(z)$ and it is easy to see that this element witnesses that $x \in A$. So $A = L$ and we have a map $TC : L \to L$ with the expected properties.

In the following we shall often confuse an element $x \in L$ with the (small) subset $\{y \in L \mid y \epsilon x\}$; by 1., this is legitimate.

Let (M, τ) be any ZF-algebra. Define the following subset of L:

$$B = \{x \in L \mid \exists! f_x : TC(x) \to M \, \forall y \epsilon TC(x)(f_x(y) = \bigvee_{z \epsilon y} \tau(f_x(z)))\}$$

We wish to apply ϵ-Induction to B. Suppose $\forall y \epsilon x (y \in B)$. We have to find $f_x : TC(x) \to M$. By construction, $TC(x) = x \vee \bigvee_{z \epsilon x} TC(z)$. Hence, by 4., $y \epsilon TC(x)$ is equivalent to $y \epsilon x \vee \exists z \epsilon x (y \epsilon TC(z))$.

For $y \epsilon x$ put $f_x(y) = \bigvee_{w \epsilon y} \tau(f_y(w))$; for $y \epsilon TC(z)$, $z \epsilon x$ put $f_x(y) = f_z(y)$. This is well-defined, because if both cases apply ($y \epsilon x$, $y \epsilon TC(z)$, $z \epsilon x$) then by the induction hypothesis $y \in B$ and consequently the uniqueness of f_y, f_y must agree with the restriction of F_z to $TC(y)$, and hence

$$\bigvee_{w \epsilon y} \tau(f_y(w)) = \bigvee_{w \epsilon y} \tau(f_z(w)) = f_z(y)$$

A similar reasoning applies if for $z, z' \epsilon x$, $y \epsilon TC(z)$ and $y \epsilon TC(z')$. Clearly, the map f_x thus defined satisfies the condition in the definition of the set B, and it is unique with this property. So $x \in B$. We have proved the hypothesis of ϵ-Induction for B, so $B = L$.

We can now define a homomorphism of ZF-algebras $\phi : L \to M$ by $\phi(x) = f_{\sigma(x)}(x)$. The verification that ϕ is a homomorphism of ZF-algebras is now straightforward, and left to the reader. ∎

Most conditions of lemma 3.5.7 are easy to check. The most problematic one is ϵ-Induction, which means that the relation ϵ is internally well-founded on L. We make the following definition.

Definition 3.5.8 Let R be a binary relation on an object X of a topos $\mathcal{E}$. The object Prog_X of 'progressive subsets of X w.r.t. R' is defined as

$$\mathrm{Prog}_X = \{Y \in \mathcal{P}(X) \mid \forall x(\forall y(R(y,x) \to y \in Y) \to x \in Y)\}$$

We write also $\mathrm{Prog}_X(Y)$ for $Y \in \mathrm{Prog}_X$.

The relation R is *internally well-founded* on X if the sentence

$$\forall Y \in \mathcal{P}(X)(\mathrm{Prog}_X(Y) \to Y = X)$$

is true in $\mathcal{E}$. R is *almost well-founded* if

$$\forall Y \in \mathcal{P}_{\neg\neg}(X)(\mathrm{Prog}_X(Y) \to Y = X)$$

holds in $\mathcal{E}$.

For $\mathcal{E}\!f\!f$ we have the following fact, first shown in [66].

Theorem 3.5.9 *For a binary relation R on an object X of $\mathcal{E}\!f\!f$ the following three assertions are equivalent:*

i) R is internally well-founded on X;

ii) R is almost well-founded on X;

iii) $\Gamma(R)$ is well-founded on $\Gamma(X)$.

Proof. i) $\Rightarrow$ ii) is trivial.

For ii) $\Rightarrow$ iii), recall that the object $\mathcal{P}_{\neg\neg}(X)$ is $\nabla(\mathcal{P}(\Gamma(X)))$; subsets of $\Gamma(X)$ are in 1-1 correspondence with $\neg\neg$-closed subobjects of X. If $Y \subseteq \Gamma(X)$ and Y is progressive w.r.t. $\Gamma(R)$ then Y corresponds to an element $\tilde{Y}$ of $\mathcal{P}_{\neg\neg}(X)$, and for this element we will have $\neg\neg\mathrm{Prog}_X(\tilde{Y})$ w.r.t. R. It is easily seen that for $\neg\neg$-closed $\tilde{Y}$, $\neg\neg\mathrm{Prog}_X(\tilde{Y})$ implies $\mathrm{Prog}_X(\tilde{Y})$; hence $\tilde{Y} = X$ by almost well-foundedness; so $Y = \Gamma(X)$ and $\Gamma(R)$ is well-founded on $\Gamma(X)$, as desired.

iii) $\Rightarrow$ i). By the recursion theorem, pick a number r such that for all e, n,

$$ren \simeq en(\langle mq \rangle rem)$$

Let $X = (X, \sim)$; suppose $P : X \to \mathcal{P}(\mathbb{N})$ represents an element of $\mathcal{P}(X)$.

Claim: if $e \in [\![\mathrm{Prog}_X(P)]\!]$ then $re \in [\![\forall x{:}X.P(x)]\!]$.

Clearly, the Claim establishes the required implication iii) $\Rightarrow$ i). Now suppose $e \in [\![\mathrm{Prog}_X(P)]\!]$.

Let $\cong$ be the equivalence relation on X given by $x \cong x'$ iff $[x \sim x'] \neq \emptyset$, so $\Gamma(X) = \{x \in X \mid E(x) \neq \emptyset\}/\cong$. Define $U \subseteq X$ by

$$U = \{x \in X \mid \forall y \in X(R(y, x) \neq \emptyset \Rightarrow \forall m \in E(y)(rem \in P(y)))\}$$

Then U is closed under $\cong$. We shall prove that $U = X$.

Since $e \in [\![\mathrm{Prog}_X(P)]\!]$, we have for all $x \in X$ and $n \in E(x)$ that $en{\downarrow}$ and

$$\forall b(b \in [\![\forall y{:}X(R(y, x) \to P(y))]\!] \Rightarrow enb{\downarrow} \wedge enb \in [\![P(x)]\!])$$

Now suppose for $x \in X$ that $\{y \in X \mid R(y, x) \neq \emptyset\}$ is a subset of U. Then

$$\forall yv \in X \forall m \in E(v)(R(y, x) \neq \emptyset \wedge R(v, y) \neq \emptyset \Rightarrow rem \in P(v))$$

so for all $y \in X$ with $R(y, x) \neq \emptyset$ we have

$$\langle mq \rangle rem \in [\![\forall v{:}X(R(v, y) \to P(v))]\!]$$

This implies that for every $y \in X$ with $R(y,x) \neq \emptyset$ we have

$$en(\langle mq \rangle rem) \in P(y)$$

which means $ren \in P(y)$ by choice of r. We conclude that $x \in U$. Therefore,

$$\forall x \in X(\{y \in X | \Gamma(R)(y,x)\} \subseteq U \Rightarrow x \in U)$$

By well-foundedness of $\Gamma(R)$, $U = X$. Hence, for all $x \in X$ and all $n \in E(x)$, $en\downarrow$ and $en(\langle mq \rangle rem) \in [\![P(x)]\!]$, i.e. $ren \in P(x)$. This means that $re \in [\![\forall x{:}X.P(x)]\!]$, as claimed.   ∎

The initial ZF-algebra in $\mathcal{E}\!f\!f$ (for the class of small maps of definition 3.5.1) will turn out to be a model of IZF that is already familiar from the literature: namely, the *McCarty realizability model* of IZF, introduced in [103] and studied further in [104, 105, 106]. In order to view this as an object of $\mathcal{E}\!f\!f$ (and actually also for definition 3.5.1 to work), we have to make a set-theoretic assumption: the existence of a strongly inaccessible cardinal.

McCarty defined sets V_α for each ordinal α, recursively as follows:

$$V_\alpha \;=\; \bigcup_{\beta < \alpha} \mathcal{P}(\mathbb{N} \times V_\beta)$$

Then he put $V = \bigcup_\alpha V_\alpha$.

Then, relations 'n realizes $a\epsilon b$' and 'n realizes $a = b$' (with n a natural number, a, b ranging over V) are defined by a simultaneous recursion:

n realizes $a\epsilon b$ if and only if there is a $c \in V$ such that
                                    $(p_0 n, c) \in b$ and $p_1 n$ realizes $a = c$
n realizes $a = b$ if and only if for all pairs (m, d) in V :
                                    if $(m, d) \in a$ then $p_0 nm$ realizes $d\epsilon b$, and
                                    if $(m, d) \in b$ then $p_1 nm$ realizes $d\epsilon a$

The reader who has seen a forcing proof in Set Theory will immediately notice the formal analogy with the definition of a generic extension $M[G]$.

The definition is now extended to 'n realizes ϕ' where ϕ is a sentence in the language of ZF with parameters from V. The clauses for $\wedge$, $\neg$, $\vee$ and $\rightarrow$ are the same as for Kleene realizability as given in section 3.1, and the clauses for $\forall$ and $\exists$ are *uniform*:

$$n \text{ realizes } \forall x \phi \quad \text{if for all } a \in V, n \text{ realizes } \phi(a)$$
$$n \text{ realizes } \exists x \phi \quad \text{if for some } a \in V, n \text{ realizes } \phi(a)$$

I call this interpretation the *McCarty model*

Theorem 3.5.10 (McCarty) *For every theorem ϕ of IZF there is a number n such that n realizes ϕ.*

In this book, I wish to connect this theorem to the Joyal-Moerdijk setup, and show that it can be seen as a consequence of theorem 3.5.6. This will follow once we have shown the following:

i)   there is an object $\mathcal{W}$ in $\mathcal{E}ff$ together with a binary relation ϵ on it, such that truth in $\mathcal{E}ff$ of sentences in the language of ZF, for the object $\mathcal{W}$, is captured exactly by McCarty's realizability definition;

ii) there is a ZF-algebra structure $(\leq, \sigma)$ on $\mathcal{W}$ such that ϵ is given by: $a\epsilon b$ iff $\sigma(a) \leq b$;

iii) this ZF-algebra is initial.

We start by defining the object $\mathcal{W}$ and the relation ϵ. Fix a strongly inaccessible cardinal κ. Then $\mathcal{W} = (V_\kappa, \sim)$, where

$$[a \sim b] = \{n \mid n \text{ realizes } a = b\}$$

and $\epsilon : V_\kappa \times V_\kappa \rightarrow \mathcal{P}(\mathbb{N})$ is given by

$$[a\epsilon b] = \{n \mid n \text{ realizes } a\epsilon b\}$$

Proposition 3.5.11 $\mathcal{W} = (V_\kappa, \sim)$ *is a well-defined object of $\mathcal{E}ff$ and ϵ is a strict relation for $\sim$.*

Proof. A quick inspection of the definition of 'n realizes $a = b$' suffices to see that if n realizes $a = b$, then $p(p_1 n)(p_0 n)$ realizes $b = a$, so $\sim$ is symmetric. So in order to prove the other properties we have to construct partial recursive functions ζ, η and θ such that for all $a, b, c \in V_\kappa$ and $n, n' \in \mathbb{N}$:

1)   if n realizes $a = b$ and n' realizes $b = c$ then $\zeta n n'$ realizes $a = c$;

2)   if n realizes $a = b$ and n' realizes $b \epsilon c$ then $\eta n n'$ realizes $a \epsilon c$;

3)   if n realizes $a = b$ and n' realizes $c \epsilon a$ then $\theta n n'$ realizes $c \epsilon b$.

We shall define these functions in one go, using the (simultaneous) recursion theorem. For readability, in this proof I write $[\,,\,]$ for pairs (but still use the projections p_0, p_1). Let s be an element which realizes the symmetry of $\sim$ (as seen above). Define ζ, η, θ such that for all n, n':

$$\begin{aligned}
\zeta n n' &\simeq [\langle m \rangle \theta n'(p_0 n m), \langle m \rangle \theta(sn)(p_1 n' m)] \\
\eta n n' &\simeq [p_0 n', \zeta n(p_1 n')] \\
\theta n n' &\simeq \eta(p_1 n')(p_0 n(p_0 n'))
\end{aligned}$$

We shall now prove the following induction hypothesis $P(\alpha)$ for $\alpha < \kappa$:

a)   For $a, b, c \in V_\alpha$, 1) holds;

b)   For $c \in V_\alpha$, $a, b \in \bigcup_{\beta < \alpha} V_\beta$, 2) holds;

c)   For $a, b \in V_\alpha$, $c \in \bigcup_{\beta < \alpha} V_\beta$, 3) holds.

Clearly it suffices to see that $P(\alpha)$ is true for all $\alpha < \kappa$. So assume that a), b), c) hold for all $\beta < \alpha$; this is the induction hypothesis.

We start by proving b) for α. So assume $c \in V_\alpha$, $a, b \in \bigcup_{\beta < \alpha} V_\beta$, and n realizes $a = b$, n' realizes $b \epsilon c$. This means that there is $e \in V$ such that $(p_0 n', e) \in c$ and $p_1 n'$ realizes $b = e$. Then both e and b are elements of $\bigcup_{\beta < \alpha} V_\beta$, so we may apply induction hypothesis a) to conclude that $\alpha n(p_1 n')$ realizes $a = e$. That implies that $[p_0 n', \alpha n(p_1 n')]$ realizes $a \epsilon c$; in other words, $\eta n n'$ realizes $a \epsilon c$, as desired.

Next we prove c) for α; so assume $a, b \in V_\alpha$, $c \in \bigcup_{\beta < \alpha} V_\beta$ and n realizes $a = b$, n' realizes $c \epsilon a$. Then there is an e such that $(p_0 n', e) \in a$

ad $p_1 n'$ realizes $c = e$. Since n realizes $a = b$ we have $p_0 n(p_0 n')$ realizes $e \epsilon b$. We have $b \in V_\alpha$ and $e, c \in \bigcup_{\beta < \alpha} V_\beta$. Therefore by b) for α, which we have already proved, we have that $\eta(p_1 n')(p_0 n(p_1 n'))$ realizes $c \epsilon b$; that is, $\theta n n'$ realizes $c \epsilon b$ as desired.

Finally we prove a) for α. Assume $a, b, c \in V_\alpha$ and n realizes $a = b$, n' realizes $b = c$. Suppose $(m, d) \in a$. Then $p_0 n m$ realizes $d \epsilon b$. Now $d \in \bigcup_{\beta < \alpha} V_\beta$, so by c) for α, already established, we conclude that $\theta n'(p_0 n m)$ realizes $d \epsilon c$. Similarly, the assumption $(m, d) \in c$ leads to the conclusion that $\theta(sn)(p_1 n'm)$ realizes $d \epsilon a$. We see that

$$\zeta n n' = [\langle m \rangle \theta n'(p_0 n m), \langle m \rangle \theta(sn)(p_1 n'm)]$$

realizes $a = c$, which is what we had to show. ∎

Proposition 3.5.12 *The object $\mathcal{W}$ is uniform.*

Proof. We use again $[,]$ for pairs. By the recursion theorem there is an index f such that for all n, $fn = [n, [f, f]]$. Let $e = [f, f]$, so for all n, $p_0 e n = [n, e]$ and $p_1 e n = [n, e]$. We prove by induction on $\alpha < \kappa$ that $e \in [a \sim a]$ for all $a \in V_\alpha$. Suppose this holds for all $\beta < \alpha$ and let $a \in V_\alpha$. If $(m, d) \in a$, then since $d \in \bigcup_{\beta < \alpha} V_\beta$, by induction hypothesis e realizes $d = d$. We have then that $p_0 e m = [m, e]$ realizes $d \epsilon a$. Similarly, $p_1 e m$ realizes $d \epsilon a$. So by definition of 'n realizes $a = b$' we see that e realizes $a = a$, i.e. $e \in [a \sim a]$. ∎

It is now clear that McCarty's realizability is exactly capturing truth in $\mathcal{E}ff$ for the structure $(\mathcal{W}, \epsilon)$. The following proposition is straightforward to prove, and left to you.

Proposition 3.5.13 *$\mathcal{W}$ satisfies the axiom of extensionality:*

$$\mathcal{W} \models \forall xy (\forall z (z \epsilon x \leftrightarrow z \epsilon y) \rightarrow x = y)$$

Theorem 3.5.14 *The object $\mathcal{W}$ admits the structure of a ZF-algebra $(\mathcal{W}, \leq, \sigma)$ such that the following properties hold:*

i) *The relation ϵ on $\mathcal{W}$ is induced from the ZF-algebra structure in the way of theorem 3.5.6;*

ii) $(\mathcal{W}, \leq, \sigma)$ *is initial.*

Proof. The successor map σ is represented by the relation

$$S(x, y) \equiv [\forall z (z \epsilon y \leftrightarrow z = x]$$

Then S is strict by uniformity of $\mathcal{W}$, relational by 3.5.11 and single-valued by 3.5.13. S is also total since for any $a \in V_\kappa$, if $a \in V_\beta$ we have $a' = \mathbb{N} \times \{a\} \in V_{\beta+1}$, and it is easy to find a canonical element of $S(a, a')$.

The order $\leq$ on $\mathcal{W}$ is the subset order: $x \leq y \leftrightarrow x \subseteq y \leftrightarrow \forall z (z \epsilon x \rightarrow z \epsilon y)$. By 3.5.13 this relation is antisymmetric.

We see that ϵ is indeed given by $x \epsilon y \leftrightarrow \sigma(x) \leq y$, so point i) of te theorem is proved once we have shown that $\mathcal{W}$ has small suprema.

Suppose $g : X \rightarrow Y$ is in $\mathcal{S}$ and $f : X \rightarrow \mathcal{W}$ is any arrow. If f is represented by F and g by G, we let $\bigvee_g(f)$ be represented by H where

$$H(y, a) = E(y) \wedge [\forall b (b \epsilon a \leftrightarrow \exists x \exists c (F(x, y) \wedge G(x, c) \wedge b \epsilon c)]$$

which is clearly strict, relational and single-valued. For totality, we have to use the fact that g is in $\mathcal{S}$, which implies that the fibres of $\Gamma(g)$ have cardinality $< \kappa$.

Given $y \in Y$, choose for every $\xi \in \Gamma(g)^{-1}([y])$ an element $a_\xi \in \Gamma(f)(\xi)$. There are $< \kappa$ many ξ's so there is a $\beta < \kappa$ such that all a_ξ's are in V_β. Now define

$$U_y = \{(n, b) \mid \exists x (p_0 n \in F(x, y) \wedge p_0(p_1 n) \in G(x, a_\xi) \wedge (p_1(p_1 n), b) \in a_{[x]})\}$$

Then $U_y \in V_\beta$ and it is straightforward to find an element of

$$\bigcap_y (E(y) \rightarrow H(y, U_y))$$

This proves that H represents an arrow $\bigvee_g(f)$ in $\mathcal{E}ff$; the check that it has the right properties of a supremum along g is straightforward. This completes the proof that $(\mathcal{W}, \leq, \sigma)$ is a ZF-algebra and that i) in the theorem holds.

We must prove that ii) holds: that $(\mathcal{W}, \leq, \sigma)$ is the initial ZF-algebra. For this we check the conditions of Lemma 3.5.7. Conditions 1 (Extensionality), 2 (Strict mono), and 4 (Irreducibility of successors) should be easy by now. For 3 (Smallness), we consider the diagram

$$
\begin{array}{ccc}
P & \xrightarrow{\ r\ } & \epsilon \\
{\scriptstyle q}\downarrow & & \downarrow{\scriptstyle \pi_2} \\
\nabla(V_\kappa) & \longrightarrow & \mathcal{W}
\end{array}
$$

where the map $\nabla(V_\kappa) \to \mathcal{W}$ is the obvious quotient, and P is the partitioned assembly of triples $\{(n, a, b) \mid (n, a) \in b\}$ with $E((n, a, b)) = \{n\}$ and $q : P \to \nabla(V_\kappa)$ sends (n, a, b) to b. The map $r : P \to \epsilon$ is induced by the function which sends (n, a, b) to (a, b); this function is tracked since if $(n, a, b) \in P$ then *pen* realizes $a \epsilon b$, if $e \in \bigcap_{a \in V_\kappa} E(a)$. It is easy to verify that r is epi, and the canonical factorization of r through the pullback of

$$
\begin{array}{c}
\epsilon \\
\downarrow{\scriptstyle \pi_2} \\
\nabla(V_\kappa) \longrightarrow \mathcal{W}
\end{array}
$$

is epi too.

The fibre $q^{-1}(b)$ is a subset of $\mathbb{N} \times V_\beta$ (if $b \in V_\beta$), and hence has cardinality $< \kappa$. So indeed $\pi_2 : \epsilon \to \mathcal{W}$ is in $\mathcal{S}$, as desired.

For the last requirement, 5 (ϵ-Induction) we invoke theorem 3.5.9 and prove that the relation $\Gamma(\epsilon)$ on $\Gamma(\mathcal{W})$ is well-founded in Set. This is easy: let $f : \Gamma(\mathcal{W}) \to \kappa$ be such that $f(\xi)$ is the least $\beta < \kappa$ such that there is an element of ξ in V_β. Obviously, if a pair (η, ξ) is in $\Gamma(\epsilon)$ then $f(\eta) < f(\xi)$. So $\Gamma(\epsilon)$ is well-founded. ■

An alternative way of building up the model $\mathcal{W}$ allows us to formulate an interesting correlation between power sets in $\mathcal{W}$ and power objects in $\mathcal{EFF}$. Define sets W_α, $\alpha < \kappa$ by:

$$
\begin{array}{rcl}
W_0 & = & \emptyset \\
W_{\alpha+1} & = & \mathcal{P}(\mathbb{N} \times W_\alpha) \\
W_\lambda & = & \bigcup_{\beta < \lambda} W_\beta \qquad (\lambda \text{ limit})
\end{array}
$$

Then clearly, $V_\kappa = \bigcup_{\alpha < \kappa} W_\alpha$. For $\alpha < \kappa$, let $\mathcal{W}_\alpha$ be the object $(W_\alpha, \sim)$ (restricted equality from $\mathcal{W}$).

Proposition 3.5.15 $\mathcal{W}_{\alpha+1}$ *is isomorphic to the power object* $\mathcal{P}(\mathcal{W}_\alpha)$, *and under this isomorphism the element relation* $\in \rightarrowtail \mathcal{W}_\alpha \times \mathcal{W}_{\alpha+1}$ *is the restriction of the relation* $\epsilon \rightarrowtail \mathcal{W} \times \mathcal{W}$ *to* $\mathcal{W}_\alpha \times \mathcal{W}_{\alpha+1}$.

Proof. This is basically a triviality, keeping in mind the proof of proposition 2.4.7. We write $\mathcal{W}_{\alpha+1}$ as $\mathcal{P}(\mathbb{N})^{\mathcal{W}_\alpha}$, and then we have for $f, g \in \mathcal{W}_{\alpha+1}$:

$$[f = g] \;=\; \bigcap_{a,b \in W_\alpha} \left([a \sim b] \to [f(a) \leftrightarrow g(b)] \right)$$

and this is clearly isomorphic to $f \sim g$.

Moreover for $b \in \mathcal{W}_\alpha$, $a \in \mathcal{W}_{\alpha+1}$ we have

$$[b \in a] \;=\; [\exists b' \in W_\alpha \, (a(b') \wedge b \sim b')]$$

which is the same as $b \epsilon a$.

From the cited proof we have that if $e \in \bigcap_{b \in W_\alpha} E(b)$ and m is such that for all n, $p_0 m n = p n e$ and $p_1 m n = p n e$, then $m \in \bigcap_{a \in W_{\alpha+1}} E(a)$. Now we see that the element e constructed in the proof of 3.5.12, is an element of $\bigcap_{\alpha < \kappa} \bigcap_{a \in W_\alpha} E(a)$. ∎

Remark. One philosophical merit of this treatment, where McCarty's model (which he calls $V(Kl)$) is embedded in $\mathcal{E}\!f\!f$, is that it answers the following point, discussed in [103] (p.135):

> We are always tempted (and, in fact, we often succumb to the temptation) to refer to $V(Kl)$ as a model or class model of IZF. It has been objected (by Solomon Feferman, among others) that this represents a serious transgression of the rules of usage among logicians. The idea behind this objection seems to be that interpretation over $V(Kl)$ is a mere interpretation and that a "real" interpretation of a language over a "real" model goes by familiar Tarski recursion on truth conditions.

The theory of general models for first order languages in toposes is well developed, and the generalization of Tarski's truth definition to arbitrary categories is the *Kripke-Joyal semantics*, which is explained in every text book on topos theory. Interpreting this semantics in $\mathcal{E}ff$ for the structure $(\mathcal{W}, \epsilon)$ gives McCarty's interpretation as we have seen, so from the point of view of $\mathcal{E}ff$ it is a fully fledged model.

I now wish to review a few elements of the set theory of $\mathcal{W}$; all this was already in [103]. We start with unordered and ordered pairs.

Define a map $\{\cdot, \cdot\}^{\wedge} : V_{\kappa} \times V_{\kappa} \to V_{\kappa}$ by

$$\{a, b\}^{\wedge} = \{(0, a), (1, b)\}$$

and define $\{a\}^{\wedge}$ as $\{a, a\}^{\wedge}$. Then define $(\cdot, \cdot)^{\wedge} : V_{\kappa} \times V_{\kappa} \to V_{\kappa}$ by

$$(a, b)^{\wedge} = \{(0, \{a\}^{\wedge}), (1, \{a, b\}^{\wedge})\}$$

Then it is easy to show that

$$\mathcal{W} \models \forall x \, (x \epsilon \{a, b\}^{\wedge} \leftrightarrow x = a \lor x = b)$$

and hence, that $(a, b)^{\wedge}$ represents the ordered pair of a and b.

Following the language of forcing, we could say that if a and b are *names* for sets ξ, η, then $(a, b)^{\wedge}$ is a name for the ordered pair (ξ, η).

We now get names for natural numbers: define for $n \in \mathbb{N}$,

$$\hat{n} = \{(k, \hat{k}) \mid k < n\}$$

and

$$\hat{\omega} = \{(n, \hat{n}) \mid n \in \mathbb{N}\}$$

Then if '$x = n$' and '$x \epsilon \omega$' denote IZF-formulas expressing that $x = n$, x is a natural number respectively, we have:

$$\mathcal{W} \models \hat{n} = n$$
$$\mathcal{W} \models \forall x \, (x \epsilon \hat{\omega} \leftrightarrow x \epsilon \omega)$$

Let $\mathcal{N} = (\hat{\omega}, \sim)$ (restricted equality from $\mathcal{W}$). Then clearly, $\mathcal{N}$ is isomorphic in $\mathcal{E}ff$ to N, the natural numbers object, and this is also an isomorphism between $(\mathcal{N}, \epsilon)$ and $(N, <)$. So if we consider sentences with parameters from $\hat{\omega}$ and all quantifiers restricted to ω, these sentences will hold in $\mathcal{W}$ if and only if the corresponding translated sentences will be true for N. This extends to a language with primitive recursive functions, so true first order arithmetic in $\mathcal{W}$ is just Kleene realizability.

McCarty lists a number of principles in his thesis [103] which hold in the model $\mathcal{W}$: CT_0, MP and some principles which follow directly from the uniformity of $\mathcal{W}$, such as (see 3.1.10):

$$
\begin{array}{ll}
\text{IP} & (\neg\phi \to \exists x\psi) \to \exists x(\neg\phi \to \psi) \\
\neg\neg\exists & \neg\neg\exists x\phi \to \exists x\neg\neg\phi \\
\text{UP}^{\mathcal{W},\omega} & \forall x\exists y \in \omega\phi \to \exists y \in \omega\forall x\phi
\end{array}
$$

Shanin's Principle should also hold.

There is also a version in $\mathcal{W}$ of the fact that every object of $\mathcal{E}\!f\!f$ is covered by a partitioned assembly. A set x is called a *base* if and only if every surjective function into x has a section (the terminology 'base' originates from Martin-Löf's type theory and is also used by P. Aczel). The *Presentation Axiom* of P. Aczel ([3]) says that every set is the surjective image of a base. If we define

$$ a^r \;=\; \{(n, (\hat{n}, b)^\wedge) \,|\, n \text{ realizes } b\epsilon a\} $$

then a^r is a well-defined element of V_κ whenever a is, and the following proposition holds:

Proposition 3.5.16 (McCarty)

  i)   *There is a number g such that for all $a \in V_\kappa$, g realizes 'a is an image of a^r';*

  ii) *There is a number e such that for all $a \in V_\kappa$, e realizes 'a^r is a base'*

Hence, the Presentation Axiom is true in $\mathcal{W}$.

There is an embedding of the classical sets (of rank $< \kappa$) into V_κ. Let us denote the κ-th element of the cumulative hierarchy by R_κ. Then we define $(-)^{\text{st}} : R_\kappa \to V_\kappa$ recursively by

$$ x^{\text{st}} \;=\; \{(0, y^{\text{st}}) \,|\, y \in x\} $$

McCarty proves that for $x, y \in R_\kappa$,

$$x = y \quad \text{iff} \quad \mathcal{W} \models x^{\text{st}} = y^{\text{st}}$$
$$x \in y \quad \text{iff} \quad \mathcal{W} \models x^{\text{st}} \epsilon y^{\text{st}}$$

Since $\mathcal{W}$ is uniform, the map $(-)^{\text{st}}$ induces an arrow $\nabla(R_\kappa) \to \mathcal{W}$ which is monic, and McCarty furthermore shows that the image of this arrow is the subobject of $\mathcal{W}$ consisting of the 'hereditarily $\neg\neg$-stable' elements of $\mathcal{W}$: a set x is hereditarily $\neg\neg$-stable if it is a $\neg\neg$-stable set of hereditarily $\neg\neg$-stable elements.

The structure $(\nabla(R_\kappa), \nabla(\in))$ is perhaps worth a closer look. It is a sheaf, and $\nabla(\in)$ is therefore $\neg\neg$-closed, hence by $\neg\neg\exists$ every formula of the language of ZF *which does not involve disjunction* is $\neg\neg$-stable. Therefore $(\nabla(R_\kappa), \nabla(\in))$ satisfies many axioms of IZF, except *Pairing* and *Infinity*. To be sure, the sentences

$$\forall xy \exists z (x \epsilon z \wedge y \epsilon z \wedge \forall w (x \epsilon w \wedge y \epsilon w \to z \subseteq w))$$
$$\exists x (\emptyset \epsilon x \wedge \forall y (y \epsilon x \to \exists z (z \epsilon x \wedge y \epsilon z)))$$

are true, but Pairing is false and there cannot be any nontrivial linear order. It looks like $\mathcal{W}$ is (in $\mathcal{E}ff$!) the extension of $(\nabla(R_\kappa), \nabla(\in))$ which *adds natural numbers*. If we think of the map $(-)^{\text{st}}$ as analogous to the functor ∇, then this should be analogous to the analysis of ∇ as given in section 3.8.1 below. But I am aware that as yet, this is not a very precise formulation.

3.5.2 The Lubarsky-Streicher-Van den Berg model for CZF

The theory CZF (for 'Constructive Zermelo-Fraenkel') was developed by J. Myhill (who called it CST;[118]) and later P. Aczel ([2, 3, 4]) with the aim of bringing Set Theory more in agreement with the philosophy behind Martin-Löf's type theory.

The main element in this philosophy is that mathematics is (and should be) *predicative*: in defining elements or subsets of a given set X, I should not use quantification over all subsets of X. For example, if A is a subset of a group G I should not define the subgroup of G generated by A as 'the intersection of all subsets of G which contain A and are closed under multiplication and inverses'.

Formally, this philosophical position is implemented by not adopting the power set axiom in set theory. Also, unrestricted separation is banned. In order to obtain a usable set theory, some other axioms are added. For an excellent introduction on CZF, see [5].

For a long time, predicative mathematics and its formalisms lived apart from categorical semantics (it must be said that a number of influential practitioners of predicative mathematics were quite reluctant to make their formal positions explicit, this despite the fact that they are logicians). This changed with two recent papers by I. Moerdijk and E. Palmgren ([112, 113]). In the first of these, they define a notion of 'ΠW-pretopos' and show that it is suitable for interpreting constructions of predicative mathematics, in the second they show how to do algebraic set theory in these categories, in order to obtain models of CZF. A lot of further work in this topic is in the recent thesis [164].

R. Lubarsky ([101]) and T. Streicher ([155]) had each, independently, constructed a nontrivial model for CZF (that is, a model which is not, for example, a model of IZF): Lubarsky's is a McCarty style realizability model, whereas Streicher's is a construction in $\mathcal{E}\!f\!f$. Van den Berg ([164]) proved that both models are isomorphic, and gave a presentation of this model in terms readers of this book can now understand: it is a definable substructure of the McCarty model $\mathcal{W}$, namely the substructure of those elements of which $\mathcal{W}$ thinks that they are *subcountable*, that is: the image of a subset of ω.

This is a very interesting result which also prompts further questions about $\mathcal{W}$. What is the axiomatic content of the result? Certainly it is not a theorem of IZF that the class of subcountable sets forms a model of CZF (for a start, the class of subcountables is not a priori closed under exponents). Which are the axioms, true in $\mathcal{W}$, which guarantee this?

3.5.3   Well-founded trees and W-Types in $\mathcal{E}\!f\!f$

An important element in the categorical semantics of predicative systems (and also occurring in our treatment of synthetic domain theory, see 3.6,3.6.4) is the notion of a W-type.

A W-type is a certain clas of well-founded trees. Here I say a few things about W-types in $\mathcal{E}ff$. I start with a general corollary of the proof of theorem 3.5.9. That proof, being entirely constructive, internalizes to give the following corollary:

Corollary 3.5.17 *Let R be a binary relation on X. Denote by $\mathcal{P}_{\mathrm{wf}}(X)$ the object of subsets Y of X such that $R \cap (Y \times Y)$ is well-founded on Y; and by $\mathcal{P}_{\neg\neg\mathrm{wf}}(X)$ the object of such Y for which it is almost well-founded. Then these two objects coincide, and $\mathcal{P}_{\mathrm{wf}}(X)$ and $\mathcal{P}_{\mathrm{wf}}(X)$ is a $\neg\neg$-closed subobject of $\mathcal{P}(X)$.*

Assuming the axiom of choice in Set, given a relation R on $(X, \sim)$, $\mathcal{P}_{\mathrm{wf}}(X, \sim)$ is the closed subobject of $\mathcal{P}(X, \sim)$ consisting of those strict relations $\alpha : X \to \mathcal{P}(\mathbb{N})$ for which there is no infinite sequence $x_0, x_1, \ldots$ in X such that for each i, both $\alpha(i)$ and $R(x_{i+1}, x_i)$ are nonempty.

Definition 3.5.18 Let $f : B \to A$ be an arrow in a locally cartesian closed category $\mathcal{E}$. The functor $P_f : \mathcal{E} \to \mathcal{E}$ is defined by

$$P_f(X) = \Sigma_A(A^*(X)^f)$$

that is, take the domain of the exponent $(A \times X \to A)^{(B \xrightarrow{f} A)}$ in $\mathcal{E}/A$.

The W-type of f is an arrow $P_f(X) \xrightarrow{a} X$ with the property that for any arrow $P_f(Y) \xrightarrow{b} Y$ there is exactly one arrow $g : X \to Y$ such that $bP_f(g) = ga$.

In a topos, W-types always exist; this was first shown by A. Blass ([26]). They can be constructed as follows.

Let X^* be the free monoid on X, the object of finite sequences of elements of X. X^* can be constructed as the set of pairs (n, f) with $f : \{k \,|\, k < n\} \to X$; that is, the domain of the exponential $(X \times N \to N)^{(<)}$ in $\mathcal{E}/N$, where $(<) \rightarrowtail N \times N \xrightarrow{\pi_2} N$ is the order relation.

An X-*labelled tree* is a subset of X^* which is closed under initial segments and contains exactly one sequence of length 1.

Given $f : B \to A$ in $\mathcal{E}$, an f-*tree* is an $(A + B)$-labelled tree t with the following properties:

1)   If $(x_1, \ldots, x_n) \in t$ then $x_i \in A$ if i is odd, and $x_i \in B$ if i is even;

2)   if $(x_1, \ldots, x_{2n}) \in t$ then there is a unique $a \in A$ such that $(x_1, \ldots, x_{2n}, a) \in t$;

3)   if $(x_1, \ldots, x_{2n+1}) \in t$ then

$$\{x \mid (x_1, \ldots, x_{2n}, x) \in t\} = \{b \in B \mid f(b) = x_{2n+1}\}$$

Then $W(f)$ is the object of *well-founded* f-trees, with respect to the relation: $R(\alpha, \beta)$ iff α extends β by one element.

Lemma 3.5.19 *Let $f : B \to A$ be an arrow in $\mathcal{E}$ with A $\neg\neg$-separated. Then every f-tree is a $\neg\neg$-closed subset of $(A + B)^*$.*

Proof. Left to you.   ∎

Hence $T(f)$, the object of f-trees, is a subobject of $\mathcal{P}_{\neg\neg}((A + B)^*)$. In $\mathcal{E}ff$, by corollary 3.5.17, $W(f)$ is a $\neg\neg$-closed subobject of $T(f)$.

In [66], an explicit construction of $T(f)$ can be found in case the codomain of f is $\neg\neg$-separated. Another construction, for general f, is in [164].

3.6   Synthetic Domain Theory in $\mathcal{E}ff$

The idea of Synthetic Domain Theory was first formulated by D. Scott in 1980. Inspired by the example of Synthetic Differential Geometry, pioneered by W. Lawvere and taken up by A. Kock, G. Reyes and I. Moerdijk ([91, 114] for expositions), he wondered whether it might be possible to do something similar for domain theory.

In order to explain the idea, I should spend a few words on what ordinary domain theory tries to achieve. Therefore subsection 3.6.1 treats some theory of complete partial orders, inasmuch it is important for semantics. Then, a short subsection, 3.6.2, is devoted to what "synthetic" is supposed to mean, with an example of synthetic differential geometry. Subsection 3.6.3 gives some axioms and axiomatic development of synthetic domain theory, and finally, 3.6.4 shows how this has models in $\mathcal{E}ff$.

3.6.1 Complete partial orders

An $(\omega\text{-})cpo$ (or cpo for short) is a poset which has least upper bounds (lubs) of $\mathbb{N}$-indexed chains $x_0 \leq x_1 \leq \cdots$ Given two cpo's X and Y, a function $f : X \to Y$ is *continuous* if it preserves these lubs. We have a category CPO of cpo's and continuous maps.

CPO is easily seen to be cartesian closed, complete and cocomplete. There is a monad ("lifting monad") L on CPO: $L(X)$ adds a new bottom element to the poset X. A cpo X has a least element, precisely when X has the structure of an algebra for the monad L, and such structure is unique if it exists.

If X has a least element $\bot$, then every continuous $f : X \to X$ has a least fixed point: it is the lub of the chain

$$\bot \leq f(\bot) \leq f^2(\bot) \cdots$$

Moreover, if X has a least element then so has X^Y for every cpo Y, and there is a continuous map fix : $X^X \to X$ assigning to every continuous map its least fixed point.

This allows an interpretation of the programming language PCF in CPO. The language PCF (see [126] for details) is a term calculus based on simply typed λ-calculus. There are two basic types B (for Boolean truth-values) and N (for natural numbers), constants t and f ('true' and 'false') of type B, constants $0, 1, 2, \ldots$ of type N, and terms of higher types which allow one to define functionals by higher-type recursion. For example, there is a cases operator

$$\text{If} \cdots \text{then} \cdots \text{else} : B \to (N \to (N \to N))$$

and for any type σ there is a fixpoint operator

$$Y_\sigma : (\sigma \to \sigma) \to \sigma$$

The *operational semantics* gives a reduction relation $\rightsquigarrow$ between such terms, for example:

$$\begin{aligned}
\text{If t then } M \text{ else } N &\rightsquigarrow M \\
\text{If f then } M \text{ then } N &\rightsquigarrow N \\
Y_\sigma M &\rightsquigarrow M(Y_\sigma M)
\end{aligned}$$

Two terms M and N of the same type are said to be in the *operational preorder*, $M \sqsubseteq N$, if whenever a term $t[M]$ reduces to a constant of type B or N, then $t[N]$ reduces to that same constant.

Denotational semantics interprets terms as arrows between cpo's with least element. It follows the standard interpretation of the simply typed λ-calculus in cartesian closed categories (for which see [95]). For the two 'ground types' B and N one takes the cpo's

$$\llbracket B \rrbracket = \quad \begin{array}{cc} t & f \\ \diagdown & | \\ & \bot \end{array} \qquad \llbracket N \rrbracket = \quad \begin{array}{ccccc} 0 & 1 & 2 & \cdots \\ \diagdown & | & \diagup \\ & \bot \end{array}$$

and hence proceeds to form $\llbracket \sigma \rrbracket$ for any type σ; a term t of type τ with free variables $x_1^{\sigma_1}, \dots, x_n^{\sigma_n}$ is then interpreted as a continuous map

$$\llbracket \sigma_1 \rrbracket \times \cdots \times \llbracket \sigma_n \rrbracket \xrightarrow{\llbracket t \rrbracket} \llbracket \tau \rrbracket$$

If M is of type $\sigma \to \sigma$ so $\llbracket M \rrbracket$ is a map into $\llbracket \sigma \rrbracket^{\llbracket \sigma \rrbracket}$, then $\llbracket Y_\sigma M \rrbracket$ will result from $\llbracket M \rrbracket$ by composing with $\mathrm{fix} : \llbracket \sigma \rrbracket^{\llbracket \sigma \rrbracket} \to \llbracket \sigma \rrbracket$.

There is a clear *denotational preorder* $\leq$ between terms M, N which are both interpreted as maps with the same domain and codomain: the pointwise order.

This interpretation of terms as maps between cpo's with bottom elements ("domains") is most useful if both preorders, the operational and the denotational, match well. One says that the interpretation is

computationally adequate if $M \leq N$ implies $M \sqsubseteq N$

fully abstract if $\sqsubseteq$ and $\leq$ coincide.

The quoted classic paper [126] had shown that an interpretation in Scott domains (a subclass of cpo's) is adequate, but not fully abstract. Milner ([110]) had proved that a fully abstract semantics always exists. However, his method was syntactic and a syntactically constructed fully abstract model does not really produce more insight than studying the operational semantics directly.

Several researchers have therefore tried to find naturally existing categories of domains which might provide fully abstract semantics for PCF or related formalisms.

Another type of semantics for which the category CPO is useful, is "solving recursive domain equations". Here we focus not on fixed points of continuous functions, but of functors. But we wish to consider functors

$$(\mathrm{CPO}^{\mathrm{op}})^n \times (\mathrm{CPO})^m \to \mathrm{CPO}$$

that is, functors ' of mixed variance', to get things like: a cpo X such that $X \cong X^X$ (a model of the untyped λ-calculus).

We consider *embedding-projection pairs* $X \underset{i}{\overset{r}{\longleftrightarrow}} Y$, maps satisfying $ri(x) = x$, $ir(y) \leq y$. It follows from these equations that if X and Y have least elements, both i and r preserve them. We have a category $\mathrm{CPO}^{\mathrm{EP}}_{\perp}$ of cpo's with least elements and embedding-projection pairs.

Theorem 3.6.1 (limit-colimit coincidence) *Given an ω-chain*

$$X_1 \underset{i_1}{\overset{r_1}{\longleftrightarrow}} X_2 \underset{i_2}{\overset{r_2}{\longleftrightarrow}} X_3 \overset{\longleftarrow}{\longrightarrow} \cdots$$

in $\mathrm{CPO}^{\mathrm{EP}}_{\perp}$. *Then there is a cpo X with least element, and embedding-projection pairs* $X_i \underset{j_i}{\overset{q_i}{\longleftrightarrow}} X$ *such that the diagram*

$$X_1 \overset{i_1}{\longrightarrow} X_2 \overset{i_2}{\longrightarrow} X_3 \longrightarrow \cdots$$

with maps j_1, j_2, j_3 to X

is a colimit in CPO, *the diagram*

$$X$$
with maps q_1, q_2, q_3 to
$$X_1 \overset{r_1}{\longleftarrow} X_2 \overset{r_2}{\longleftarrow} X_3 \qquad \cdots$$

is a limit in CPO, *and the diagram of embedding-projection pairs*

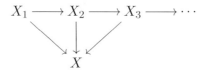

is a colimit in $\mathrm{CPO}_{\perp}^{\mathrm{EP}}$.

Theorem 3.6.2 *Suppose* $F : (\mathrm{CPO}_{\perp}^{\mathrm{op}})^n \times (\mathrm{CPO}_{\perp})^m \to \mathrm{CPO}$ *is locally continuous, that is: preserves lubs of chains of maps. Then there is a functor*

$$\tilde{F} : (\mathrm{CPO}_{\perp}^{\mathrm{EP}})^{m+n} \to \mathrm{CPO}_{\perp}^{\mathrm{EP}}$$

which preserves colimits of ω-chains and moreover has the same action on objects as F.

Note that for such a functor $\tilde{F}$ there are always objects X for which $\tilde{F}(X) \cong X$. This can be applied, for example, to the functor $F(Y, X) = X^Y$, which is locally continuous. Passing to $\mathrm{CPO}_{\perp}^{\mathrm{EP}}$ and composing with the diagonal embedding we find that there is a cpo X such that $X \cong X^X$.

3.6.2   The synthetic approach

The idea of working 'synthetically' is, that instead of *constructing* objects with certain properties by set-theoretic means, one imposes the wanted properties by postulates.

In the 19th century, 'synthetic' was the antonym of 'analytic'. Doing geometry synthetically meant for example: reasoning about manifolds without mentioning local coordinates, charts or atlases. A quick glance at modern synthetic differential geometry may give you an idea of how one works. The following very rough sketch is based on [91].

The *line R* is *given* to us, together with two specified points 0 and 1. The operations of multiplication, addition, subtraction and division by a non-zero natural number, are given to us by geometric constructions. So, R is a $\mathbb{Q}$-algebra. Define

$$D = \{x \in R \mid x^2 = 0\}$$

D can be geometrically pictured as the intersection of the circle with radius 1 and center $(0, 1)$, and the x-axis.

The basic axiom is now:

Axiom. For every function $f : D \to R$ there is a *unique* element $b \in R$ satisfying for all $d \in D$:

$$f(d) = f(0) + bd$$

As immediate consequences of the Axiom, we have that $D \neq \{0\}$ (by the uniqueness requirement), and that classical logic *fails* (we cannot define a function f on D such that $f(0) = 0$ and $f(x) = 1$ if $x \neq 0$).

Another quick corollary is, that for any function $f : R \to R$ we can, for every $x \in R$, apply the Axiom to $f_x : D \to R$ defined by $f_x(d) = f(x + d)$, to obtain an element $f'(x)$ which satisfies

$$f_x(d) = f(x) + f'(x)d$$

It is straightforward to derive the properties $(f + g)'(x) = f'(x) + g'(x)$, $(fg)'(x) = f(x)g'(x) + f'(x)g(x)$ and the Chain rule $(f \circ g)'(x) = f'(g(x))g'(x)$. From that, one goes on to derive Taylor series and a lot of basic calculus, then defines manifolds, integration, flows...

You see: we *postulate* a certain world to exist without further ado ('the line R', which also in Brouwer's view is the primordial intuition of *time*), then we impose axioms which may be more special.

3.6.3 Elements of Synthetic Domain Theory

Our postulate for Synthetic Domain Theory (SDT) is that every set comes equipped with a notion of 'open' subset, which system satisfies the following requirements (we write $U \subset_o X$ for: U is an open subset of X):

i) If $f : X \to Y$ is any function and $U \subset_o Y$, then $f^{-1}(U) \subset_o X$

ii) There is a set Σ which classifies open subsets: there is an open subset $T \subset_o \Sigma$ such that for every $U \subset_o X$ there is a unique classifying map $\chi_U : X \to \Sigma$ with the property that $\chi_U^{-1}(T) = U$

iii)   For every set X we have $X \subset_o X$

iv)   For every chain $U \subset_o X \subset_o Y$ we have $U \subset_o Y$.

If we work in a topos, our 'sets' are objects etc., then requirement ii) implies that Σ is a subobject of Ω and together with iii) we have that the 'generic open' $T \subset \Sigma$ is the factorization of $\mathsf{true} : 1 \to \Omega$ through Σ.

Requirements iii) and iv) are equivalent to the following properties of Σ (given that $\Sigma \subset \Omega$):

a) $\mathsf{true} \in \Sigma$

b) $(p \in \Sigma \land p \to (q \in \Sigma)) \to ((p \land q) \in \Sigma)$

A subobject Σ of Ω with these properties is called a *dominance* (Rosolini, [136, 137]). Note that in particular, any dominance is closed under $\land$.

The following lemma gives a method to construct dominances.

Lemma 3.6.3 *Suppose A is an object with partial map classifier $\tilde{A}$. Let* $\mathsf{s} : \tilde{A} \to \Omega$ *classify* $A \rightarrowtail \tilde{A}$*, so $\mathsf{s}(\alpha)$ is the proposition $\exists x(x \in \alpha)$. Suppose Φ is a subset of A satisfying the conditions:*

i) $\exists a(a \in \Phi)$

ii)   *For all $a \in A$ and $U \subseteq A$: if $(a \in \Phi \to \exists b(b \in U))$ then there is an $\alpha \in \tilde{A}$ such that*

$$(a \in \Phi \to \mathsf{s}(\alpha) \land \alpha \subset U)$$

iii)   *For all $a \in A$ and $\alpha \in \tilde{A}$, if $(a \in \Phi \to \mathsf{s}(\alpha))$ then there is a $b \in A$ such that*

$$((a \in \Phi \land \alpha \subset \Phi) \leftrightarrow b \in \Phi)$$

Then the subobject $\Sigma \subset \Omega$ defined by

$$\Sigma \; = \; \{p \in \Omega \,|\, \exists a(p \leftrightarrow a \in \Phi)\}$$

is a dominance.

Proof. Certainly, by i), true $\in \Sigma$. For the other requirement, suppose $p \in \Sigma$ and $p \rightarrow (q \in \Sigma)$. Let a be such that $p \leftrightarrow a \in \Phi$. Then we have

$$a \in \Phi \rightarrow \exists b(q \leftrightarrow b \in \Phi)$$

By ii) there is $\alpha \in \tilde{A}$ such that

$$a \in \Phi \rightarrow \mathsf{s}(\alpha) \wedge (q \leftrightarrow \alpha \subset \Phi)$$

(taking $\{b \mid q \leftrightarrow b \in \Phi\}$ for U in ii)). By iii) there is $b \in A$ such that

$$((a \in \Phi \wedge \mathsf{s}(\alpha)) \leftrightarrow b \in \Phi)$$

It follows that $p \wedge q \leftrightarrow b \in \Phi$, so $p \wedge q \in \Sigma$. ∎

An example of an A as in the lemma is: let A be a set of computations of some type, and $\Phi \subset A$ the set of terminating computations.
  In $\mathcal{E}ff$, the main example we shall study is:

$$A = N^N$$
$$\Phi = \{f \in N^N \mid \exists n(f(n) = 0)\}$$

Then the dominance resulting from this is the r.e. subobject classifier of section 3.2.7.
  As our first axiom, we take

Axiom 1. *For every* X, *$\emptyset \subset_o X$. Equivalently,* false $\in \Sigma$.

Given a dominance Σ, we define a functor L which is going to mimick the 'lift monad'. For an object X, $L(X)$ is the subobject of $\tilde{X}$ defined by

$$L(X) \; = \; \{\alpha \in \tilde{X} \mid \mathsf{s}(\alpha) \in \Sigma\}$$

where, as before, $\mathsf{s} : \tilde{X} \rightarrow \Omega$ classifies $X \rightarrowtail \tilde{X}$.
  We have maps $\eta_X : X \rightarrow L(X)$, $\eta_X(x) = \{x\}$, and $\mu_X : L^2(X) \rightarrow L(X)$, $\mu_X(A) = \bigcup A$.
  In order to see that μ_X is well-defined (that $\mu_X(A) \in L(X)$), note that $\mathsf{s}(\mu_X(A))$ is equivalent to

$$\exists \alpha \in L(X)(\alpha \in A) \; \wedge \; \forall \alpha \in L(X)(\alpha \in A \rightarrow \exists x \in X(x \in \alpha))$$

The first conjunct is in Σ since $A \in L^2(X)$, and it implies that the second is in Σ. By requirement b) in the definition of dominance, the conjunction is in Σ.

The object $L(X)$ classifies partial maps into X with open domain. That is, there is a natural bijection between maps $Y \to X$ and maps $U \to X$ with $U \subset_o Y$.

Definition 3.6.4 An *object with* $\perp$ is an algebra for the monad L. A *strict map* between objects with $\perp$ is an L-algebra homomorphism.

A *Lambek algebra*[1] for L is just an arrow $L(X) \xrightarrow{\alpha} X$. A morphism of Lambek algebras $(L(X) \xrightarrow{\alpha} X) \to (L(Y) \xrightarrow{\beta} Y)$ is an arrow $f : X \to Y$ such that $\beta L(f) = f\alpha$. Analogously, we have Lambek *coalgebras* $X \xrightarrow{\alpha} L(X)$ and coalgebra morphisms.
Lambek's Lemma says that every *initial* Lambek algebra is an isomorphism; similarly, every *final* (terminal) Lambek coalgebra is an isomorphism.

In Posets, the initial Lambek algebra for the lift functor is the poset $\omega = \{0 < 1 < 2 < \cdots\}$ and the terminal Lambek coalgebra for that functor is the poset $\omega + 1 = \{0 < 1 < 2 < \cdots < \omega\}$. A poset X is a cpo if every arrow $\omega \to X$ can be uniquely extended to a continuous map $\omega + 1 \to X$. In view of this, we are interested in initial Lambek algebras and final Lambek coalgebras for L.

Theorem 3.6.5 *The initial Lambek algebra and the final Lambek coalgebra for L exist.*

Proof. Let $F = \{\psi \in \Sigma^N \mid \forall n(\psi(n+1) \to \psi(n))\}$. Define $\tau : F \to L(F)$ by

$$\tau(\psi) = \{\lambda n.\psi(n+1) \mid \psi(0)\}$$

Then τ is well-defined, and I claim that (F, τ) is a final Lambek coalgebra for L: given a coalgebra $(X \xrightarrow{\sigma} L(X)$, let $f : X \to F$ be defined by

$$f(x)(0) = \mathsf{s}(\sigma(x))$$
$$f(x)(n+1) = \mathsf{s}(\sigma(x)) \wedge f(y)(n)$$

---

[1] The term 'Lambek algebra' for 'algebra for a functor' was suggested to me by Peter Freyd

where, given $\mathsf{s}(\sigma(x))$, y is the unique element of $\sigma(x)$.

The initial Lambek algebra for L is a subobject of F. Define

$$I \;=\; \{\psi \in F \,|\, \forall \phi \in \Omega[\forall n \in N((\psi(n) \to \phi) \to \phi) \to \phi]\}$$

This formula was given by M. Jibladze in [79], and is called *Jibladze's formula*. I leave it to you to check, or look up in, e.g. [174], that τ^{-1} : $L(F) \to F$ maps $L(I)$ into I, giving a Lambek algebra structure σ on I.
∎

Let $\iota : I \to F$ be the canonical map from (I, σ) to (F, τ^{-1}).

Definition 3.6.6 An object X is *complete* if $X^{\iota} : X^F \to X^I$ is an isomorphism.

Note that completeness is an orthogonality property. Therefore, given a diagram of complete objects its limit, if it exists, is again complete. The terminal object 1 is complete, and if Y is complete, so is Y^X for any X.

An object which is *not* complete is I. It is not hard to derive that were I complete, we would have $I = F$ (completeness of I would give that I is a retract of F, and then use the final coalgebra property of F). However, $\lambda n.\mathsf{true}$ is certainly an element of F, but it cannot be in I (take $\phi = \mathsf{false}$ in Jibladze's formula).

Theorem 3.6.7 *Suppose X is a complete object with $\bot$. Then every arrow $g : X \to X$ has a fixed point.*

Proof. See, e.g., [174], theorem 1.13. ∎

This was surprising; on the basis of just one axiom we can prove the analogue of the fixed point property for cpo's for general complete objects with $\bot$. Shouldn't this make us a bit suspicious? It should indeed; the theory so far is, from a classical point of view, not inconsistent, but *totally empty*: $\Sigma \cong 2$, an object with $\bot$ is a set with a specified element, and the only complete object is 1. Intuitionistically, however, we can go further. The next axiom takes us outside classical logic.

Axiom 2. Σ *is complete.*

Since Σ is a retract of F, and F a retract of Σ^N (which is complete when Σ is), this axiom is equivalent to the statement that F is complete.

Note that Σ is isomorphic to $L(1)$ and hence has the structure of a (free) L-algebra; thus Σ is an object with $\perp$. Hence Axiom 2 implies that we can apply theorem 3.6.7 to Σ: ever map $g : \Sigma \to \Sigma$ has a fixed point. It follows, for example, that Σ, as subobject of Ω, can not be closed under the negation map $\neg : \Omega \to \Omega$.

For an object X we may consider the map $\eta_X : X \to \Sigma^{\Sigma^X}$ given by $\eta_X(x)(P) = P(x)$. Also on X, we can define a relation $\sqsubseteq_X$ by: $x \sqsubseteq y$ iff $\forall U \subseteq_o X(x \in U \to y \in U)$. Clearly, this is a preorder on X, called the Σ-*preorder*. The object X is called a Σ-*poset* if this is a partial order, i.e. if the relation $\sqsubseteq_X$ is antisymmetric. This is equivalent to: the map η_X is monic (the Σ-preorder is analogous to the specialization preorder for topoogical spaces; see e.g.[81]. Under this analogy, the property of being a Σ-poset corresponds to the T_1-property for spaces). We call X a *regular* Σ-*poset* if the map η_X is a $\neg\neg$-closed monic.

The limit-colimit coincidence was the result of *constructing* a category out of the category of cpo's, with the property that many functors of mixed variance defined on it, have (parametrized) fixed points. By contrast, the following definition, given by P. Freyd in [46], is completely in the synthetic spirit and simply *imposes* the required property for a category (in a very strong way).

Definition 3.6.8 (Freyd) A category $\mathcal{C}$ is called *algebraically compact* if for every functor $T : \mathcal{C} \to \mathcal{C}$ there exist an initial Lambek algebra $T(I) \xrightarrow{\sigma} I$ and a final Lambek coalgebra $F \xrightarrow{\tau} T(F)$, and moreover the canonical map

$$
\begin{array}{ccc}
T(I) & \xrightarrow{\ T(\iota)\ } & T(F) \\
{\scriptstyle\sigma}\downarrow & & \downarrow{\scriptstyle\tau^{-1}} \\
I & \xrightarrow{\ \ \iota\ \ } & F
\end{array}
$$

of Lambek algebras, which exists by Lambek's lemma and initiality of σ, is an isomorphism.

This is a very strong definition. It follows at once that the property of being algebraically compact is self-dual: if $\mathcal{C}$ is algebraically compact, then so is $\mathcal{C}^{\mathrm{op}}$. Furthermore, Freyd proved the nontrivial theorem that if $\mathcal{A}$ and $\mathcal{B}$ are algebraically compact, so is $\mathcal{A} \times \mathcal{B}$. Hence, if $\mathcal{A}$ is algebraically compact, so is $(\mathcal{A}^{\mathrm{op}})^n \times \mathcal{A}^m$. As proved by M. Fiore in his thesis ([43]), this implies that recursive domain equitions can be solved in any algebraically compact category.

Note that every algebraically compact category has a *zero object* (an object which is both initial and terminal); apply the definition to the identity functor.

Now assume we work in a topos $\mathcal{E}$ where we have defined a dominance Σ and associated lift monad L. By a *category of predomains* we shall mean a full internal subcategory $\mathcal{C}$ of $\mathcal{E}$ which consists of complete objects and is closed under L. The associated category of domains then will be the Eilenberg-Moore category of L-algebras on $\mathcal{C}$. We can now formulate:

> **Axiom 3**. *There is a category of predomains such that its associated category of domains is complete and algebraically compact.*

Again, axiom 3 is impossible to satisfy non-trivially in a classical world. As Freyd pointed out, every algebraically compact preorder is trivial (it must have a zero object); at the same time, classically every complete, algebraically compact category must be a preorder.

However, in non-Boolean toposes several candidates for categories of predomains have been identified.

The oldest notion is that of a *replete* object (Taylor-Phoa-Hyland:[156, 122, 72]). A map $g : P \to Q$ is called Σ-equable if $\Sigma^g : \Sigma^Q \to \Sigma^P$ is an isomorphism. An object A is *replete* if for any Σ-equable map $g : P \to Q$, any map $P \to A$ extends uniquely via g to a map $Q \to A$. By Axiom 2, the map $\iota : I \to F$ is Σ-equable so every replete object is complete. In [72] there is a proof that the replete objects are closed under L, and since repleteness is an orthogonality property, the replete objects form a complete category.

A second category is advocated in [100]. An object X is *well-complete* if $L(X)$ is complete. Well-complete implies complete, and if X is well-complete the so is $L(X)$ (it is *not* true that if X is complete, so is $L(X)$!). In [100] the authors prove that also well-completeness is an orthogonality property.

Thirdly, in [174] there is a proof (under the assumption that the dominance Σ is $\neg\neg$-separated) that if X is a complete, regular Σ-poset, so is $L(X)$.

So, we have (at least if Σ is $\neg\neg$-separated) three candidate notions of predomains:

1)   The replete objects

2)   The well-complete objects

3)   The regular Σ-posets

Of these three, the notion 'well-complete' has been the most successful. The most important research in synthetic domain theory was carried out in three centres, in three stages in time: the initial step forward was made by Scott and Rosolini at CMU (Pittsburgh); then the topic was taken up by Hyland and Taylor (and Hyland's student Phoa) in Cambridge; after that, the centre was Edinburgh, where Longley and Simpson worked. In particular Simpson has pushed the subject a long way forward, and has also achieved important applications (see e.g. [149, 150]).

The following proposition gives another characterization of I and F, and is useful for determining them in $\mathcal{E}ff$.

Proposition 3.6.9 *Let* true $: 1 \to \Sigma$ *be the evident map. Then in the notation of section 3.5.3, F is isomorphic to $T(\text{true})$, the object of* true-*trees, and under this isomorphism the subobject $I \subset F$ corresponds to $W(\text{true})$, the object of well-founded* true-*trees.*

Proof. According to the definition of f-trees in 3.5.3, a true-tree t is a set of sequences $(x_1, \ldots, x_n)$ with the following properties:

i) $x_i \in \Sigma$ if and only if i is odd, and $x_i = *$ ($*$ is the only element of 1) if i is even;

ii)   if $(x_1, \ldots, x_{2n}) \in t$ then there is a unique $x_{2n+1} \in \Sigma$ such that $(x_1, \ldots, x_{2n}, x_{2n+1}) \in t$, for all $n \geq 0$;

iii)   if $(x_1, \ldots, x_{2n+1}) \in t$ then $(x_1, \ldots, x_{2n+1}, *) \in t \leftrightarrow x_{2n+1}$.

Of course, t is also a tree, that is: closed under initial segments. But we see that t does not really branch. Note that for $n \geq 0$ we have $x_{2n+3} \to x_{2n+1}$.

Define a map $\alpha : T(\text{true}) \times N \to \Omega$ (written $t, n \mapsto \alpha_t(n)$) recursively as follows: $\alpha_t(0) = x$ for the unique x (by ii) of the definition of t) such that $(x) \in t$; if $\alpha_t(0), \ldots, \alpha_t(n)$ have been defined let

$$\alpha_t(n+1) \;=\; \exists u[(\alpha_t(0), *, \ldots, *, \alpha_t(n), *, u) \in t \;\wedge\; u]$$

We prove the following two properties by induction on n:

1) $\alpha_t(n) \in \Sigma$;

2) $\alpha_t(n) \leftrightarrow \exists v[(\alpha_t(0), *, \ldots, *, \alpha_t(n), *, v) \in t]$

For $n = 0$, both 1) and 2) hold by definition of t. Suppose they hold for $\alpha_t(n)$. Now $\alpha_t(n+1)$ is equivalent to the proposition

$$\exists u[(\alpha_t(0), *, \ldots, *, \alpha_t(n), *, u) \in t] \;\wedge \\ \forall v[(\alpha_t(0), *, \ldots, *, \alpha_t(n), *, v) \in t \to v]$$

which we write as $p \wedge q$. By induction hypothesis, $p \leftrightarrow \alpha_t(n)$ so $p \in \Sigma$. Now if u satisfies p, that is: $(\alpha_t(0), *, \ldots, *, \alpha_t(n), *, u) \in t)$, then $u \in \Sigma$ and $q \leftrightarrow u$, hence $q \in \Sigma$. So $p \to (q \in \Sigma)$. By axiom b) for a dominance, we have $p \wedge q \in \Sigma$, i.e. $\alpha_t(n+1) \in \Sigma$ which completes the induction step for 1).

For 2), suppose $\alpha_t(n+1)$, say u satisfies

$$(\alpha_t(0), *, \ldots, *, \alpha_t(n), *, u) \in t \;\wedge\; u$$

Then both $\alpha_t(n+1)$ and u, so $u = \alpha_t(n+1)$ and we have

$$(\alpha_t(0), *, \ldots, *, \alpha_t(n+1)) \in t \;\wedge\; \alpha_t(n+1)$$

By definition of t we have $\exists v[(\alpha_t(0), *, \ldots, *, \alpha_t(n+1), *, v) \in t]$. So we have

$$\alpha_t(n+1) \to \exists v[(\alpha_t(0), *, \ldots, *, \alpha_t(n+1), *, v) \in t]$$

The converse implication follows at once from the definition of t, whic proves 2).

We conclude that we have a map

$$\alpha : T(\text{true}) \to \Sigma^N$$
$$t \mapsto (\alpha_t(0), \alpha_t(1), \dots)$$

which clearly factors through F. There is also a map in the other direction. Define $\beta : F \to T(\text{true})$ as follows: let $\beta(\psi)$ be the tree generated by

$$\{(\psi(0))\} \cup \bigcup_{n \geq 0} \{(\psi(0), *, \dots, *, \psi(n+1)) \mid \psi(n)\}$$

Then β is an inverse for α, as is left to you.

That under the isomorphism $F \simeq T(\text{true})$, I corresponds to $W(\text{true})$ is straightforward, and also left to you.   ∎

3.6.4   Models for SDT in $\mathcal{E}ff$

In $\mathcal{E}ff$, we shall consider the dominance

$$\Sigma = \{p \in \Omega \mid \exists f{:}N^N(p \leftrightarrow \exists x(f(x) = 0))\}$$

which we saw already in section 3.2.7 and which was first considered by Mulry and Rosolini ([136]). It is easy to verify (for example, using 3.6.3) that Σ is a dominance. It is by no means the *only* dominance in $\mathcal{E}ff$; for example,

$$\Sigma' = \{p \subset \Omega \mid \exists f{:}N^{N \times N}(p \leftrightarrow \exists x \forall y f(x,y) = 0)\}$$

is also a dominance.

But for the Rosolini dominance Σ it is straightforward to show that we can satisfy the axioms of synthetic domain theory.

In section 3.2.7 we saw that Σ is $\neg\neg$-separated and can be represented by the assembly $(\{\bot, \top\}, E_\Sigma)$ with $E_\Sigma(\top) = K$, the standard set, and $E_\Sigma(\bot) = \bar{K}$, the complement of K.

I restrict the description of the lift monad L to the category of assemblies, because all models we shall see will be subcategories of Ass.

For an assembly (X, E), the lift $L(X, E)$ is the object $(X_\perp, E_\perp)$, defined by

$$
\begin{aligned}
X_\perp &= X \cup \{\perp_X\} \qquad &\perp_X \text{ is a new element, not in } X \\
E_\perp(x) &= \{n \mid nn \in E(x)\} \\
E_\perp(\perp_X) &= \bar{K}
\end{aligned}
$$

In order to see that this is a correct representation, you should recall that $L(X)$ classifies partial maps into X with open (which is now: semidecidable) domain. In proposition 3.2.28 we have seen a characterization of semidecidable subobjects of assemblies. This should suffice to work out the representation of L given above.

Let us look at the initial Lambek algebra and final Lambek coalgebra for L. The final coalgebra was defined internally by

$$
F \;=\; \{\psi \in \Sigma^N \mid \forall n(\psi(n+1) \to \psi(n))\}
$$

From this definition we see that since Σ is $\neg\neg$-separated, F is a $\neg\neg$-closed subobject of Σ^N, i.e. a subassembly of (RE, W) in the notation of proposition 3.2.28: RE being the set of r.e. subsets of $\mathbb{N}$, and $W(R)$ the set of indices of R as r.e. set.

Under this representation of Σ^N, F is then the subassembly of those r.e. sets which are initial segments of $\mathbb{N}$. That is: F is isomorphic to the object $(\omega + 1, E_F)$ given by

$$
\begin{aligned}
E_F(n) &= \{e \mid W_e = \{m \mid m < n\}\} \\
E_F(\omega) &= \{e \mid W_e = \mathbb{N}\}
\end{aligned}
$$

About I, we know from the theory in the previous section that

$$
\{\psi \in F \mid \exists n \neg \psi(n)\} \subseteq I \subseteq \{\psi \in F \mid \neg\neg \exists n \neg \psi(n)\}
$$

But we have also seen in 3.6.9 that the inclusion $I \subset F$ is (up to ismorphism) the inclusion $W(\text{true}) \subset T(\text{true})$. In section 3.5.3 we have seen that this inclusion is $\neg\neg$-closed in $\mathcal{E}ff$. Hence I is a subassembly of F and can be presented as (ω, E_F) (restrict E_F to ω).

We should verify that our axioms (the axioms 1,2,3 from the previous section) are true in $\mathcal{E}ff$. Axiom 1 needs no comment; certainly false $\in \Sigma$

holds. As for axiom 2, the completeness of Σ, this follows from the Rice-Shapiro theorem in a way similar to 3.2.30. The object Σ^F is the assembly of r.e. subobjects of F; such a subobject is completely determined by its intersection with I.

From the construction of L on assemblies it is immediate that if X is modest, so is $L(X)$. This means that L can also be viewed as an internal monad on the internal category $\mathcal{P}$ of 'internal modest sets' (see section 3.4.1). That is the place where we are going to look for an algebraically compact category of domains. In fact, there seem to be two such:

a) The internal category of *well-complete modest sets with* $\perp$ is algebraically compact in $\mathcal{E}ff$ ([100]).

b) The regular Σ-posets in $\mathcal{P}$ are studied in [47] under the name 'extensional PERs'. In [46], Freyd claims that [47] proves that the complete regular Σ-posets with $\perp$ in $\mathcal{P}$ form an algebraically compact category.

3.7 Synthetic Computability Theory in $\mathcal{E}ff$

In studying the effective topos, we have of course been using a lot of basic recursion theory. And we have seen that some theorems of recursion theory can be reformulated to state categorical properties of certain objects of $\mathcal{E}ff$; for example, the Rice and Rice-Shapiro theorems in section 3.2.7. On the other hand, study of the effective topos should also prompt new questions in recursion theory. The effective topos should be a podium where category theory and recursion theory play together to mutual benefit. However, we have not seen many nontrivial examples of this.

A new approach to the question of how the study of $\mathcal{E}ff$ can be useful to guide research in recursion theory, has recently been formulated by A. Bauer in his paper on 'Synthetic Computability Theory' ([13]). Using ideas from synthetic domain theory, a theory of sets and functions is presented, completely free of any consideration of machine models such as Turing machines, or definition schemes for recursive functions; yet yielding theorems which can be interpreted in $\mathcal{E}ff$, which interpretation then turns out to give theorems of recursion theory.

Part of Bauer's motivation is apparently in the following quote:

> *Descriptions of Turing machines and numerous uses of Gödel encodings give classical computability theory its distinguishing flavor, which many "main-stream" mathematicians find unpalatable.*

Of course, one can argue with this, and debate whether the need to reason intuitionistically and adopt axioms which are classically inconsistent, makes life better for the classical mathematician. My view is essentially that recursion theory is often criticized for not being what it cannot be. Recursion theory is a piece of *intensional mathematics*: it is a theory not about sets and functions, but about *names* for these things.

Be that as it may, it is surprising to see quite a bit of basic recursion theory being developed out of one simple non-logical axiom, which is why I devote this section to a sketch of Bauer's ideas.

The setup is a topos in which the natural numbers object N is projective and internally projective, every $\neg\neg$-stable subobject of an (internally) projective object is (internally) projective, and in which Markov's Principle holds. Examples include Set (assuming Choice) and $\mathcal{E}ff$.

We use the r.e. subobject classifier Σ.

The following easy observation is due to Lawvere.

Proposition 3.7.1 *Suppose $A \to B^A$ is a surjection. Then every map $B \to B$ has a fixed point.*

Proof. For $f : B \to B$ let $x \in A$ be such that for all $y \in A$, $e(x)(y) = f(e(y)(y))$. Then $e(x)(x)$ is a fixed point for f. ∎

Proposition 3.7.1 can be seen as a constructive diagonal argument. It implies that there cannot be surjections $N \to N^N$, $N \to 2^N$ etc.

Definition 3.7.2 Call an object A *enumerable* if there is a decidable subobject D of N and a surjection $D \to A$.

The only non-logical axiom we introduce is now:

Axiom. *The object Σ^N is enumerable*

It follows at once that Σ and Σ^N have the fixed point property, by proposition 3.7.1. And hence, that $2 \subsetneq \Sigma \subsetneq \Omega_{\neg\neg}$.

Note, that for subobjects of N, the notions of semidecidable and enumerable coincide.

Let L be the lift functor as in section 3.6.3. $L(N)^N$ is the object of partial functions $N \rightharpoonup N$ with semidecidable domain.

Proposition 3.7.3 $L(N)^N$ *is enumerable.*

Proof. It is not hard to prove the statement that every binary relation on N with semidecidable domain contains a partial function defined on that domain. Now let $V_{(-)} : N \to \Sigma^{N \times N}$ be an enumeration. Since N is projective, there is a map $\varphi_{(-)} : N \to L(N)^N$ such that for each n, φ_n is a partial function contained in V_n and with the same domain. But then $\varphi_{(-)} : N \to L(N)^N$ is an enumeration. ∎

Using proposition 3.7.3 we can prove the statement which corresponds to the theorem in recursion theory on the existence of disjoint, inseparable r.e. sets. Let $A_i = \{n \mid \varphi_n(n) = i\}$, for $1 = 0, 1$.

Proposition 3.7.4 *For every decidable subobject D of N, there is an $n \in N$ such that $n \in A_0 \cap D$ or $n \in A_1 - D$.*

Proof. Let $d : N \to N$ be the characteristic function of D: $d(k) = 0$ if $k \in D$ and $d(k) = 1$ otherwise. There is an n such that $d = \varphi_n$. For this n, if $d(n) = 0$ then $n \subset A_0 \cap D$, and if $d(n) = 1$ then $n \in A_1 - D$. ∎

As a consequence of 3.7.4, we can, just as in section 3.2.7, build a Kleene tree and construct an isomorphism between 2^N and N^N.

Next, we consider objects which are algebras for L as a pointed functor, that is, objects A together with a map $\epsilon : L(A) \to A$ such that the diagram

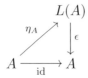

commutes. We call such objects *focal* (although an object may have
more than one focal structure); the map ϵ is called the focal map. It
is easy to see that the focal objects form an exponential ideal: if X is
focal, so is X^Y for any Y. Hence if A is focal and enumerable, so is A^N:
if $e : N \to A$ is an enumeration and $\epsilon L(A) \to A$ the focal map, then by
3.7.3 and internal projectivity of N, we have a surjection

$$N \xrightarrow{\varphi_{(-)}} L(N)^N \xrightarrow{L(e)^N} L(A)^N \xrightarrow{\epsilon^N} A^N$$

We obtain a generalization of Rice's Theorem:

Proposition 3.7.5 *If A is focal, then the diagonal map $2 \to 2^A$ is an
isomorphism.*

Since Σ, and hence also Σ^N, are focal, this generalizes 3.2.29.

Proposition 3.7.6 *Let A be enumerable and focal. Then for every total
binary relation R on A there is $x \in A$ such that $(x, x) \in R$.*

Proof. Let $e : N \to A$ the enumeration and $\epsilon : L(A) \to A$ be the focal
map. So $\epsilon(\{x\}) = x$.
    We have $\forall k \in N \exists m \in N (e(k), e(m)) \in R$ by totality of R, so by
number choice let $c \in N^N$ be such that $\forall k{:}N\, (e(k), e(c(k))) \in R$. It
suffices to find a k satisfying $e(c(k)) = e(k)$.
    We have $\forall m{:}N \exists n{:}N\, \epsilon(L(ec)(\varphi_m(m))) = e(n)$, so again by number
choice let $g{:}N^N$ satisfy $\epsilon(L(ec)(\varphi_m(m))) = e(g(m))$. Choose j such that
$g = \varphi_j$, and let $k = g(j)$. Then

$$e(k) = e(g(j)) = \epsilon(L(ec)(\varphi_j(j))) = e(c(g(j))) = e(c(k))$$

as desired.   ∎

As a corollary, we get the Recursion theorem:

Corollary 3.7.7 *For every $f{:}N^N$ there is $n{:}N$ such that $\varphi_n = \varphi_{f(n)}$.*

Proof. Apply 3.7.6 to the relation

$$R = \{(u, v) \in L(N)^N \times L(N)^N \mid \exists n{:}N(u = \varphi_n \wedge v = \varphi_{f(n)})\}$$

and recall that $L(N)^N$ is focal and enumerable.   ■

In [13], there are also theorems corresponding to the Rice-Shapiro and Myhill-Shepherdson theorems. Time will tell how far this development will go.

3.8   General Comments about the Effective Topos Construction

The effective topos construction is still, after 30 years, puzzling logicians and topos theorists. Whereas for Grothendieck toposes there exists a large body of theory, with representation theorems such as in the classic [86], the theory of classifying topoi and the whole field of generalized topogy, toposes like the effective topos offer few handles for understanding.

What is its place in the 2-category of toposes and geometric morphisms?

Or maybe we should look for another context in which to study it. Maybe more basic (and therefore harder) questions should be answered: which category-theoretic or otherwise general construction yields the category of subsets of $\mathbb{N}$ and partial recursive functions? Or, does the monoid of total recursive functions have any significant characterizing properties among monoids? We can say something about $\mathcal{K}_1$, as pca (it is pseudo-initial with respect to decidable applicative morphisms), but then what do we know about partial combinatory algebras?

What are the subtoposes (in the geometric sense of section 2.5.1) of $\mathcal{E}ff$, equivalently what are the local operators $j : \Omega \to \Omega$? We have seen (at some length) the $\neg\neg$-operator and corresponding subtopos Set, and we know that for any Turing degree there is a corresponding subtopos (2.6.4). We have seen that the Lifschitz tripos (2.6.8) is a subtripos of the effective tripos, and we shall see that it is not a standard realizability tripos (see section 4.4 below), so it is of a different shape than the other examples.

Just as little do we know about internal *locales* in $\mathcal{E}ff$. In short, we know awfully little about geometric morphisms into $\mathcal{E}ff$. As an illustration, the following question was asked at my Ph.D. defence in 1991. It is still unanswered:

> **Question** (Moerdijk) Is Set the only Grothendieck topos that is a subtopos of $\mathcal{E}ff$, or are there others?

just as little do we know about possible geometric morphisms out of $\mathcal{E}ff$, apart from the trivial observation that we can never have a geometric morphism to a Grothendieck topos.

By far the best investigated functor into $\mathcal{E}ff$ is $\nabla : \text{Set} \to \mathcal{E}ff$. In section 3.8.1, I have tried to give an account of how category theorists (most notably E. Robinson and G. Rosolini) have studied ∇ from an abstract point of view.

Maybe surprisingly, when we start studying maps out of $\mathcal{E}ff$, we soon meet ∇ again. In section 3.8.2 we study a bit the question whether $\mathcal{E}ff$ has a small dense subcategory, which allows a nice (non-geometric) embedding of $\mathcal{E}ff$ into a Grothendieck topos. The answer is seen to depend on what sort of filtered colimits are preserved by ∇.

The last section of this chapter discusses A. Pitts' *effective monad* and some material pertaining to the question whether Troelstra's proof-theoretic 'idempotence' of realizabiity has a semantic counterpart.

3.8.1 Analogy between ∇ and the Yoneda embedding

In his seminal paper [70], M. Hyland makes the following remark:

> *André Joyal has pointed out thet ∇ is analogous to the Yoneda embedding: it is cartesian, full and faithful and (so) preserves exponentiation. But I do not understand the force of this analogy.*

Of course, the analogy does go a little further than that (as Hyland undoubtedly knew): assume that $\mathcal{C}$ is a small category with finite limits, then the image of $y : \mathcal{C} \to \text{Set}^{\mathcal{C}^{\text{op}}}$ consists (up to isomorphism) of the *indecomposable projective* objects of $\text{Set}^{\mathcal{C}^{\text{op}}}$. Recall that an object is indecomposable if it cannot be written as a nontrivial coproduct.

The same holds for ∇: every projective object is isomorphic to a partitioned assembly, i.e. a set X together with a function $p : X \to \mathbb{N}$.

If the function p is nonconstant, say $p^{-1}(0) \neq \emptyset$ and $p^{-1}(\mathbb{N} - \{0\}) \neq \emptyset$ then (X, p) is isomorphic to a coproduct $\nabla(p^{-1}(0)) + Y$ where Y is the object $(p^{-1}(\mathbb{N} - \{0\}), p)$. If p is constant, then (X, p) is isomorphic to $\nabla(X)$.

A serious attempt to stretch the analogy as far as it goes, was made in the paper [134]. We start with the observation, that like $\mathcal{E}ff$, the category $\text{Set}^{\mathcal{C}^{\text{op}}}$ is an exact completion (at least if $\mathcal{C}$ has finite limits): the projective objects in $\text{Set}^{\mathcal{C}^{\text{op}}}$ are sums of representables. They are closed under finite limits, and every presheaf is covered by a projective, by standard presheaf theory. Another way of defining the category of projectives is as a category we have seen before: the category $\text{Fam}(\mathcal{C})$.

Is there any kind of similarity between $\text{Fam}(\mathcal{C})$ and the category of partitioned assemblies? After all, since we explore the analogy between $y : \mathcal{C} \rightarrow \text{Set}^{\mathcal{C}^{\text{op}}}$ and $\nabla : \text{Set} \rightarrow \mathcal{E}ff$, we should have an analogy between the subcategories of projectives of both target categories, since both are exact completions.

Now the category $\text{Fam}(\mathcal{C})$ is itself a completion construction: it is the *coproduct completion* of $\mathcal{C}$. That means the following: we have an evident functor $\eta : \mathcal{C} \rightarrow \text{Fam}(\mathcal{C})$ with the following properties:

i)   The category $\text{Fam}(\mathcal{C})$ has all small coproducts;

ii) For any functor $\mathcal{C} \xrightarrow{F} \mathcal{D}$ where $\mathcal{D}$ is a category which has all small coproducts, there is an essentially unique factorization

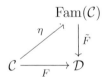

by a coproduct-preserving functor $\tilde{F} : \text{Fam}(\mathcal{C}) \rightarrow \mathcal{D}$.

Pushing our analogy leads us to ask: is the category of partitioned assemblies maybe also a coproduct completion, and then (naturally, since Set is the source of ∇) a coproduct completion of Set?

The answer in [134] is *yes*, provided we take a bit of care. Because at this point it is useful to have a look at the limitations of the analogy too. The category $\mathrm{Set}^{\mathcal{C}^{\mathrm{op}}}$ is also the *colimit completion* of $\mathcal{C}$ w.r.t. y: any functor from $\mathcal{C}$ to a cocomplete category $\mathcal{D}$ factors essentially uniquely through a colimit preserving functor (left Kan extension) from $\mathrm{Set}^{\mathcal{C}^{\mathrm{op}}}$ to $\mathcal{D}$. Now the fact that this is a *free* colimit completion means that the Yoneda embedding y preserves almost *no* colimits which may exist in $\mathcal{C}$: y preserves no coproducts at all (in particular, not initial objects), and only those epis which are preserved by every functor: the split ones. By contrast, ∇ does preserve the initial object and all epis.

Let us switch attention to the similarities between $\nabla : \mathrm{Set} \to \mathrm{PAss}$ (where PAss denotes the category of partitioned assemblies) and $\eta : \mathcal{C} \to \mathrm{Fam}(\mathcal{C})$. The functor η preserves epis but not the initial object. Now if $\mathcal{C}$ has a *strict* initial object (recall that this means: initial, and every arrow into it is an isomorphism) we can easily modify η a bit so that it does preserve the initial object. Let $\mathrm{Fam}_*(\mathcal{C})$ be the full subcategory of $\mathrm{Fam}(\mathcal{C})$ on those objects $(X, (C_x)_{x \in X})$ such that for all $x \in X$, C_x is non-initial in $\mathcal{C}$. We have a functor $\eta_* : \mathcal{C} \to \mathrm{Fam}_*(\mathcal{C})$ defined by:

$$\eta_*(C) = \begin{cases} (\{*\}, C) & \text{if } C \text{ is non-initial} \\ (\emptyset, \emptyset) & \text{otherwise} \end{cases}$$

(note, that the strictness of the initial object is needed for η_* to be a functor). Then η_* preserves epis and the initial object, $\mathrm{Fam}_*(\mathcal{C})$ has all coproducts, and every functor F from $\mathcal{C}$ to a category $\mathcal{D}$ such that $\mathcal{D}$ has all coproducts and F preserves the initial object, factors essentially uniquely through a coproduct-preserving functor $F_* : \mathrm{Fam}_*(\mathcal{C}) \to \mathcal{D}$ via η_*. We call $\mathrm{Fam}_*(\mathcal{C})$ the *nonempty coproduct completion* of $\mathcal{C}$.

Note that in $\mathrm{Fam}(\mathcal{C})$ and in $\mathrm{Fam}_*(\mathcal{C})$ the new, artificially added coproducts come from the coproducts in Set. We speak about the free completion of $\mathcal{C}$ by (nonempty) Set-indexed coproducts.

Now suppose that we want to turn this around, and wish to consider 'the free completion of Set by (nonempty) $\mathcal{C}$-indexed coproducts'? A real conceptual analysis of what this might mean involves concepts of enriched category theory which lie beyond the scope of this book. However, the discussion above suggests that if we write the free coproduct completions of $\mathcal{C}$ as $\mathrm{Fam}^{\mathrm{Set}}(\mathcal{C})$ and $\mathrm{Fam}^{\mathrm{Set}}_*(\mathcal{C})$, we now look at $\mathrm{Fam}^{\mathcal{C}}(\mathrm{Set})$ and $\mathrm{Fam}^{\mathcal{C}}_*(\mathrm{Set})$.

Suppose $\mathcal{C}$ is a subcategory of Set which contains $\emptyset$ as initial object. Let $\mathrm{Fam}^{\mathcal{C}}(\mathrm{Set})$ be the category of families of sets $(X_i)_{i\in A}$ indexed by an object A of $\mathcal{C}$, with as arrows $(X_i)_{i\in A} \to (Y_j)_{j\in B}$ pairs $(f,(\phi_i)_{i\in A})$ with $f : A \to B$ an arrow in $\mathcal{C}$ and $\phi_i : X_i \to Y_{f(i)}$ a function. Equivalently, objects are arrows $X \to A$ with A an object of $\mathcal{C}$, and arrows are commutative squares

$$
\begin{array}{ccc}
X & \xrightarrow{\ \phi\ } & Y \\
\downarrow & & \downarrow \\
A & \xrightarrow[\ f\ ]{} & B
\end{array}
$$

with f in $\mathcal{C}$. That is, $\mathrm{Fam}^{\mathcal{C}}(\mathrm{Set})$ is the comma category $\mathrm{Set}/\mathcal{C}$. And $\mathrm{Fam}^{\mathcal{C}}_*(\mathrm{Set})$ then, is the full subcategory of $\mathrm{Set}/\mathcal{C}$ on the *surjective* functions $X \to A$.

Now let us further assume that $\mathcal{C}$ has a terminal object which is also terminal in Set, say $\{*\}$. Then we have an embedding $\mathrm{Set} \to \mathrm{Fam}^{\mathcal{C}}(\mathrm{Set})$ sending X to $X \to \{*\}$, and an embedding $\mathrm{Set} \to \mathrm{Fam}^{\mathcal{C}}_*(\mathrm{Set})$ which sends X to $X \to \{*\}$ if X is nonempty, and $\emptyset$ to $\emptyset \to \emptyset$.

The point is now, that if we consider the category $\mathbf{R}$ of subsets of $\mathbb{N}$ and partial recursive functions (an arrow $A \to B$ in $\mathbf{R}$ is a partial recursive function which is defined on A and maps A into B) in the role of $\mathcal{C}$, we easily see that $\mathrm{Fam}^{\mathbf{R}}_*(\mathrm{Set})$ is isomorphic to PAss. We summarize this in the following slogan:

> *The category of partitioned assemblies is the free cocomple-*
> *tion of* Set *by nonempty, recursively indexed coproducts*

I hope this discussion renders, in a language as naive as possible, the essential point of [134]. In that paper, the authors use the language of fibrations. There are fibrations $\mathrm{Set} \to \mathbf{R}$ and $\mathrm{PAss} \to \mathbf{R}$, and the latter is the free completion of the former under 'adding left adjoints to the reindexing functors along surjections in $\mathbf{R}$, which left adjoints must satisfy the Beck-Chevalley condition'.

For another view on the construction of $\mathcal{E}ff$ and related categories, also based on the exact completion idea, see [133].

3.8.2 Small dense subcategories in $\mathcal{E}ff$

A fundamental question is: how does $\mathcal{E}ff$ compare to Grothendieck topoi? Is it possible to embed $\mathcal{E}ff$ into a Grothendieck topos in a nice way? In [136], a functor from $\mathcal{E}ff$ into the "recursive topos" of Mulry ([116]) is defined, but this functor does not preserve a lot of structure (it is, for example, not an embedding).

Nice embeddings can be obtained by considering small full dense subcategories of $\mathcal{E}ff$. Recall that for every category $\mathcal{E}$, a subcategory $\mathcal{C} \subset \mathcal{E}$ is *dense* if for every object X of $\mathcal{E}$, the natural cocone with vertex X for the diagram $\mathcal{C}{\downarrow}X \overset{\text{dom}}{\to} \mathcal{C} \to \mathcal{E}$ is colimiting. If this is the case, and J is the Grothendieck topology on $\mathcal{C}$ induced by the canonical topology on $\mathcal{E}$, then the left Kan extension of the Yoneda embedding on $\mathcal{C}$, the functor from $\mathcal{E}$ to $[\mathcal{C}^{\mathrm{op}}, \text{Sets}]$ which sends X to $\mathcal{E}(-, X)$, factors through the sheaf topos $\text{Sh}(\mathcal{C}, J)$ and this factorisation is full and faithful, cartesian closed, and preserves all limits and colimits of $\mathcal{E}$; hence also the natural numbers object. This is standard topos theory; see [83] or [102].

Since $\mathcal{E}ff$ is an exact completion, if a small full dense subcategory $\mathcal{C}$ of $\mathcal{E}ff$ exists, we may assume that $\mathcal{C}$ consists of projective objects of bounded cardinality (given a small dense subcategory, by taking projective covers of all objects one can construct a small dense subcategory on a set of projective objects). It seems natural to suppose that the countable projective objects form a dense subcategory; it certainly is true that whenever $X \overset{f}{\underset{g}{\rightrightarrows}} Y$ is a parallel pair of arrows in $\mathcal{E}ff$ and $f \neq g$, then there is a countable projective object A and a map $a : A \to X$ such that $fa \neq ga$.

Basically, this section contains two theorems: theorem 3.8.2 states an equivalent condition for the full subcategory of λ-small (i.e., having underlying set of cardinality less than λ) projectives to be dense in $\mathcal{E}ff$, relating this to the preservation by ∇ of λ-filtered colimits. Then, after a few folklore results included for completeness' sake, theorem 3.8.5 states that ∇ does not preserve ω_1-filtered colimits.

I recall the definition from [83], D2.3.1: a category is λ-small if its class of arrows has cardinality $< \lambda$. A category is called λ-filtered if every diagram in it, indexed by a λ-small category, has a cocone.

The following characterization of the projective objects appears in
[134]. Let $\eta_N : N \to \nabla(\mathbb{N})$ be the unit of the adjunction $\Gamma \dashv \nabla$ at N,
and $\eta_N^* : \mathcal{E}ff/\nabla(\mathbb{N}) \to \mathcal{E}ff/N$ the pullback functor. There is a functor
$\nabla_N : \mathrm{Sets}/\mathbb{N} \to \mathcal{E}ff/N$ obtained by composing with η_N^*. Furthermore
denote, as usual, the forgetful (domain) functor $\mathcal{E}ff/N \to \mathcal{E}ff$ by Σ_N.
Then:

Lemma 3.8.1 (Robinson, Rosolini) *An object of $\mathcal{E}ff$ is projective if
and only if it is isomorphic to one in the image of $\Sigma_N \circ \nabla_N$.*

Theorem 3.8.2 *Let $\lambda > \omega$ be a regular cardinal. Then the following
two assertions are equivalent:*

i)   The full subcategory of $\mathcal{E}ff$ on the λ-small projectives is dense.

ii) $\nabla : \mathrm{Set} \to \mathcal{E}ff$ preserves λ-filtered colimits.

For $\lambda = \omega$, the implication i)$\Rightarrow$ii) still holds.

Proof. i)$\Rightarrow$ii): First observe that, since ∇ preserves epi-mono factorizations, statement ii) is equivalent to saying that for any set X, $\nabla(X)$ is
the vertex of a colimiting cocone for the diagram consisting of all $\nabla(Y)$
for $Y \subseteq X$ λ-small, and (∇-images of) inclusions. Now since for any X,
any cocone to $\nabla(X)$ for a diagram of λ-small projectives also yields a
cocone for a diagram of ∇'s of λ-small subsets of X (by sheafification),
it is clear that i) implies ii).

For ii)$\Rightarrow$i), observe that if $\nabla : \mathrm{Set} \to \mathcal{E}ff$ preserves λ-small colimits then
the same is true for the functor $\nabla/\mathbb{N} : \mathrm{Set}/\mathbb{N} \to \mathcal{E}ff/\nabla(\mathbb{N})$ because the
forgetful functors $\Sigma_{\mathbb{N}} : \mathrm{Set}/\mathbb{N} \to \mathrm{Set}$ and $\Sigma_{\nabla(\mathbb{N})} : \mathcal{E}ff/\nabla(\mathbb{N}) \to \mathcal{E}ff$ preserve and create colimits. Since the pullback functor $\eta_N^* : \mathcal{E}ff/\nabla(\mathbb{N}) \to
\mathcal{E}ff/N$ has a right adjoint, the composite functor $\nabla_N : \mathrm{Set}/\mathbb{N} \to \mathcal{E}ff/N$
preserves λ-filtered colimits too.
  In order to prove i), it clearly suffices to prove that every projective
object X is a colimit of its λ-small sub-projectives. So suppose that for
every λ-small sub-projective Y of X we are given a map $\phi_Y : Y \to (Z, =)$
in $\mathcal{E}ff$, such that for $Y' \subset Y$, $\phi_Y \upharpoonright Y' = \phi_{Y'}$. Each such projective Y is a
set Y together with a map $e : Y \to \mathbb{N}$; equivalently, an $\mathbb{N}$-indexed family

of sets $(Y_n)_{n\in\mathbb{N}}$. Any map $(Y_n)_{n\in\mathbb{N}} \to (Z,=)$ is represented by a function $f : Y \to Z$ such that for some partial recursive function p we have that for all n such that $Y_n \neq \emptyset$, $p(n)$ is defined and

$$p(n) \in \bigcap_{y\in Y_n} [f(y) = f(y)]$$

In such a case, one says that p *tracks* f. Two such functions $f, g : Y \to Z$ represent the same morphism iff there is a partial recursive function q such that for all n with $Y_n \neq \emptyset$, $q(n) \in \bigcap_{y\in Y_n} [f(y) = g(y)]$.

Now I claim that for some partial recursive function p, it holds that for $Y \subset X$ λ-small, *every* ϕ_Y has a representative which is tracked by p; for otherwise choose for every p a λ-small $Y_p \subset X$ for which no representative tracked by p exists; since there are only countably many partial recursive functions the union $\bigcup_p Y_p$ is still λ-small (since $\lambda > \omega$); a contradiction is easily obtained.

Fix such a p as in the previous paragraph. Construct an object $(Z', =')$ from $(Z,=)$ by putting

$$Z' = \{(n, z) \,|\, p(n) \text{ is defined and } p(n) \in [z = z]\}$$

and

$$[(n, z) =' (m, z)] = \begin{cases} \{n\} \wedge [z = z'] & \text{if } n = m \\ \emptyset & \text{otherwise} \end{cases}$$

Recall that $\{n\} \wedge [z = z']$ is $\{\langle n, a\rangle \,|\, a \in [z = z']\}$, where $\langle -, -\rangle$ is a recursive bijection $\mathbb{N}^2 \to \mathbb{N}$.

The object Z' comes with maps $Z' \xrightarrow{\pi_1} N$ and $Z' \xrightarrow{\pi_2} Z$ such that every $\phi_Y : Y \to Z$ factors through some $\phi'_Y : Y \to Z'$ which has the property that if one regards $Y = (Y_n)_{n\in\mathbb{N}}$ as an object of $\mathcal{E}ff/N$, ϕ'_Y is a map over N.

We have therefore a cocone for the λ-filtered diagram of sub-projectives of X, regarded as objects of $\mathcal{E}ff/N$, with vertex the object $Z' \xrightarrow{\pi_1} N$. Since the diagram is in the image (under ∇_N) of a λ-filtered diagram in Sets/$\mathbb{N}$ and ∇_N preserves λ-filtered colimits, its colimit is the projective X (as object of $\mathcal{E}ff/N$), and there is a unique mediating map $X \to Z'$

over N. But then the composite $X \to Z$ is the unique mediating map for the original cocone of the ϕ_Y's.   ∎

It is worth noting that this result also applies to other realizability toposes based on partial combinatory algebras A, provided (for the implication ii)$\Rightarrow$i)) one replaces ω by $|A|$.

So, we are led to study the preservation of λ-filtered colimits by ∇.

  Clearly, if $\nabla :$ Set $\to \mathcal{E}ff$ preserves λ-filtered colimits then so does $\nabla :$ Set $\to$ Ass.

Proposition 3.8.3 $\nabla :$ Set $\to$ Ass *does not preserve filtered colimits.*

Proof. Let $e \mapsto [e] : \mathbb{N} \to \mathcal{P}_{\text{fin}}(\mathbb{N})$ be a bijective coding of finite subsets of $\mathbb{N}$. Let A be the assembly $(\mathbb{N}, E)$ where $E(n) = \{e \,|\, n \in [e]\}$. Then for any finite subset $[e]$ of $\mathbb{N}$ there is a map of assemblies $\nabla([e]) \to A$, tracked by the function which is constant e; and this system of maps is clearly a cocone for the diagram of ∇'s of finite subsets of $\mathbb{N}$ and inclusions between them. But there is no mediating map: $\nabla(\mathbb{N}) \to A$. ∎

Proposition 3.8.4 $\nabla :$ Set $\to$ Ass *preserves ω_1-filtered colimits.*

Proof. Easy.   ∎

Theorem 3.8.5 *The functor* $\nabla :$ Set $\to \mathcal{E}ff$ *does not preserve ω_1-filtered colimits.*

Proof. Let D be the ω_1-filtered diagram of countable subsets of ω_1 and inclusions between them; clearly, in Sets, the cocone $D \to \omega_1$ is colimiting. We shall see that $\nabla(D) \to \nabla(\omega_1)$ is not colimiting in $\mathcal{E}ff$.

  Recall the necessary ingredients of the construction of an ω_1-*Aronszajn tree* (see [94] for the full story). If α is a countable ordinal and $s, t : \alpha \to \omega$, we write $s \sim t$ if the set $\{\xi \in \alpha \,|\, s(\xi) \neq t(\xi)\}$ is finite. If $s \sim t$, let $d(s, t)$ be the cardinality of this set.

  It is possible to construct a sequence $\{s_\alpha : \alpha \in \omega_1\}$ such that for each α, s_α is a 1-1 function from α into ω, and such that for $\alpha < \beta$, $s_\alpha \sim (s_\beta \restriction \alpha)$.

Let T^* consist of all injective functions $s : \alpha \to \omega$, defined on some countable α, such that $s \sim s_\alpha$. Note that for each $\alpha \in \omega_1$, the set $L_\alpha = \{s \in T^* \,|\, \mathrm{dom}(s) = \alpha\}$ is countable.

Equip T^* with the structure of an object of $\mathcal{Eff}$, by defining

$$[s = t] \;=\; \begin{cases} \emptyset & \text{if } \mathrm{dom}(s) \neq \mathrm{dom}(t) \\ \{n \,|\, d(s,t) \leq n\} & \text{otherwise} \end{cases}$$

Clearly, if $n \in [s = t]$ and $m \in [t = u]$ then $m + n \in [s = u]$, so this is a well-defined equality relation. $(T^*, =)$ is a uniform object since $0 \in \bigcap_{s \in T^*} [s = s]$.

For each $\alpha \in \omega_1$ let $\phi_\alpha : \alpha \to T^*$ be defined by

$$\phi_\alpha(\beta) = s_\alpha {\restriction} \beta$$

Then for each pair $\alpha < \alpha'$ in ω_1 we have that

$$d(s_\alpha, s_{\alpha'} {\restriction} \alpha) \in \bigcap_{\beta \in \alpha} [\phi_\alpha(\beta) = \phi_{\alpha'}(\beta)]$$

which means that the functions ϕ_α and $\phi_{\alpha'} {\restriction} \alpha$ define the same morphism from $\nabla(\alpha)$ to $(T^*, =)$ in $\mathcal{Eff}$; we shall denote this morphism also by ϕ_α.

If $A \subset \omega_1$ is a countable set, let $\phi_A : A \to T^*$ be the restriction of ϕ_α to A, where $\alpha = \sup\{\beta + 1 \,|\, \beta \in A\}$. Clearly then, the system

$$\{\phi_A : \nabla(A) \to (T^*, =) \,|\, A \subset \omega_1 \text{ countable}\}$$

defines a cocone on $\nabla(D)$ with vertex $(T^*, =)$. I claim that this cocone does not factor through $\nabla(\omega_1)$.

Suppose, to the contrary, that there is a morphism $\Phi : \nabla(\omega_1) \to (T^*, =)$ such that for each $\alpha \in \omega_1$, $\Phi \circ \nabla(\iota_\alpha) = \phi_\alpha$, where ι_α is the inclusion of α in ω_1. Then $\Phi : \omega_1 \to T^*$ has the property that for every α there is an $n \in \omega$ such that

$$n \in \bigcap_{\beta \in \alpha} [\phi_\alpha(\beta) = \Phi(\beta)]$$

Then there must be a number n such that the set

$$A_n \;=\; \{\alpha \in \omega_1 \,|\, n \in \bigcap_{\beta \in \alpha} [\phi_\alpha(\beta) = \Phi(\beta)]\}$$

is *unbounded* in ω_1. Fix such an n for the rest of the proof. If $\alpha < \alpha'$ are elements of A_n, then

$$2n \in \bigcap_{\beta \in \alpha} [\phi_\alpha(\beta) = \phi_{\alpha'}(\beta)]$$

So for each $\beta < \alpha$ there are at most $2n$ ordinals $\xi \in \beta$ such that $s_\alpha(\xi) \neq s_{\alpha'}(\xi)$; it follows that $2n + 1 \in [s_\alpha = s_{\alpha'} \restriction \alpha]$.

However, this is a contradiction once we have proved the following

CLAIM 1. Let A be unbounded in ω_1; then there exist, for each $k \in \omega$, elements $\alpha < \alpha'$ of A such that $d(s_\alpha, s_{\alpha'} \restriction \alpha) \geq k$.
Proof of Claim 1: first observe that if $A \subseteq \omega_1$ is unbounded, then for each $\xi \in \omega_1$ there is at least one n such that the set

$$A_{\xi,n} = \{\alpha \in A \mid \alpha > \xi \text{ and } s_\alpha(\xi) = n\}$$

is unbounded.

CLAIM 2. Let A be unbounded. Then for each $\eta \in \omega_1$ there is a $\xi > \eta$ such that there are n, m with $n \neq m$ and both $A_{\xi,n}$ and $A_{\xi,m}$ unbounded.
Proof of Claim 2: suppose Claim 2 is false; then by the remark preceding it, there is $\eta \in \omega_1$ such that for each $\xi > \eta$ there is exactly one n such that $A_{\xi,n}$ is unbounded. Then for every $\xi > \eta$ there is a $\beta_\xi \in A$ such that for all $\alpha, \alpha' \in A$ that are $\geq \beta_\xi$, $s_\alpha(\xi) = s_{\alpha'}(\xi)$. But then the function $\xi \mapsto s_{\beta_\xi}(\xi)$ is easily seen to be a 1-1 function from $\{\xi \mid \eta < \xi\}$ to ω, which is impossible.

Proof of Claim 1, continued: we construct, for each $k \in \omega$, sequences $(\xi_1, \dots, \xi_k)$ and $((n_1, m_1), \dots, (n_k, m_k))$ with $\xi_1 < \cdots < \xi_k < \omega_1$, $n_i, m_i \in \omega$ such that $n_i \neq m_i$ and the sets

$$A_{\vec{\xi},\vec{n}} = \{\alpha \in A \mid \alpha > \xi_k \text{ and } \forall i \leq k (s_\alpha(\xi_i) = n_i)\}$$
$$B_{\vec{\xi},\vec{m}} = \{\alpha \in A \mid \alpha > \xi_k \text{ and } \forall i \leq k (s_\alpha(\xi_i) = m_i)\}$$

are both unbounded.

For $k = 1$ simply apply Claim 2. Inductively, suppose $(\xi_1, \dots, \xi_k)$ and $((n_1, m_1), \dots, (n_k, m_k))$ have been defined satisfying the conditions.

Apply Claim 2 with $A = A_{\vec{\xi},\vec{n}}$ and $\eta = \xi_k$. One finds $\xi_{k+1} > \xi_k$ and $a \neq b$ such that both $A_{\xi_{k+1},a}$ and $A_{\xi_{k+1},b}$ are unbounded.

If $B_{\vec{\xi},\xi_{k+1},\vec{m},a}$ is unbounded, let $n_{k+1} = b, m_{k+1} = a$. If $B_{\vec{\xi},\xi_{k+1},\vec{m},b}$ is unbounded, let $n_{k+1} = a, m_{k+1} = b$. If neither of these two, let $n_{k+1} = a$ and pick m_{k+1} arbitrary, such that $B_{\vec{\xi},\xi_{k+1},\vec{m},m_{k+1}}$ is unbounded. ∎

3.8.3 Idempotence of realizability

Soon after Kleene presented his definition of realizability for first order arithmetic, he and his student D. Nelson ([119]) worked out how to formalize the interpretation: to any formula φ of intuitionistic arithmetic (or 'Heyting Arithmetic', the system is usually called HA) a formula $x \mathbf{r} \varphi$ was assigned (with x a fresh variable) which expresses that x is a number which realizes φ. The theorem was that whenever φ is a theorem of HA, so is $\exists x(x \mathbf{r} \varphi)$; thus one obtains an interpretation of HA into itself (or into PA).

This led automatically to the questions:

1) What is the realizability theory of HA? What is the set of sentences φ for which $\exists x(x \mathbf{r} \varphi)$ is provable in HA?

2) What happens if we iterate the interpretation? How do the formulas $\exists x(x \mathbf{r} \varphi)$ and $\exists y(y \mathbf{r} \exists x(x \mathbf{r} \varphi))$ relate to each other?

These questions are somewhat related. The Dragalin-Troelstra analysis ([37, 160, 161]) of formalized realizability noted that every formula $x \mathbf{r} \varphi$ is (up to equivalence in HA) almost negative, and the axiom scheme ECT_0 has the following properties:

i) $HA + ECT_0 \vdash \varphi \leftrightarrow \exists x(x \mathbf{r} \varphi)$

ii) $HA \vdash \exists x(x \mathbf{r} \varphi) \Leftrightarrow HA + ECT_0 \vdash \varphi$

It follows that the formulas $\exists x(x \mathbf{r} \varphi)$ and $\exists y(y \mathbf{r} \exists x(x \mathbf{r} \varphi))$ are equivalent in HA. In the words of Troelstra: realizability is 'idempotent'.

Does this idempotence extend to the semantic world of the effective topos? Is there, in $\mathcal{E}ff$, an internal notion of realizability such that we have an equivalence $\phi \leftrightarrow \exists x(x \mathbf{r} \phi)$ in $\mathcal{E}ff$?

The answer is yes, provided we take into account that realizability, as Kleene intended it to be, is an interpretation of intuitionistic reasoning into a *classical* world (which, in the formalized version, is reflected by the fact that the formula x **r** φ is almost negative, which means that it is true classically precisely when it is true intuitionistically).

Another approach to the idempotence question was investigated by A. Pitts in [123]. On any topos $\mathcal{E}$ with natural numbers object N, one can construct an 'effective topos over $\mathcal{E}$', which we call $e\mathcal{E}$. Define a tripos over $\mathcal{E}$ whose value at an object X of $\mathcal{E}$ is the set of arrows $\mathcal{E}(X, \mathcal{P}(N))$, ordered as follows: $\phi \leq \psi$ if there is an arrow $1 \xrightarrow{n} N$ in $\mathcal{E}$ such that the sentence

$$\forall x{:}X \forall m \in \phi(x)\,(nm{\downarrow} \wedge nm \in \psi(x))$$

is true in $\mathcal{E}$.

The topos $e\mathcal{E}$ is then the topos constructed out of this tripos. Many of the results we have seen about $\mathcal{E}ff$, hold more generally for $e\mathcal{E}$, for example $\nabla : \mathcal{E} \to e\mathcal{E}$ is the direct image of a geometric inclusion (although, of course, $\mathcal{E}$ is no longer in general the category of $\neg\neg$-sheaves in $e\mathcal{E}$).

Now in particular, this construction can be carried out for $\mathcal{E} = \mathcal{E}ff$. Is this 'realizability construction' (up to equivalence) idempotent?

The investigation of $e\mathcal{E}ff$ is greatly facilitated by the iteration theorem 2.7.1. Since $e\mathcal{E}ff$ results by a tripos-to-topos construction on $\mathcal{E}ff$, which itself arises out of a tripos on Set, this theorem tells us that $e\mathcal{E}ff$ results from a tripos on Set whose value at a set X is the set of arrows $\mathcal{E}ff(\nabla(X), \mathcal{P}(N))$, ordered by: $\phi \leq \psi$ iff there is a number n such that

$$\mathcal{E}ff \models \forall x{:}\nabla(X) \forall m \in \phi(x)\,(nm{\downarrow} \wedge nm \in \psi(x))$$

Now we know from section 3.1.1 (Shanin's Principle) that $\mathcal{P}(N)$ is covered by $\mathcal{P}_{\neg\neg}(N)$ by a map which is internally defined as $A \mapsto \{p_0 n \,|\, n \in A\}$.

Since $\nabla(X)$ is projective, every $\phi : \nabla(X) \to \mathcal{P}(N)$ factors through a map $\phi' : \nabla(X) \to \mathcal{P}_{\neg\neg}(N)$ via this covering. Then saying that $\phi \leq \psi$ means for the factorizations ϕ', ψ': there is a number n such that

$$\mathcal{E}ff \models \forall x{:}\nabla(X) \forall m\,(\exists k(pmk \in \phi'(x) \to nm{\downarrow} \wedge \exists l(p(nm)l \in \psi'(x))))$$

By ECT, this is equivalent to

$$\mathcal{E}\!f\!f \models \forall x{:}\nabla(X)\exists g\forall mk\,(pmk \in \phi'(x) \rightarrow nm{\downarrow}\wedge gmk{\downarrow}\wedge p(nm)(gmk) \in \psi'(x))$$

Now using the uniformity principle for $\nabla(X)$ and the fact that 1 is projective in $\mathcal{E}\!f\!f$, we see that $\phi \leq \psi$ iff there are numbers n, g such that

$$\mathcal{E}\!f\!f \models \forall x{:}\nabla(X)\forall mk\,(pmk \in \phi'(x) \rightarrow p(nm)(gmk) \in \psi'(x))$$

Taking into account the interpretation of the element relation between N and $\mathcal{P}_{\neg\neg}(N)$, this means that $e\mathcal{E}\!f\!f$ is constructed out of a tripos on Set whose value at a set X is $\mathcal{P}(\mathbb{N} \times \mathbb{N})^X$, with $\phi \leq \psi$ iff for some numbers n, g we have: for all $x \in X$ and all $(m, k) \in \phi(x)$, $nm{\downarrow}$ and $gmk{\downarrow}$ and $(nm, gmk) \in \psi(x)$.

That is, $e\mathcal{E}\!f\!f$ is $\mathsf{RT}(\mathbb{N} \ltimes \mathbb{N})$, where $\ltimes$ is as in example 1.4.11. The inclusion $\mathcal{E}\!f\!f \rightarrow e\mathcal{E}\!f\!f$ corresponds to the applicative morphism $\mathbb{N} \ltimes \mathbb{N} \rightarrow \mathbb{N}$ given at the end of section 2.6.3. This morphism is not an equivalence.

Pitts proves in [123] that the construction $\mathcal{E} \mapsto e\mathcal{E}$ gives a *monad* on a subcategory of the category of toposes and geometric morphisms: the *effective monad*. I give the main definitions and statements; leaving proofs to the reader.

Throughout, we consider toposes with natural numbers object; if $\mathcal{E}$ is such a topos, the NNO is denoted $N_{\mathcal{E}}$.

Definition 3.8.6 A finite limit preserving functor L is called *exact* if L is regular and preserves finite colimits.

It is not hard to show that a regular functor between toposes is exact precisely when it preserves the NNO.

For any finite limit preserving functor $L : \mathcal{E} \rightarrow \mathcal{F}$ we have a comparison morphism $\lambda : N_{\mathcal{F}} \rightarrow L(N_{\mathcal{E}})$ such that the diagram

$$
\begin{array}{ccccc}
1 & \xrightarrow{\;0\;} & N_{\mathcal{F}} & \xrightarrow{\;s\;} & N_{\mathcal{F}} \\
{\scriptstyle\simeq}\big\downarrow & & \big\downarrow{\scriptstyle\lambda} & & \big\downarrow{\scriptstyle\lambda} \\
L(1) & \xrightarrow[L(0)]{} & L(N_{\mathcal{E}}) & \xrightarrow[L(s)]{} & L(N_{\mathcal{E}})
\end{array}
$$

commutes.

Let $\mathrm{App}_{\mathcal{E}}$ be the partial recursive application relation in $\mathcal{E}$:

$$\mathrm{App}_{\mathcal{E}} \;=\; \{(n,m,k)\,|\,\exists y(T(n,m,y)\wedge U(y)=k)\}$$

Then $L(N_{\mathcal{E}})$ with application relation $L(\mathrm{App}_{\mathcal{E}})$ is a pca in $\mathcal{F}$; we write the application on $L(N_{\mathcal{E}})$ as $(x,y)\mapsto x^{L}y$. Then in $\mathcal{F}$, the sentence

$$\forall nmk{:}N\,(nm=k\to(\lambda n)^{L}(\lambda m)=\lambda k)$$

is true.

The functor L is said to *conserve application*, if

$$\mathcal{F}\models\forall nm((\lambda n)^{L}(\lambda m)\!\downarrow\;\to\;nm\!\downarrow\wedge\,(\lambda n)^{L}(\lambda m)=\lambda(nm))$$

The following properties hold for functors $\mathcal{E}\xrightarrow{L}\mathcal{F}\xrightarrow{K}\mathcal{G}$ which preserve finite limits:

i)   If L and K conserve application, so does KL;

ii)   if L and KL conserve application, so does K;

iii) if L is exact, it conserves application.

Furthermore: for any topos $\mathcal{E}$ with NNO, the functor $\nabla_{\mathcal{E}}:\mathcal{E}\to e\mathcal{E}$ conserves application.

The topos $e\mathcal{E}$ has a universal property w.r.t. exact functors and regular functors which conserve application:

Proposition 3.8.7 *Let $L:\mathcal{E}\to\mathcal{F}$ be a regular functor which conserves application. Then there is an exact functor $\bar{L}:e\mathcal{E}\to\mathcal{F}$ such that the diagram*

commutes up to isomorphism; and $\bar{L}$ is unique up to isomorphism with this property.

From this proposition it follows that if L is regular and conserves application, there is an exact functor $eL : e\mathcal{E} \to e\mathcal{F}$ such that $(eL)\nabla_{\mathcal{E}} \simeq \nabla_{\mathcal{F}}L$. So we have a functor $\mathcal{E} \to e\mathcal{E}$ defined on the category of toposes with NNO, and regular functors which conserve application; and a natural transformation from the identity to this functor.

Now consider a geometric morphism $f : \mathcal{F} \to \mathcal{E}$. Since $\nabla_{\mathcal{F}}$ and $f^* : \mathcal{E} \to \mathcal{F}$ are regular functors which conserve application, by proposition 3.8.7 we have an essentially unique exact functor $e\mathcal{E} \to e\mathcal{F}$, which we would like to call $(ef)^*$; it is essentially unique with the property that $(ef)^*\nabla_{\mathcal{E}} \simeq \nabla_{\mathcal{F}}f^*$.

Say that the geometric morphism f conserves application, if the functor f_* does.

Theorem 3.8.8 *If $f : \mathcal{F} \to \mathcal{E}$ is a geometric morphism which conserves application, then $(ef)^*$ has a right adjoint $(ef)_*$, and we have a geometric morphism $ef : e\mathcal{F} \to e\mathcal{E}$ such that the diagram*

$$
\begin{array}{ccc}
\mathcal{F} & \xrightarrow{\ f\ } & \mathcal{E} \\
{\scriptstyle \eta_{\mathcal{F}}}\big\downarrow & & \big\downarrow{\scriptstyle \eta_{\mathcal{E}}} \\
e\mathcal{F} & \xrightarrow[\ ef\ ]{} & e\mathcal{E}
\end{array}
$$

commutes (here $\eta_{\mathcal{F}}$ is the inclusion, i.e. $(\eta_{\mathcal{F}})_* = \nabla_{\mathcal{F}}$).

So, the construction $e(-)$ is also a functor on the category of toposes with NNO and geometric morphisms which conserves application. This functor turns out to admit a *monad structure*. Pitts calls this the 'effective monad'.

Now if $\mathcal{E} = \mathsf{RT}(A)$, then (by a similar reasoning as applied to $\mathcal{E}ff$ above), $e\mathcal{E} = \mathsf{RT}(\mathbb{N} \ltimes A)$. The construction $\mathbb{N} \ltimes (-)$ is certainly functorial on PCA: if $\gamma : A \to B$ is an applicative morphism, then we have an applicative morphism $\mathbb{N} \ltimes \gamma : \mathbb{N} \ltimes A \to \mathbb{N} \ltimes B$ defined by

$$(n, a) \mapsto \{(n, b) \mid b \in \gamma(a)\}$$

The functor $\mathbb{N} \ltimes (-)$ admits a *comonad structure* on PCA with counit $\varepsilon : \mathbb{N} \ltimes A \to A$ given by $(n, a) \mapsto p\bar{n}a$, and comultiplication $\delta : \mathbb{N} \ltimes A \to \mathbb{N} \ltimes (\mathbb{N} \ltimes A)$ sending (n, a) to $(n, (n, a))$.

About idempotence of the effective topos construction: we may also consider a construction $e_{\neg\neg}(-)$: for a topos $\mathcal{E}$ form the tripos which assigns to an object X the set of maps $\mathcal{E}(X, \mathcal{P}_{\neg\neg}(N))$, with the same preorder. Since Set is Boolean, $e_{\neg\neg}(\text{Set})$ is the effective topos, and $e_{\neg\neg}(\mathcal{E}ff) = \mathcal{E}ff$, as follows by a similar iteration argument as we have seen before.

This can be turned into an internal realizability interpretation in $\mathcal{E}ff$ as follows. The following treatment is taken from [169].

Proposition 3.8.9 *Suppose $\mathcal{L}$ is a relational language in many-sorted predicate logic, and $[\![\cdot]\!]$ an interpretation of $\mathcal{L}$ in $\mathcal{E}ff$ (for each sort σ of $\mathcal{L}$, $[\![\sigma]\!]$ is an object of $\mathcal{E}ff$, and for each relation symbol $R \subseteq \sigma_1 \times \cdots \times \sigma_n$, $[\![R]\!]$ is a subobject of $[\![\sigma_1]\!] \times \cdots \times [\![\sigma_n]\!]$).*
    Then there is an extension $\mathcal{L}'$ of $\mathcal{L}$ containing a sort ν of natural numbers, an extension $[\![\cdot]\!]'$ of $[\![\cdot]\!]$ to $\mathcal{L}'$, such that $[\![\nu]\!]'$ is the natural numbers object of $\mathcal{E}ff$, and a syntactical translation of $\mathcal{L}'$ into itself:

$$\varphi \mapsto x \, \mathbf{r} \, \varphi$$

(x a variable of sort ν, not occurring in φ), which has the same inductive clauses as Kleene's realizability, such that:

- $\neg\neg x \, \mathbf{r} \, \varphi \to x \, \mathbf{r} \, \varphi$

- $\varphi \leftrightarrow \exists x (x \, \mathbf{r} \, \varphi)$ *(for sentences φ)*

are both true in $\mathcal{E}ff$.

Proof. The proof depends on $[\![\cdot]\!]$. I start by considering the case that all sorts σ of $\mathcal{L}$ are interpreted by *separated* objects $[\![\sigma]\!]$ of $\mathcal{E}ff$. As usual, $a : \mathcal{E}ff \to \mathcal{E}ff$ is the sheafification functor $\nabla \circ \Gamma$.
    The familiar surjection $\nabla(\mathcal{P}(\mathbb{N})) \overset{q}{\twoheadrightarrow} \Omega$ from section 3.1.1 has the property that every map $(A, \sim) \overset{f}{\to} \Omega$ with (A, sim) separated, factors through q as $q \circ f'$ for some $(A, sim) \overset{f'}{\to} \nabla(\mathcal{P}(\mathbb{N}))$. Since $\nabla(\mathcal{P}(\mathbb{N}))$ is a sheaf, we have:

> For any separated (A, sim) and subobject $\varphi \rightarrowtail (A, sim)$, there is a function $F : \Gamma(A, sim) \to \mathcal{P}(\mathbb{N})$ in Sets such that the classifying map $\tilde{\varphi} : (A, sim) \to \Omega$ factors as $q \circ \nabla(F) \circ \eta$.

Now $\mathcal{L}'$ is defined as follows:

- for any sort σ of $\mathcal{L}$, add a new sort $l(\sigma)$;

- add sorts ν and $\Pi(\nu)$;

- for any sort σ of $\mathcal{L}$ add a function symbol $E_\sigma : l(\sigma) \to \Pi(\nu)$;

- For any relation symbol $R \subseteq \sigma_1 \times \cdots \times \sigma_n$ of $\mathcal{L}$, add a function symbol $f_R : l(\sigma_1) \times \cdots \times l(\sigma_n) \to \Pi(\nu)$;

- add a relation symbol $\in \subseteq \nu \times \Pi(\nu)$;

- add a constant $\mathbf{0} \in \nu$, a relation symbol $T \subseteq \nu^3$, and function symbols $\langle \cdot, \cdot \rangle : \nu^2 \to \nu$, $U : \nu \to \nu$ and $(\cdot)_0, (\cdot)_1 : \nu \to \nu$.

The realizability definition is as follows. We work relative to an *assignment of variables*, which is a 1-1 function assigning to every variable x of sort σ of $\mathcal{L}$, a variable x' of sort $l(\sigma)$. Whenever x and x' are mentioned it is tacitly assumed that they correspond to each other under this assignment.

Now define:

$$
\begin{array}{lll}
x \, \mathbf{r} \, R(y_1, \ldots, y_n) & \equiv & x \in f_R(y_1', \ldots, y_n') \\
x \, \mathbf{r} \, t \in A & \equiv & x = t \wedge t \in A \qquad \text{\textit{A} a term of} \\
& & \qquad\qquad\qquad\quad \text{sort } \Pi(\nu) \\
x \, \mathbf{r} \, t = s & \equiv & x = t \wedge t = s \qquad \text{\textit{t, s} terms of} \\
& & \qquad\qquad\qquad\quad \text{sort } \nu \\
x \, \mathbf{r} \, \varphi \wedge \psi & \equiv & (x)_0 \, \mathbf{r} \, \varphi \wedge (x)_1 \, \mathbf{r} \, \psi \\
x \, \mathbf{r} \, \varphi \to \psi & \equiv & \forall y^\nu (y \, \mathbf{r} \, \varphi \to \\
& & \quad \exists z^\nu (T(x, y, z) \wedge U(z) \, \mathbf{r} \, \psi) \\
x \, \mathbf{r} \, \varphi \vee \psi & \equiv & ((x)_0 = \mathbf{0} \to (x)_1 \, \mathbf{r} \, \varphi) \wedge \\
& & \quad ((x)_0 \neq \mathbf{0} \to (x)_1 \, \mathbf{r} \, \psi) \\
x \, \mathbf{r} \, \exists y^\sigma \varphi & \equiv & \exists y'^{l(\sigma)} ((x)_0 \in E_\sigma(y') \wedge (x)_1 \, \mathbf{r} \, \varphi) \\
x \, \mathbf{r} \, \forall y^\sigma \varphi & \equiv & \forall y'^{l(\sigma)} \forall z^\nu (z \in E_\sigma(y') \to \\
& & \quad \exists w^\nu (T(x, z, w) \wedge U(w) \, \mathbf{r} \, \varphi)) \\
x \, \mathbf{r} \, \exists y^\nu \varphi & \equiv & (x)_1 \, \mathbf{r} \, \varphi[(x)_0/y] \\
x \, \mathbf{r} \, \forall y^\nu \varphi & \equiv & \forall y^\nu \exists z^\nu (T(x, y, z) \wedge U(z) \, \mathbf{r} \, \varphi) \\
x \, \mathbf{r} \, \exists/\forall y^\tau \varphi & \equiv & \exists/\forall y^\tau (x \, \mathbf{r} \, \varphi) \qquad \text{τ among the} \\
& & \qquad\qquad\qquad\quad \text{sorts } l(\sigma) \text{ or } \Pi(\nu)
\end{array}
$$

The interpretation $[\![\,\cdot\,]\!]'$ of $\mathcal{L}'$ in $\mathcal{E}\!f\!f$ is straightforward:

- $[\![\, l(\sigma) \,]\!]' = a([\![\,\sigma\,]\!])$, $[\![\,\nu\,]\!]' = N$, $[\![\,\Pi(\nu)\,]\!]' = \nabla(\mathcal{P}(\mathbb{N}))$. The symbols $\mathbf{0}$, U, T, $(\cdot)_0$, $(\cdot)_1$ and $\langle \cdot, \cdot \rangle$ have their expected meaning. $\in \,\subseteq\, \nu \times \Pi(\nu)$ is interpreted as the element relation $\in \rightarrowtail N \times \nabla(\mathcal{P}(\mathbb{N}))$;

- for f_R, choose a morphism

$$[\![\, f_R \,]\!]' : a([\![\,\sigma_1\,]\!]) \times \cdots \times a([\![\,\sigma_n\,]\!]) \to \nabla(\mathcal{P}(\mathbb{N}))$$

  such that the classification of $[\![\,R\,]\!] \rightarrowtail [\![\,\sigma_1\,]\!] \times \cdots \times [\![\,\sigma_n\,]\!]$ factors as $q \circ [\![\, f_R \,]\!]' \circ \eta$;

- for E_σ: choose a morphism $[\![\, E_\sigma \,]\!]' : a([\![\,\sigma\,]\!]) \to \nabla(\mathcal{P}(\mathbb{N}))$ such that the classification of $[\![\,\sigma\,]\!] \rightarrowtail a([\![\,\sigma\,]\!])$ factors as $q \circ [\![\, E_\sigma \,]\!]'$.

The fact that $\neg\neg x \; \mathbf{r} \; \varphi \to x \; \mathbf{r} \; \varphi$ holds under $[\![\,\cdot\,]\!]'$, follows by induction; for the induction step involving existential quantifiers, use property $\neg\neg\exists$. For the equivalence $\varphi \leftrightarrow \exists x (x \; \mathbf{r} \; \varphi)$:
Let $i_\sigma : \sigma \to l(\sigma)$ be extra function symbols, interpreted by the morphisms $\eta : [\![\,\sigma\,]\!] \to a([\![\,\sigma\,]\!])$. Let φ be a formula of $\mathcal{L}'$ with free $\mathcal{L}$-variables $y_1^{\sigma_1}, \ldots, y_n^{\sigma_n}$ and variables $\vec{z}$ not in $\mathcal{L}$, say A is the interpretation of the product of the sorts in $\vec{z}$. By comprehension (in $\mathcal{E}\!f\!f$) for $\nabla(\mathcal{P}(\mathbb{N}))$ w.r.t. $\neg\neg$-stable formulas with a free ν-variable, there is a map:

$$[\![\,\sigma_1\,]\!] \times \cdots \times [\![\,\sigma_n\,]\!] \times A \xrightarrow{f_\varphi} \nabla(\mathcal{P}(\mathbb{N}))$$

defined in $\mathcal{E}\!f\!f$ by

$$(y_1, \ldots, y_n, \vec{z}) \mapsto \{ x \mid (x \; \mathbf{r} \; \varphi)[i_{\sigma_1}(y_1)/y_1', \ldots, i_{\sigma_n}(y_n)/y_n'] \}$$

It follows from the description of the internal logic of $\mathcal{E}\!f\!f$, that the classification of $[\![\,\varphi\,]\!] \rightarrowtail [\![\,\sigma_1\,]\!] \times \cdots \times [\![\,\sigma_n\,]\!] \times A$ factors as $q \circ f_\varphi$. But since q classifies the *inhabited* $\neg\neg$-closed subsets of N, we have

$$\varphi(y_1, \ldots, y_n, \vec{z}) \leftrightarrow \exists x (x \; \mathbf{r} \; \varphi)[i_{\sigma_1}(y_1)/y_1', \ldots, i_{\sigma_n}(y_n)/y_n']$$

whence for sentences φ:

$$\varphi \leftrightarrow \exists x (x \; \mathbf{r} \; \varphi)$$

In the case that not every $[\![\sigma]\!]$ is separated, one does the following. Choose a separated cover $A_\sigma \twoheadrightarrow [\![\sigma]\!]$ for each σ. For $R \subseteq \sigma_1 \times \cdots \times \sigma_n$ let $\overline{R}$ be the pullback

$$
\begin{array}{ccc}
\overline{R} & \rightarrowtail & \prod_{i=1}^{n} A_{\sigma_i} \\
\downarrow & & \downarrow \\
[\![R]\!] & \rightarrowtail & \prod_{i=1}^{n} [\![\sigma_i]\!]
\end{array}
$$

Interpret $l(\sigma)$ by $a(A_\sigma)$ and f_R by a map:

$$
a(\prod_{i=1}^{n} A_{\sigma_i}) \cong \prod_{i=1}^{n} L(A_{\sigma_i}) \rightarrow \nabla(\mathcal{P}(\mathbb{N}))
$$

such that the classification of $\overline{R} \rightarrowtail \prod_{i=1}^{n} A_{\sigma_i}$ is $q \circ [\![f_R]\!] \circ \prod_{i=1}^{n} \eta_{\sigma_i}$ (here $\eta_{\sigma_i} : A_{\sigma_i} \rightarrow a(A_{\sigma_i})$ is the universal map). The interpretation of E_σ is likewise. The realizability interpretation remains the same; again, $\neg\neg x \mathbf{r} \varphi \rightarrow x \mathbf{r} \varphi$ holds.

For the equivalence $\varphi \leftrightarrow \exists x (x \mathbf{r} \varphi)$: if $g_\sigma : A_\sigma \rightarrow [\![\sigma]\!]$ are the chosen separated covers, and $\varphi \equiv \varphi(y_1^{\sigma_1}, \ldots, y_n^{\sigma_n}, \vec{z})$, then just as in the separated case

$$
\forall w_1 \in A_{\sigma_1} \cdots \forall w_n \in A_{\sigma_n} [\bigwedge_{i=1}^{n} g_{\sigma_i}(w_i) = y_i \rightarrow
$$
$$
(\varphi \leftrightarrow \exists x (x \mathbf{r} \varphi)[\eta_{\sigma_1}(w_1)/y_1', \ldots \eta_{\sigma_n}(w_n)/y_n'])]
$$

holds in $\mathcal{E}ff$, again giving

$$
\varphi \leftrightarrow \exists x (x \mathbf{r} \varphi)
$$

for sentences φ. ∎

Chapter 4

Variations

4.1 Extensional Realizability

Suppose a realizes a statement of the form $\forall x(A(x) \to \exists y B(y))$. Then a codes a function which assigns to each x and realizer for $A(x)$, a y and a realizer for $B(y)$. Now if we have a realizer b for

$$\forall x(A(x) \to \exists y B(y)) \to C$$

then b acts on such realizers a for the premiss, but need not respect a's behaviour as a function.

Extensional realizability is the name for a number of interpretations which do take into account the functional behaviour of realizers. The formal treatment defines for every formula φ a notion 'x is equivalent to x' as realizers of φ', and a realizer for an implication $\varphi \to \psi$ will have to send equivalent realizers of φ to equivalent realizers of ψ.

Here I treat two (inequivalent) ways to do this, for the language of first-order arithmetic. The first notion defines, for every φ, a *partial* equivalence relation on the set of Kleene realizers of φ (as defined in section 3.1); we shall denote this relation by $\sim_\varphi$. The inductive definition is as follows, where it is assumed throughout that $a \sim_\varphi b$ implies that a and b are Kleene realizers of φ:

1) If φ is an atomic sentence, then $a \sim_\varphi b$ iff $a = b$;

2) $a \sim_{\varphi \wedge \psi} b$ iff a and b code pairs (a_0, a_1), (b_0, b_1) respectively, and $a_0 \sim_\varphi b_0$ and $a_1 \sim_\psi b_1$;

3) $a \sim_{\varphi \vee \psi} b$ iff again a and b code pairs, and either $a_0 = b_0 = 0$ and $a_1 \sim_\varphi b_1$, or $a_0 \neq 0$, $b_0 \neq 0$ and $a_1 \sim_\psi b_1$;

4) $a \sim_{\varphi \to \psi} b$ iff for all pairs c, d such that $c \sim_\varphi d$, $ac{\downarrow}$ and $bd{\downarrow}$ and $ac \sim_\psi bd$

   (Note that here the partiality comes in: not every realizer a of $\varphi \to \psi$ will satisfy $a \sim_{\varphi \to \psi} a$);

5) $a \sim_{\exists x \varphi(x)} b$ iff a and b code pairs, $a_0 = b_0$ and $a_1 \sim_{\varphi(a_0)} b_1$;

6) $a \sim_{\forall x \varphi(x)} b$ iff for all n, $an{\downarrow}$ and $bn{\downarrow}$ and $an \sim_{\varphi(n)} bn$.

We then say that a is an *extensional realizer* of φ, and write $a \, \mathbf{r}_e \, \varphi$, if $a \sim_\varphi a$.

The second notion defines by recursion on φ, simultaneously a set of realizers for φ (we shall write $a \, \mathbf{e} \, \varphi$), and a *total* equivalence relation on this set, which we denote $a =_\varphi b$:

1) If φ is an atomic sentence, then $a \, \mathbf{e} \, \varphi$ iff φ is true, and $a =_\varphi b$ iff $a = b$;

2) $a \, \mathbf{e} \, \varphi \wedge \psi$ iff a codes (a_0, a_1), $a_0 \, \mathbf{e} \, \varphi$ and $a_1 \, \mathbf{e} \, \psi$;

   $a =_{\varphi \wedge \psi} b$ iff $a_0 =_\varphi b_0$ and $a_1 =_\psi b_1$;

3) $a \, \mathbf{e} \, \varphi \vee \psi$ iff a codes (a_0, a_1), $a_0 = 0$ and $a_1 \, \mathbf{e} \, \varphi$, or $a_0 \neq 0$ and $a_1 \, \mathbf{e} \, \psi$;

   $a =_{\varphi \vee \psi} b$ iff $a_0 = b_0 = 0$ and $a_1 =_\varphi b_1$, or $a_0 \neq 0$, $b_0 \neq 0$ and $a_1 =_\psi b_1$;

4) $a \, \mathbf{e} \, \varphi \to \psi$ iff for all b and b': if $b =_\varphi b'$ then $ab{\downarrow}$, $ab'{\downarrow}$ and $ab =_\psi ab'$;

   $a =_{\varphi \to \psi} b$ iff for all c, if $c \, \mathbf{e} \, \varphi$ then $ac =_\psi bc$;

5) $a \, \mathbf{e} \, \exists n \varphi$ iff a codes (a_0, a_1) and $a_1 \, \mathbf{e} \, \varphi(a_0)$;

   $a =_{\exists n \varphi} b$ iff $a_0 = b_0$ and $a_1 =_{\varphi(a_0)} b_1$;

6) a **e** $\forall n\varphi$ iff for all n, $an\downarrow$ and an **e** $\varphi(n)$;

   $a =_{\forall n\varphi} b$ iff for all n, $an =_{\varphi(n)} bn$.

If you are familiar with the two extensional type structures (constructed out of indices of partial recursive functions) HRO^E and HEO, both 'extensionalisations' of the intensional type structure HRO (see [161] for definitions), you will see that $\mathbf{r}_e$ is similar to HRO^E, and **e** to HEO (and Kleene realizability to HRO).

   However, whereas it was shown by Bezem ([23]) that the models HRO^E and HEO are isomorphic, we shall see that the realizability definitions $x\ \mathbf{r}_e\ \varphi$ and $x\ \mathbf{e}\ \varphi$ are *not* equivalent.

   In fact, you may already have guessed this. Evidently, if there is no number a such that a **e** φ, then 0 **e** $\neg\varphi$. On the other hand, if $a\ \mathbf{r}_e\ \varphi$ then a is a Kleene realizer for φ. It may be the case that $\varphi \to \psi$ is Kleene realizable, yet not $\mathbf{r}_e$-realizable; but in that case $\neg(\varphi \to \psi)$ is not $\mathbf{r}_e$-realizable either. Let us see the relavent example (taken from [171]) right away.

Lemma 4.1.1 *The following sentence of* **HA** *is neither* $\mathbf{r}_e$- *nor* **e**-*realizable:*

$$\forall e[\forall x\exists y(\neg\neg\exists z T(e, x, z) \to T(e, x, y)) \to$$

$$\exists v\forall x\exists u(T(v, x, u) \wedge (\neg\neg\exists y T(e, x, y) \to T(e, x, U(u))))]$$

Proof. The proof is similar for both realizabilities; I give it for **e**-realizability. The reasoning is informal; but can be carried out in **HA**+MP.

   Let A denote the sentence in the statement of the lemma, and suppose for contradiction that w **e** A. Then w codes a total recursive function. I remark:

i) If e codes the empty function, then $\langle f\rangle p_0(wef)$ is an effective operation of type 2 (i.e. sends codes for the same total recursive function to the same number), for every code of a total recursive function will realize $\forall x\exists y(\neg\neg\exists z T(e, x, z) \to T(e, x, y))$, and these realizers are equivalent if they code the same function.

ii) If k realizes $\forall x \exists y(\neg\neg\exists z T(e, x, z) \rightarrow T(e, x, y))$, then $p_1(wek)$ realizes the formula

$$\forall x \exists u(T(p_0(wek), x, u) \wedge (\neg\neg\exists y T(e, x, y) \rightarrow T(e, x, U(u))))$$

which is equivalent to an almost negative formula, and therefore holds. So in this case we always have:

$$\forall x[p_0(wek)x\downarrow \wedge (\neg\neg\exists y T(e, x, y) \rightarrow T(e, x, p_0(wek)x))]$$

Let $B(e, k, n, x)$ be an abbreviation for the expression $p_0((wS_1^2(e, k, n))(\langle y \rangle 0))x$ (where S_1^2 is from the Smn theorem).

Using the recursion theorem we can find an index e such that the partial recursive function φ_e of three variables satisfies:

$$\varphi_e(k, n, x) \simeq \begin{cases} \text{undefined} & \text{if not } T(n, n, x) \\ & \text{if } T(n, n, x): \\ \text{undefined} & \text{if } B(e, k, n, x) \\ & \text{is undefined} \\ 0 & \text{if } B(e, k, n, x) \\ & \text{is defined and not} \\ & T(S_1^2(e, k, n), x, B(e, k, n, x)) \\ U(B(e, k, n, x)) + 1 & \text{else} \end{cases}$$

Again some remarks:

iii) If $T(n, n, x)$, then $B(e, k, n, x)$ is always defined. For if not, $S_1^2(e, k, n)$ would code the empty function, and see i)-ii).

iv) If $T(n, n, x)$, then never $T(S_1^2(e, k, n), x, B(e, k, n, x))$. For were this the case we would have:

$$\begin{aligned} S_1^2(e, k, n)x &= U(B(e, k, n, x)) \\ \varphi_e(k, n, x) &= U(B(e, k, n, x)) + 1 \end{aligned}$$

which is contradictory.

Let $C(k, n)$ be an abbreviation for the expression $S_1^2(e, S_1^1(k, n), n)$.

Again using the recursion theorem, with e as just defined, we take an index k for a partial recursive function of two variables, such that:

$$\varphi_k(n, x) \simeq \begin{cases} 0 & \text{if not } T(n, n, x) \\ p(\mu z.T(C(k, n), x, z))(\langle y \rangle 0) & \text{else} \end{cases}$$

Then $S_1^1(k, n)$ always realizes

$$\forall x \exists y (\neg\neg \exists z T(C(k, n), x, z) \to T(C(k, n), x, y))$$

Furthermore:

If nn is undefined then $S_1^1(k, n)$ codes the constant zero function and $C(k, n)$ the empty function, so

$$(*) \quad p_0(wC(k, n)S_1^1(k, n)) = p_0(wC(k, n)(\langle y \rangle 0))$$

If nn is defined, say $T(n, n, x)$, then (see remark ii))

$$p_0(wC(k, n)S_1^1(k, n))x$$

is defined, and

$$T(C(k, n), x, p_0(wC(k, n)S_1^1(k, n))x)$$

holds. By remarks iii)-iv) we have that

$$p_0(wC(k, n)(\langle y \rangle 0))x = B(e, S_1^1(k, n), n, x)$$

is defined and *not*

$$T(C(k, n), x, p_0(wC(k, n)S_1^1(k, n))x)$$

Therefore in this case:

$$(**) \quad p_0(wC(k, n)S_1^1(k, n)) \neq p_0(wC(k, n)(\langle y \rangle 0))$$

(Note, that both sides are always defined!)

Now $(*)$ and $(**)$ give us a decision procedure for the question: "is nn defined?", and the contradiction is obtained. ∎

Corollary 4.1.2 $\mathbf{r}_e$- *and* **e**-*realizability are not equivalent.*

Proof. For the sentence A of lemma 4.1.1 we clearly have that $\neg A$ is
e-realizable. However, the sentence A is an instance of Church's Thesis
CT_0 so Kleene-realizable; it follows that $\neg\neg A$ is $\mathbf{r}_e$-realizable. These
facts are provable in **HA**+MP, where MP denotes Markov's Principle.■

Corollary 4.1.3 *The open schema*

$$B \to \exists x(x \ \mathbf{e} \ B)$$

is not **e**-*realizable.*

Proof. Take for B the formula $\forall x \exists y(\neg\neg\exists z T(e,x,z) \to T(e,x,y))$.
Then $\exists v(v \ \mathbf{e} \ B)$ is equivalent to

$$\exists v \forall x \exists u(T(v,x,u) \wedge (\neg\neg\exists z T(e,x,z) \to T(e,x,U(u))))$$

and apply lemma 4.1.1.   ■

For a syntactical treatment of the realizability notion $a \ \mathbf{e} \ \varphi$ (and an
axiomatization, formalized in a conservative extension of HA+MP), see
[171]. We now turn to toposes for the two extensional realizabilities.

A topos for **e**-realizability was briefly indicated in section 2.6.6; this
topos occurred first in [123]. One takes the set PER of partial equiv-
alence relations on $\mathbb{N}$. For two functions $\phi, \psi : X \to$ PER say $\phi \leq \psi$
iff there is a partial recursive function f which maps, for each x, $\phi(x)$
equivariantly into $\psi(x)$. Then $\text{PER}^{(-)}$ defines a tripos on Set, and the
topos corresponding to this tripos is denoted Ext.

In 2.6.6 we have seen that Ext is a subtopos of the topos $\text{RT}(T(\mathcal{K}_1))$.

There is also a relation with $\mathcal{E}ff$: in the category of toposes and
geometric morphisms, $\mathcal{E}ff$ is a retract of Ext. For, we have a forgetful
map $U :$ PER $\to \mathcal{P}(\mathbb{N})$ which sends a partial equivalence relation to
its field. The map U induces a transformation of triposes which has
both adjoints. The left adjoint is induced by the map $\mathcal{P}(\mathbb{N}) \overset{i}{\to}$ PER
which sends A to the minimal equivalence relation on A, and the right
adjoint is induced by a similar map $\mathcal{P}(\mathbb{N}) \overset{r}{\to}$ PER, now sending A to the
maximal equivalence relation on A. The left adjoint plainly preserves

finite meets, so we have a retraction diagram of geometric morphisms of triposes, and hence a retraction of toposes.

It is not hard to prove (you can also see [171]) that if $(A, \sim)$ is an assembly in $\mathcal{E}ff$, then $(A, r(\sim))$ is its image in Ext under the geometric inclusion. Also, this map preserves the natural numbers object. Since the direct image of a geometric inclusion always preserves exponents, the whole finite type structure over N is preserved.

The requirement that equivalence between realizers be preserved, makes statements of the form $\forall x(A(x) \rightarrow \exists y B(x, y))$ very strong. In fact, for the finite type hierarchy over N in Ext and the language of arithmetic in all finite types, we have that the axiom of choice

$$\mathrm{AC}_{\sigma,\tau} \quad \forall x^\sigma \exists y^\tau \varphi \rightarrow \exists z^{\sigma \rightarrow \tau} \forall x^\sigma \varphi(x, zx)$$

holds in Ext.

We can now revisit the principles CT, WCN and BP from section 3.1, and recall from the proof of 3.1.7 that WCN and BP are equivalent under $\mathrm{AC}_{\sigma,\tau}$.

Proposition 4.1.4 CT *and* WCN *(and hence* BP*) fail in* Ext.

Proof. CT, together with $\mathrm{AC}_{\sigma,\tau}$, implies that there is an effective operation which assigns to every total recursive function an index; but this is impossible in view of the continuity of effective operations given by the Kreisel-Lacombe-Shoenfield theorem. For BP we would need an effective operation which assigns to every $F{:}N^{N^N}$ and $f{:}N^N$ a modulus of continuity for F at f; but this cannot be done extensionally in codes, as proved in [162]. ∎

However, weakenings of CT and BP (putting $\neg\neg$ for the existential quantor) hold in Ext.

The failure of CT also has consequences for analysis in Ext, as compared to $\mathcal{E}ff$. A careful analysis of the relations between various continuity principles in the context of intuitionistic mathematics was carried out by P. Lietz in his thesis ([97]). On the basis of his results, Bauer and Simpson proved ([15], example 4.12):

Proposition 4.1.5 *In* Ext, *the statement that every function* $R \to R$ *is* sequentially continuous *(meaning: preserves limits of converging sequences), is true. However, "Brouwer's theorem" that every such function is* ε, δ-*continuous, fails.*

4.1.1 Ext as exact completion?

In [171], there is a characterization of the projective objects in Ext.

Proposition 4.1.6 *In* Ext,

i) *an object is projective if and only if it is isomorphic to an object* $(X, \sim)$ *for which* $x \sim y$ *is empty whenever* $x \neq y$, *and* $x \sim x$ *is the maximal equivalence relation on a set with at most two elements;*

ii) *every object is covered by a projective object;*

iii) *the full subcategory on the projective objects is not closed under finite products in* Ext.

From proposition 4.1.6 it follows that Ext is not an exact completion in the sense of section 3.2.4. However, A. Carboni and E. Vitale (see [33]) have given a definition of 'exact completion over a category with weak finite limits'. Their conditions hold for Ext.

Ext is, as remarked, a subtopos of $\mathsf{RT}(T(\mathcal{K}_1))$. Recall that $T(\mathcal{K}_1)$ is the order-pca of nonempty subsets of $\mathcal{K}_1$.

A lot of the theory of $\mathcal{E}\!f\!f$ carries over to arbitrary toposes $\mathsf{RT}(A)$ for order-pca's A; in particular the exact completion result.

Generally, in such a topos $\mathsf{RT}(A)$, an object is projective if and only if it is isomorphic to an object $(X, \sim)$ for which $x \sim y$ is empty if $x \neq y$, and $x \sim x$ is a *principal downset* of A, i.e. a set of the form $\downarrow a = \{u \in A \mid u \leq a\}$ for some $a \in A$.

Just as for $\mathcal{E}\!f\!f$, the projective objects are closed under finite limits and every object is covered by a projective object, so $\mathsf{RT}(A)$ is an exact completion.

For $\mathsf{RT}(T(\mathcal{K}_1))$ the projectives form a category we are already familiar with:

Proposition 4.1.7 *The full subcategory of* $\mathsf{RT}(T(\mathcal{K}_1))$ *on the projective objects is equivalent to the category of assemblies on* $\mathcal{K}_1$. *Hence* $\mathsf{RT}(T(\mathcal{K}_1)) = \mathrm{Ass}_{\mathrm{ex/lex}}$.

I should point out that some time after this proposition had appeared (in [171],3.21), M. Menni arrived at the same result by a different method: by analysing the conditions under which the ex/lex completion of a category is a topos ([108, 109]).

To conclude this section, a remark on $\mathbf{r}_e$-realizability. Define a variation on the tripos underlying Ext, as follows. By a *partial PER* on $\mathbb{N}$ we mean a subset A of $\mathbb{N}$ together with a partial equivalence relation $\sim$ on A (so the field of $\sim$ is a subset of A). Call the set of these pairs PPER. Given two functions $\phi, \psi : X \to$ PPER, let us write $(A_x, \sim_x)$ for $\phi(x)$ and $(B_x, \approx_x)$ for $\psi(x)$. Then define $\phi \leq \psi$ to hold if there is a number a such that for all x:

a) if $n \in A_x$ then $an\downarrow$ and $an \in B_x$;

b) if $n \sim_x m$ then $an \approx_x am$

Then the assignment $X \mapsto$ PPER^X defines a tripos on Set. The topos represented by this tripos is called Ext$'$ in [171], where it is shown that it is a topos for $\mathbf{r}_e$-realizability.

   Clearly, the effective tripos is an *open* subtripos of the tripos PPER$^{(-)}$ in the sense of section 2.6.10: for any X, the sub-preorder of PPER^X on those functions ϕ such that $\phi \leq \lambda x.(\mathbb{N}, \emptyset)$ is isomorphic to the value of the effective tripos at X. Therefore, $\mathcal{E}\!f\!f$ is an open subtopos of Ext$'$. Since inverse image functors of open inclusions are logical functors, this generalizes our remark that $\mathbf{r}_e$-realizability implies Kleene realizability.

4.2 Modified Realizability

Modified realizability arose as a straightforward interpretation of a system of arithmetic in all finite types, HA$^\omega$. To any formula φ one assigns a type $\tau(\varphi)$, and realizers for φ are terms of type $\tau(\varphi)$. The type $\tau(\varphi)$ depends on the logical structure of φ only, and is straightforwardly defined:

$\tau(\varphi \wedge \psi) = \tau(\varphi) \times \tau(\psi); \ \tau(\varphi \to \psi) = \tau(\varphi) \to \tau(\psi), \ \tau(\exists x^\sigma \varphi) = \sigma \times \tau(\varphi)$
etc. This definition was given by Kreisel ([93], in a footnote). Troelstra
([161]) turned this into an interpretation of HA, by first interpreting the
statements $x^{\tau(\varphi)} \ \mathbf{r} \ \varphi$ in the type structure HRO, which is a model of
HA^ω; and then interpreting HRO, which is all about recursive indices,
into HA. The resulting interpretation, when restricted to firstorder arithmetic, assigns, in its informal, semantical form, to every sentence ϕ *two*
sets of natural numbers: a set D_ϕ of *potential* realizers and a set of *actual* realizers of ϕ, which is a subset of D_ϕ. The set D_ϕ is what remains
(after the double re-interpretation) of the type $\tau(\phi)$. We have:

$D_\phi = \mathbb{N}$ if ϕ is an atomic sentence;

$D_{\phi \wedge \psi}$ is the set of coded pairs $\{pnm \,|\, n \in D_\phi, m \in D_\psi\}$;

$D_{\phi \to \psi} = \{n \,|\, \forall m \in D_\phi(nm{\downarrow} \wedge nm \in D_\psi)\}$;

$D_{\exists x \phi} = \{pnm \,|\, n \in \mathbb{N}, m \in D_\phi\}$;

$D_{\forall x \phi} = \{n \,|\, \forall m(nm{\downarrow} \wedge nm \in D_\phi)\}$

(For simplicity I have left out a clause for $\vee$, which is no real loss since
in arithmetic, $\vee$ is a definable connective)

For each ϕ then, out of D_ϕ the actual realizers $x \ \mathbf{mr} \ \phi$ are selected,
as follows:

For ϕ atomic, $n \ \mathbf{mr} \ \phi$ iff ϕ is true;

$n \ \mathbf{mr} \ \phi \wedge \psi$ if $n \in D_{\phi \wedge \psi}$, $p_0 n \ \mathbf{mr} \ \phi$ and $p_1 n \ \mathbf{mr} \ \psi$;

$n \ \mathbf{mr} \ \phi \to \psi$ if $n \in D_{\phi \to \psi}$ and for all m satisfying $m \ \mathbf{mr} \ \phi$,
$nm \ \mathbf{mr} \ \psi$;

$n \ \mathbf{mr} \ \exists x \phi$ if $n \in D_{\exists x \phi}$ and $p_1 n \ \mathbf{mr} \ \phi(p_0 n)$;

$n \ \mathbf{mr} \ \forall x \phi$ if $n \in D_{\forall x \phi}$ and for all m, $nm \ \mathbf{mr} \ \phi(n)$.

Every D_ϕ is nonempty. Actually we can find a canonical element in this
set and, modulo a bit of recoding, an element which belongs to *all* D_ϕ.
Namely, by the recursion theorem we can find a number e such that for

all n, $en = e$. Choosing a suitable coding of pairs and of partial recursive functions, we may assume $e = 0$ and $pee = e = 0$. Then $0 \in \bigcap_\phi D_\phi$.

Salient features of this realizability notion are that the principles CT_0 and IP are **mr**-realizable. The reason for the **mr**-realizability of IP is that any **mr**-realizer of an implication $\neg A \rightarrow B$ must also be defined at every *potential* realizer of the premiss, hence at 0; and if A has no **mr**-realizer then 0 is an **mr**-realizer of $\neg A$.

As a consequence, the principles ECT_0 and MP are *not* **mr**-realizable, because these principles clash with $CT_0 + IP$ (see [161]).

The modified realizability tripos M, as given in section 2.6.7, assigns to every set X the set of functions ϕ on X such that for every $x \in X$, $\phi(x)$ is a pair (A_x, D_x) of subsets of $\mathbb{N}$ such that $A_x \subseteq D_x$ and $0 \in D_x$ (of course, we work now with the assumption that $p00 = 0$ and for all n, $0n = 0$).

In section 2.6.7 we also saw that M is a closed subtripos of the tripos R of functions ϕ where $\phi(x)$ is an arbitrary inclusion $A_x \subseteq D_x$. This latter tripos R can be analyzed as follows. Consider the category $\mathrm{Set}^\rightarrow$ which has functions $X \rightarrow Y$ as objects, and commutative squares as arrows. Let $\Delta : \mathrm{Set} \rightarrow \mathrm{Set}^\rightarrow$ be the diagonal functor so $\Delta(X) = (X \overset{\mathrm{id}}{\rightarrow} X)$. Δ preserves the natural numbers object (it has both adjoints), and a function ϕ on a set X as in the tripos R, i.e. such that $\phi(x)$ is an inclusion $A_x \subseteq D_x$ of subsets of $\mathbb{N}$, is nothing but a subobject of $\Delta(X) \times N$ (N denoting as usual the NNO of $\mathrm{Set}^\rightarrow$); that is, a map $\Delta(X) \rightarrow \mathcal{P}(N)$ in $\mathrm{Set}^\rightarrow$. Such maps define the effective tripos on $\mathrm{Set}^\rightarrow$. Now $\mathrm{Set}^\rightarrow$ itself arises out of a tripos-to-topos construction on Set for which the constant objects functor is Δ, so by Pitts' iteration theorem (theorem 2.7.1) we have that the topos Set[R] is the effective topos on $\mathrm{Set}^\rightarrow$, which is $e(\mathrm{Set}^\rightarrow)$ in the notation of section 3.8.3.

So the topos represented by the modified realizability tripos M, from now on the topos Mod, is a closed subtopos of $e(\mathrm{Set}^\rightarrow)$.

Now $\mathrm{Set}^\rightarrow$ is the category of sheaves on Sierpinski space (the two-point space with one open point), and there are two geometric morphisms from Set to $\mathrm{Set}^\rightarrow$, corresponding to the two points $0 \leq 1$ (1 is the open point). We have

$$
\begin{aligned}
0_*(X) &= (X \xrightarrow{!} 1) \\
0^*(f) &= \mathrm{dom}(f) \\
1_*(X) &= \Delta(X) = (X \xrightarrow{\mathrm{id}} X) \\
1^*(f) &= \mathrm{cod}(f)
\end{aligned}
$$

Consequently there are two geometric morphisms from Set to $e(\mathrm{Set}^{\rightarrow})$ but only one of them factors through Mod. In order to get the full picture it is necessary to observe that, of course, the effective tripos is also a subtripos of the tripos R, so the effective topos is also a subtopos of $e(\mathrm{Set}^{\rightarrow})$. The following proposition was proved in [172]:

Proposition 4.2.1 *We have commutative diagrams of geometric morphisms*

$$
\begin{array}{ccc}
\mathrm{Set} \xrightarrow{\ 0\ } \mathrm{Set}^{\rightarrow} & \mathrm{Set} \xrightarrow{\ 1\ } \mathrm{Set}^{\rightarrow} & \mathrm{Set} \\
\downarrow{\scriptstyle\nu} \qquad \downarrow{\scriptstyle\eta^{\rightarrow}} & \downarrow{\scriptstyle\eta} \qquad \downarrow{\scriptstyle\eta^{\rightarrow}} & \swarrow \qquad \downarrow \\
\mathrm{Mod} \xrightarrow[m]{} e(\mathrm{Set}^{\rightarrow}) & \mathcal{E}\!f\!f \xrightarrow[e]{} e(\mathrm{Set}^{\rightarrow}) & \mathrm{Mod} \longrightarrow \mathcal{E}\!f\!f
\end{array}
$$

and the squares are pullbacks in the category of toposes and geometric morphisms.

Mod lies, as subtopos of $e(\mathrm{Set}^{\rightarrow})$, over the closed point 0 of $\mathrm{Set}^{\rightarrow}$, whereas $\mathcal{E}\!f\!f$ lies over the open point; and Mod is the closed complement of $\mathcal{E}\!f\!f$ as subtoposes of $e(\mathrm{Set}^{\rightarrow})$. There is some more analysis of this situation, and of the local operators in $e(\mathrm{Set}^{\rightarrow})$ associated to it, in [172].

Here we notice that the constant objects functor for the modified realizability tripos, $\nabla_{\mathsf{M}} : \mathrm{Set} \to \mathrm{Mod}$, is *not* isomorphic to the direct image of the geometric inclusion $\nu : \mathrm{Set} \to \mathrm{Mod}$. Let $\Phi : \mathsf{M} \to \mathsf{R}$ be the geometric inclusion of triposes. Then Φ^+ is induced by the map which sends an inclusion (A, D) to the pair $(A^+, \{0\} \cup D^+)$, where A^+ denotes $\{n + 1 \mid n \in A\}$.

We have that $\nabla_{\mathsf{M}}(X)$ is the object $(X, \exists_{\delta}^{\mathsf{M}}(\top_X^{\mathsf{M}}))$ where $\exists^{\mathsf{M}}$ is existential quantification in M. Since Φ^+ preserves the top element and existential quantification, we have

$$\exists_\delta^M(\top_X^M) \simeq \exists_\delta^M(\Phi_X^+(\top_X^R)) \simeq \Phi_{X\times X}^+(\exists_\delta^R(\top_X^R))$$

and that means that $\nabla_M(X)$ is given as $(X, \sim_M)$ where

$$[x \sim_M x'] = \begin{cases} (\mathbb{N}^+, \mathbb{N}) & \text{if } x = x' \\ (\emptyset, \{0\}) & \text{otherwise} \end{cases}$$

On the other hand, by the commuting squares of proposition 4.2.1 and the fact that m is an inclusion, we have

$$\nu_*(X) \simeq m^* m_* \nu_*(X) \simeq m^*(\eta^\rightarrow)_* 0_*(X)$$

In $\mathrm{Set}^\rightarrow$, the power object $\mathcal{P}(N)$ is the second projection from $\{(U, V) \in \mathcal{P}(\mathbb{N})^2 \,|\, U \subseteq V\}$ to $\mathcal{P}(\mathbb{N})$ and

$$(\eta^\rightarrow)_*(X \xrightarrow{f} Y)_0(x, x') = (\{n \,|\, x = x'\}, \{n \,|\, f(x) = f(x')\})$$
$$(\eta^\rightarrow)_*(X \xrightarrow{f} Y)_1(y, y') = (\{n \,|\, y = y'\})$$

So $(\eta^\rightarrow)_*(0_*(X))_0(x, x') = (\{n \,|\, x = x'\}, \mathbb{N})$. It follows that $\nu_*(X) = (X, \sim_\nu)$ with

$$[x \sim_\nu x'] = \begin{cases} (\mathbb{N}, \mathbb{N}) & \text{if } x = x' \\ (\emptyset, \mathbb{N}) & \text{otherwise} \end{cases}$$

It is easy to see that the predicates $\sim_M$ and $\sim_\nu$ are not isomorphic in $M(X \times X)$ and that the functors ∇_M and ν_* are not naturally isomorphic.

For the logic of Mod, the functor ν_* is the more basic one, because it embeds Set as $\neg\neg$-sheaves in Mod. It is straightforward to show, as was stated in [75] and written out in [172], that the full subcategory of Mod on the $\neg\neg$-separated objects (subobjects of objects $\nu_*(X)$), which we call *modified assemblies*, can be presented as follows:

A modified assembly is a triple (X, E, B) with X a set, B a subset of $\mathbb{N}$ containing 0, and $E : X \to \mathcal{P}(\mathbb{N})$ a function which assigns to every x a nonempty subset of B;

an arrow $(X, E, B) \to (Y, E', B')$ is a function $f : X \to Y$ which is tracked by a number a in the sense that a maps every element of B to an element of B', and for every x, every element of $E(x)$ to an element of $E'(f(x))$.

In the category of modified assemblies, there is also an interesting model of Synthetic Domain Theory, see [174] for details.

Another notion of 'modified assemblies' is defined in [153]; this is a category more related to subobjects of objects $\nabla_M(X)$. For a precise connection, see [172]. In the latter paper, there is furthermore a generalization of the Independence of Premiss principle, valid in $e(\text{Set}^{\rightarrow})$, which implies the principle IP in Mod. Also, there is a characterization of the projective objects in Mod, and a proof that Mod is an exact completion.

In [75] and [120], there is a more general definition of 'modified realizability toposes on conditional pca's with a right-absorptive subset' (that is, a subset $\Theta \subset A$ such that for all $a \in \Theta$ and $b \in A$, $ab \in \Theta$). The aim is to apply the construction to get a strong normalization proof for the Calculus of Constructions. For a critical note on this, see the final pages of [97]. There, Lietz also suggests a variation on the construction of the modified realizability tripos: take those inclusions $A \subseteq D$ of subsets of $\mathbb{N}$ satisfying $A = \emptyset \Rightarrow D = \emptyset$ and $A \neq \emptyset \Rightarrow 0 \in D$. This suggestion seems worth working out.

For an amalgamation of the ideas of modified realizability and relative realizability, see [25].

4.3 Function Realizability

Of the host of realizability toposes of the form $\mathsf{RT}(A)$, I single out $\mathsf{RT}(\mathcal{K}_2)$ for more detailed treatment.

In every topos $\mathsf{RT}(A)$ we have a natural numbers object: by the theory in section 1.3.1, let $\{\bar{n} \mid n \in \mathbb{N}\}$ be the Curry numerals in A. Then since we have primitive recursion in A with arbitrary parameters from A (1.3.5), it is straightforward that the object $(\mathbb{N}, \sim)$ with $[n \sim m] = \{\bar{n} \mid n = m\}$ is an NNO in $\mathsf{RT}(A)$. The Curry numerals are not always the easiest representation of the natural numbers; in many cases one can find an isomorphic object with very simple elements.

For example in $\mathcal{K}_2$ we can take just as well the constant functions $\mathbb{N} \to \mathbb{N}$ as representatives for the natural numbers. Write $[n]$ for the constant function with value $[n]$. So, from now on N denotes the object $(\mathbb{N}, \sim)$ with $[n \sim m] = \{[n] \mid n = m\}$.

We consider also the 'object of realizers' in $\mathsf{RT}(\mathcal{K}_2)$: it is $\mathcal{K}_2$ itself, viewed as the partitioned assembly $\mathcal{K}_2, \mathrm{id} : \mathcal{K}_2 \to \mathcal{K}_2)$. I write also $\mathcal{K}_2$ in, order to denote this object.

Proposition 4.3.1 *The object $\mathcal{K}_2$ is isomorphic to N^N in $\mathsf{RT}(\mathcal{K}_2)$.*

We see at once from this proposition that the object N^N is projective in $\mathsf{RT}(\mathcal{K}_2)$. The treatment of projective and internally projective objects does not differ essentially from that in $\mathcal{E}ff$; as in every topos $\mathsf{RT}(A)$ we have that the notions of projective and internally projective coincide. Hence:

Proposition 4.3.2 *The principles of countable and dependent choices and choice over N^N hold in $\mathsf{RT}(\mathcal{K}_2)$.*

Let us have a short look at first order arithmetic in $\mathsf{RT}(\mathcal{K}_2)$. It is governed by what is generally called 'function realizability', introduced by Kleene in 1965 ([89]), as an interpretation of a language for the types N^N and N. I omit the clauses, which are completely straightforward analogues of the clauses for Kleene realizability for numbers.

Suppose ϕ is a formula of first order arithmetic, with free variables $x_1, \ldots, x_k$. Clearly, reasoning classically there is a function $\alpha_\phi \in \mathbb{N}^{\mathbb{N}}$ with the property that for every k-tuple $n_1, \ldots, n_k$ of natural numbers

$$\begin{aligned}
\alpha_\phi[\langle n_1, \ldots, n_k \rangle] &= [0] \quad \text{if } \phi(n_1, \ldots, n_k) \text{ is true} \\
\alpha_\phi[\langle n_1, \ldots, n_k \rangle] &= [1] \quad \text{if } \phi(n_1, \ldots, n_k) \text{ is false}
\end{aligned}$$

(note, that the left hand side denotes application in $\mathcal{K}_2$).

From this it is easy to derive

Proposition 4.3.3 *First order arithmetic in $\mathsf{RT}(\mathcal{K}_2)$ is classically true arithmetic.*

Proposition 4.3.3 does not extend to the theory of N^N. The nature of the pca, with its partial continuous maps, imposes some continuity principles on us which are not classically true. First, let us define what 'almost negative' means for formulas in our extended language. We have variables $x, y, \ldots$ for numbers and $\alpha, \beta, \ldots$ for type N^N; primitive recursive function symbols, terms $\alpha(x)$ and $\bar{\alpha}x = \langle\alpha(0),\ldots,\alpha(x-1)\rangle$. The expression $\alpha\beta\downarrow$ abbreviates $\exists x(\alpha(\bar{\beta}x) > 0)$ and $\alpha\beta(n) = m$ stands for

$$\exists x(\alpha(\langle n\rangle * \bar{\beta}x) = m + 1 \wedge \forall y < x\alpha(\langle n\rangle * \bar{\beta}x) = 0)$$

An *almost negative formula* is then a formula where (just as in section 3.1) disjunction only occurs between atomic formulas, and the quantifiers $\exists x$ and $\exists\alpha$ also only directly before atomic formulas. In complete analogy to the role of the principle ECT_0 we have the principle GC of 'Generalized Continuity'

GC $\forall\alpha(A(\alpha) \rightarrow \exists\beta B(\alpha,\beta)) \rightarrow \exists\gamma\forall\alpha(A(\alpha) \rightarrow \gamma\alpha\downarrow \wedge B(\alpha,\gamma\alpha))$

in which the formula $A(\alpha)$ must be almost negative.

The principle GC is as much a choice principle as a principle asserting continuity of functions. It was shown by Troelstra ([161]) to characterize formalized function realizability in the formal system EL.

Proposition 4.3.4 *The principles* BP *and* WCN *hold in* $\mathrm{RT}(\mathcal{K}_2)$.

Proof. By proposition 4.3.1, $N^{(N^N)}$ is the assembly of functions $\mathcal{K}_2 \rightarrow \mathbb{N}$ which are tracked by some element of $\mathcal{K}_2$. Note that F is such a function and ϕ tracks F, then for every $\alpha \in \mathcal{K}_2$ we have that $F(\alpha) = \phi\alpha(0)$.

Now the function Γ which assigns to each α and β the least x such that $\alpha(\langle 0\rangle * \bar{\beta}x) > 0$ is then defined on all α which track an element of $N^{(N^N)}$ and all $\beta \in \mathcal{K}_2$, and is partial continuous, so represented by a $\gamma \in \mathcal{K}_2$. From such a γ it is easy to find a realizer in $\mathcal{K}_2$ for the statement

$$\forall F{:}N^{(N^N)}\forall f{:}N^N\exists x\forall g{:}N^N(\bar{f}x = \bar{g}x \rightarrow F(f) = F(g))$$

which is BP. By the remark in the proof of corollary 3.1.7 and corollary 4.3.2, WCN follows.   ∎

For 2^N we have an even stronger continuity axiom which holds in $\mathrm{RT}(\mathcal{K}_2)$, namely uniform continuity:

Proposition 4.3.5 *In* $\mathrm{RT}(\mathcal{K}_2)$, *every function from* 2^N *to* N *is uniformly continuous:*

$$\forall F{:}N^{(2^N)}\exists n\forall fg{:}2^N(\bar{f}n = \bar{g}n \rightarrow F(f) = F(g))$$

Proof. Since 2^N is a $\neg\neg$-closed subobject of N^N, proposition 4.3.1 tells us that 2^N is isomorphic to the regular subassembly of $\mathcal{K}_2$ on the functions which take values in $\{0, 1\}$. Suppose $F{:}2^N \to N$ is tracked by ϕ. Then there is a finite set A_ϕ of finite $0, 1$-sequences σ such that $\phi(\sigma) > 0$ for every $\sigma \in A_\phi$, and such that every $\alpha \in 2^N$ has an initial segment in A_ϕ. Taking

$$n = \max\{\mathsf{lh}(\sigma) \,|\, \sigma \in A_\phi\}$$

we have that if $\bar{f}n = \bar{g}n$, then $F(f) = F(g)$. It is easily seen that n can be obtained continuously in ϕ, given that ϕ tracks a function $2^N \to N$. ∎

We see from 4.3.5 that the analogue of proposition 3.2.26 (2^N and N^N are isomorphic in $\mathcal{E}ff$) fails in $\mathsf{RT}(\mathcal{K}_2)$; certainly not every $F{:}N^{N^N}$ is uniformly continuous (for example, let $F(\alpha) = \sum_{i \leq \alpha(0)} \alpha(i)$).

The Uniformity Principle holds in $\mathsf{RT}(\mathcal{K}_2)$ as it does in any topos $\mathsf{RT}(A)$. Recall the remark made in section 3.1.1 that this principle has no non-classical first order consequences.

The category of modest sets over $\mathcal{K}_2$ is interesting, due to the topological nature of the pca $\mathcal{K}_2$. It is related to the category Equ of 'equilogical spaces', promoted in 1996 by D. Scott ([148, 14]) as a good category for semantics of different kinds. The connection we briefly mention here is due to A. Bauer ([12]).

Definition 4.3.6 An *equilogical space* is a T_0-topological space X, with a countable basis, together with an equivalence relation on it (no relationship between the topology and the equivalence relation is required). A *map* of equilogical spaces is an equivalence class of continuous, equivalence-preserving maps, where two such maps are equivalent if for every element of the domain, their images are equivalent. There is a category Equ of equilogical spaces.

Definition 4.3.7 (Bauer) The full subcategory of Equ on those objects whose underlying space is 0-dimensional , is called $\mathsf{0Equ}$. Recall that a space is 0-dimensional if it has a basis consisting of clopen sets.

Theorem 4.3.8 (Bauer) *The category* OEqu *is equivalent to the category of modest sets on* $\mathcal{K}_2$.

Proof. Recall that a modest set is a separated discrete object; every modest set is isomorphic to an assembly on $\mathcal{K}_2$ with the property that $E(x) \cap E(y) = \emptyset$ whenever $x \neq y$. Equivalently, a modest set is an equivalence relation on a subset of $\mathcal{K}_2$; viewed in this way, an arrow between modest sets is an equivalence class of equivariant maps which are tracked by some element of $\mathcal{K}_2$. So we can define a functor from the modest sets on $\mathcal{K}_2$ to OEqu by sending an equivalence relation on $A \subseteq \mathcal{K}_2$ to itself, but now as an equivalence relation on the sub*space* A of $\mathcal{K}_2$. Then A is a 0-dimensional space with a countable basis, so we have a well-defined object of OEqu. If a map between modest sets is equivariant and tracked by an element of $\mathcal{K}_2$, its tracking is continuous, so its equivalence class is an arrow in OEqu.

The functor thus defined is clearly faithful. It is full because if A and B are subspaces of $\mathcal{K}_2$ then by the remark at the end of example 1.4.3, every continuous map $A \to B$ is given by some element of $\mathcal{K}_2$.

Finally the functor is essentially surjective on objects because every 0-dimensional T_0-space with a countable basis is a subspace of $\mathcal{K}_2$: if $\{U_n \mid n \in \mathbb{N}\}$ is a countable basis of clopen sets then define $F : A \to \mathcal{K}_2$ by

$$F(x)(n) = \begin{cases} 0 & \text{if } x \in U_n \\ 1 & \text{otherwise} \end{cases}$$

It is easy to check that F is an embedding.   ∎

Another result by Bauer ([11],4.1.3) is that Equ itself is equivalent to the category of modest sets on $\mathcal{P}(\omega)$ (Example 1.4.6). Recall the applicative morphisms $\gamma : \mathcal{P}(\omega) \to \mathcal{K}_2$ and $\iota : \mathcal{K}_2 \to \mathcal{P}(\omega)$ from the examples in section 1.5, which were shown in example i) of section 2.5.3 to induce a geometric morphism of toposes $\mathsf{RT}(\mathcal{P}(\omega)) \to \mathsf{RT}(\mathcal{K}_2)$ which is a surjection. Now both these applicative morphisms have the property that their images of distinct elements are disjoint sets. This means that the adjunction between the respective categories of assemblies restricts to a similar adjunction between the categories of modest sets. Hence we have the result, also noted by Bauer, that OEqu is a coreflective (full, because $\gamma\iota \simeq \mathrm{id}_{\mathcal{K}_2}$) subcategory of Equ.

For more on the topos $\mathsf{RT}(\mathcal{P}(\omega))$, see [11].

The topos $\mathsf{RT}(\mathcal{K}_2)$ has an interesting subtopos, which is analogous to Lifschitz realizability (see sections 2.6.8 above, and 4.4 below). Let us use an easy coding of pairs for elements of $\mathcal{K}_2$ and write $p_i\alpha$ for the function $n \mapsto p_i(\alpha(n))$, $i = 0, 1$. Define

$$V_\alpha = \{\beta \leq p_1\alpha \mid (p_0\alpha)\beta{\uparrow}\}$$

We have the following counterparts of the propositions in section 2.6.8:

Proposition 4.3.9 *There is no $\gamma \in \mathcal{K}_2$ with the property that for all α, if $V_\alpha \neq \emptyset$ then $\gamma\alpha{\downarrow}$ and $\gamma\alpha \in V_\alpha$.*

Proposition 4.3.10 *There is an element $\zeta \in \mathcal{K}_2$ such that whenever $\beta\gamma{\downarrow}$ for every $\gamma \in V_\alpha$, $\zeta\alpha\beta{\downarrow}$ and $V_{\zeta\alpha\beta} = \{\beta\gamma \mid \gamma \in V_\alpha\}$.*

Proposition 4.3.11 *There is an element $\zeta \in \mathcal{K}_2$ such that for all α, $\zeta\alpha{\downarrow}$ and $V_{\zeta\alpha} = \bigcup\{V_\beta \mid \beta \in V_\alpha\}$.*

Proposition 4.3.12 *There is an element $\beta \in \mathcal{K}_2$ such that for all α, $\beta\alpha{\downarrow}$ and $V_{\beta\alpha} = \{\alpha\}$.*

In complete analogy with the Lifschitz tripos, we have a subtripos of the realizability tripos on $\mathcal{K}_2$: let $K = \{\alpha \mid V_\alpha \neq \emptyset\}$. Define Σ as the set of those subsets H of K which have the property that whenever $\alpha \in H$ and $\emptyset \subsetneq V_\beta \subseteq V_\alpha$, then $\beta \in H$.

For functions $\phi, \psi : X \to \Sigma$ define $\phi \leq \psi$ iff $\phi \leq \psi$ in the realizability tripos on $\mathcal{K}_2$.

The realizability notion which this tripos generalizes was investigated from a syntactical point of view in [165]. It is shown there that this notion refutes the schema WCN.

For a result about continuity principles in realizability toposes over domain models, see [41].

4.4   Lifschitz Realizability

Recall the Lifschitz realizability tripos P_L from section 2.6.8. The topos represented by this tripos will be called Lif. From the geometric inclusion of P_L into the effective tripos we know that Lif is a subtopos of $\mathcal{E}\!f\!f$. In this section we explore this subtopos a bit.

The local operator in $\mathcal{E}\!f\!f$ for which Lif is the category of sheaves, is the map $\Omega \to \Omega$ induced by $A \mapsto \{e \mid V_e \neq \emptyset \wedge V_e \subseteq A\}$.

The natural numbers object in Lif is the object $(\mathbb{N}, \sim)$ where $[n \sim m] = \emptyset$ if $n \neq m$, and $[n \sim n] = \{e \mid V_e = \{n\}\}$.

First order arithmetic in Lif is governed by *Lifschitz realizability*, which can be formulated as follows. The notion is $x \; \mathbf{r}_L \; \phi$, '$x$ Lifschitz-realizes ϕ', for a number x and a sentence ϕ.

If ϕ is an atomic sentence then $x \; \mathbf{r}_L \; \phi$ iff $V_x \neq \emptyset$ and ϕ is true;

$x \; \mathbf{r}_L \; (\phi \wedge \psi)$ iff $V_x \neq \emptyset$ and for all $y \in V_x$, $p_0 y \; \mathbf{r}_L \; \phi$ and $p_1 y \; \mathbf{r}_L \; \psi$;

$x \; \mathbf{r}_L \; (\phi \to \psi)$ iff $V_x \neq \emptyset$ and for all $y \in V_x$ and all a such that $a \; \mathbf{r}_L \; \phi$, $ya\!\downarrow$ and $ya \; \mathbf{r}_L \; \psi$;

$x \; \mathbf{r}_L \; \exists n\phi(n)$ iff $V_x \neq \emptyset$ and for all $y \in V_x$, $p_1 y \; \mathbf{r}_L \; \phi(p_0 y)$;

$x \; \mathbf{r}_L \; \forall n\phi(n)$ iff $V_x \neq \emptyset$ and for all $y \in V_x$ and all n, $yn\!\downarrow$ and $yn \; \mathbf{r}_L \; \phi(n)$.

By a *bounded Σ_2^0-formula* or *$B\Sigma_2^0$-formula* I mean a formula of the form $\exists y \leq t \forall x A$, where A is a quantifier-free formula and y does not occur in the term t. *Markov's Principle for $B\Sigma_2^0$-formulas* or *$B\Sigma_2^0$-MP* is the schema $\neg\neg\psi \to \psi$ for $B\Sigma_2^0$-formulas ψ.

If we use the expression $V_e \neq \emptyset$ also as an abbreviation for the formula $\neg\forall y \leq p_1 e \exists w T(p_0 e, y, w)$ and $I(V_e)$ for the positive statement $\exists y \leq p_1 e \forall w \neg T(p_0 e, y, w)$, then it is clear that the schema $B\Sigma_2^0$-MP is equivalent to the sentence

$$\forall e(V_e \neq \emptyset \to I(V_e))$$

The principle ECT_L, which bears the same relationship to Lif as the principle ECT_0 to $\mathcal{E}ff$, is

$$\forall x(A(x) \to \exists y B(x,y)) \to \exists e \forall x(ex{\downarrow} \wedge I(V_{ex}) \wedge \\ \forall y \in V_{ex} B(x,y))$$

where $A(x)$ must be a $B\Sigma_2^0$-formula.

Proposition 4.4.1 *The principles* MP, $B\Sigma_2^0$-MP *and* ECT_L *are Lifschitz realizable.*

Actually, as shown in [165], the principle ECT_L characterizes a formalized version of Lifschitz realizability in the system $\mathrm{HA}+\mathrm{MP}+B\Sigma_2^0{-}\mathrm{MP}$. The following lemma and proposition appear in Lifschitz' original paper [98].

Lemma 4.4.2 *There is a partial recursive function F such that whenever V_e is a singleton, $F(e)$ is defined and is an element of V_e.*

Proposition 4.4.3 *i)* CT_0 *is not* $\mathbf{r}_L$-*realizable;*

ii) *The principle* $\mathrm{CT}_0!$ *is* $\mathbf{r}_L$-*realizable, where* $\mathrm{CT}_0!$ *is the schema*

$$\forall x \exists! y A(x,y) \to \exists e \forall x \exists w (T(e,x,w) \wedge A(x,U(w)))$$

Proof. For i), let G be the function from the proof of proposition 2.6.3. Any realizer for the instance of CT_0 with the formula $y \in V_{G(x)}$ in the place of A, would contradict that proposition.
  ii) follows more or less directly from lemma 4.4.2. ∎

Now actually the schema CT_0 is an amalgam of the statement CT that every function is recursive, and a choice principle which states that every total relation contains a function. In fact we have:

Proposition 4.4.4 *In Lif,* CT *holds but countable choice fails. In fact there is a total Π_1^0-relation on N which does not contain a function.*

Proof. For CT, you use lemma 4.4.2; for failure of choice you use the relation $\{(n,m) \mid m \in V_{G(n)}\}$ where G is the function in the proof of 2.6.3. ∎

Proposition 4.4.5 Lif *is not equivalent to a topos of the form* $\mathsf{RT}(A)$ *for an (order-)pca A.*

Proof. For in such toposes, N is $(\mathbb{N}, \sim)$ with $[n \sim m] = \downarrow\{\bar{n} \,|\, n = m\}$, $\bar{n}$ as usual denoting the Curry numeral corresponding to n. Thus N is always projective. ∎

As demonstrated in [170], there is a logical characterization of Lif among subtoposes of $\mathcal{E}\!f\!f$. Namely, Lif is the *largest* subtopos $\mathcal{E}$ of $\mathcal{E}\!f\!f$ such that $\mathcal{E} \models (O)$, where (O) is the statement

$$\forall ef \in T\,[\forall xy(ex = 0 \vee fy = 0) \to \forall x(ex = 0) \vee \forall y(fy = 0)]$$

Here T is the subobject of N of indices of total recursive functions.

Since this is a somewhat peculiar result (in general, there is no construction of a 'best' subtopos satisfying a logical principle), I expand on it a little. In general, given a monic arrow $U \rightarrowtail V$ in a topos, there is a least local operator j such that sheafification w.r.t. j turns $U \to V$ into an isomorphism. However, if U and V are interpretations of logical formulas, it is not given that sheafification will preserve these interpretations.

The construction of the least j as in the above paragraph, is given in [80], chapter 3:

$$j(p) \;=\; \forall q[\forall x{:}V((x \in U \to q) \to q) \to ((p \to q) \to q)]$$

In our example of the principle (O), let T^2 denote the subobject of N consisting of pairs of indices of total recursive functions. Define the following subobjects of N:

$$
\begin{aligned}
A &= \{e \,|\, e \in T^2 \wedge \forall xy(p_0ex = 0 \vee p_1ey = 0)\} \\
B_0 &= \{e \,|\, e \in T^2 \wedge \forall x(p_0ex = 0)\} \\
B_1 &= \{e \,|\, e \in T^2 \wedge \forall x(p_1x = 0)\}
\end{aligned}
$$

Then A, B_0 and B_1 are defined by almost negative formulas, and $B_0 \vee B_1 \leq A$ in the lattice of subobjects of N; the principle (O) says that the converse inequality also holds.

We have the following two propositions:

Proposition 4.4.6 *Suppose U, V_1, V_2 are subobjects of N in $\mathcal{E}ff$, defined by almost negative formulas ϕ, ψ_1, ψ_2 respectively; and $V_1 \vee V_2 \leq U$. Suppose j is a local operator in $\mathcal{E}ff$ with associated sheaf functor $a : \mathcal{E}ff \to \mathrm{Sh}_j(\mathcal{E}ff)$. Then $a(V_1 \vee V_2 \to U)$ is an isomorphism in $\mathrm{Sh}_j(\mathcal{E}ff)$ if and only if the formula*

$$\forall x{:}N(\phi(x) \to \psi_1(x) \vee \psi_2(x))$$

is true in $\mathrm{Sh}_j(\mathcal{E}ff)$.

Proposition 4.4.7 *For the objects A, B_1, B_2 given, the least local operator in $\mathcal{E}ff$ for which the associated sheaf functor maps the inclusion $B_1 \vee B_2 \to A$ to an isomorphism, is the local operator defining* Lif.

Clearly, these two propositions together imply the logical characterization of Lif given above.

A second-order principle which is true in $\mathcal{E}ff$ but fails in Lif, is discussed in [167] and named "Richman's Principle" there. It says: *for every decidable subset X of N which has the property that for every decidable subset Y of N, either $X \subseteq Y$ or $X \cap Y = \emptyset$, there is an n such that $X = \{n\}$.* The question had been raised by Richman (as reported in [27]) to what extent this is a constructive principle: would it be a consequence of constructive logic, and if not, might it be provable from principles such as CT and MP? In [27], Blass and Scedrov present a sheaf topos in which the principle is not true (however its negation is false), but in that topos, MP and CT are not true either. In Lif, as shown in [167], the principle is false; and in Lif, CT and MP hold.

4.5 Relative Realizability

'Relative realizability' was the name coined by the Logic and Computability group at CMU (Scott, Awodey, Bauer, Birkedal) for a number of realizability interpretations which arise from an *elementary* inclusion of pca's (see section 2.6.9): that is, we have pca's $A' \subset A$ such that for $a, a' \in A'$, aa' is defined in A if and only if it is defined in A', and in this case the results are the same; and moreover there are elements k and s in A' which satisfy the axioms of theorem 1.1.3 both w.r.t. A and A'.

Examples are the inclusions of $\mathcal{P}(\omega)^{\mathrm{re}} \subset \mathcal{P}(\omega)$ and $\mathcal{K}_2^{\mathrm{rec}} \subset \mathcal{K}_2$. Another example is that of a Σ_1-elementary extension of two models of Peano Arithmetic: such a model M is a pca by putting $ab = c$ iff $M \models \exists y(T(a,b,y) \wedge U(y) = c)$; an extension $M \subset N$ is Σ_1-elementary if for every Σ_1-sentence ϕ with parameters from M, $M \models \phi$ iff $N \models \phi$.

Given such an inclusion, one can define, besides the realizability triposes P_A and $\mathsf{P}_{A'}$ on A and A' respectively, a realizability tripos $\mathsf{P}_{A',A}$ as follows: elements of $\mathsf{P}_{A',A}(X)$ are maps $X \to \mathcal{P}(A)$, but the preorder is realized by elements from A', so $\phi \leq \psi$ iff there is an $a \in A'$ such that for all x and all $b \in \phi(x)$, $ab{\downarrow}$ and $ab \in \psi(x)$.

There are connections between the triposes $\mathsf{P}_{A'}$, P_A and $\mathsf{P}_{A',A}$. First of all, the Heyting prealgebras $\mathsf{P}_{A',A}(X)$ and $\mathsf{P}_A(X)$ have the same underlying set, the triposes have the same generic element (the identity function on $\mathcal{P}(A)$), and all constructions of the tripos structure are the same: also in $\mathsf{P}_{A',A}(X)$, the implication is defined by $(\phi \to \psi)(x) = \{a \in A \mid \forall b \in \phi(x)(ab{\downarrow} \wedge ab \in \psi(x))\}$, and also for $f : X \to Y$ and $\phi \in \mathsf{P}_{A',A}(X)$, we have that universal quantification along f in $\mathsf{P}_{A',A}$ is given by

$$\forall_f(\phi)(y) = \{a \in A \mid \forall b \in A \forall x \in f^{-1}(y)(ab{\downarrow} \wedge ab \in \phi(x))\}$$

It follows that also all constructions in the topos represented by $\mathsf{P}_{A',A}$, which I denote by $\mathsf{RT}(A', A)$, are the same as in $\mathsf{RT}(A)$.

An object of $\mathsf{RT}(A', A)$ is an object $(X, \sim)$ of $\mathsf{RT}(A)$ such that for $\sim$, there are realizers in A' witnessing the symmetry and transitivity; similarly, an arrow $(X, \sim) \to (Y, \sim)$ in $\mathsf{RT}(A', A)$ is represented by a function $F : X \times Y \to \mathcal{P}(A)$ such that there are elements of A' which realize that F is strict, relational, single-valued and total.

However, the exponential $(Y, \sim)^{(X, \sim)}$ is just as in $\mathsf{RT}(A)$; just as the subobject classifier. In other words, we have a *logical* functor (a functor preserving the topos structure) from $\mathsf{RT}(A', A)$ to $\mathsf{RT}(A)$.

There are two geometric morphisms connecting $\mathsf{RT}(A', A)$ to $\mathsf{RT}(A')$. On the level of triposes we have transformations $\delta_!$ and δ_* from $\mathsf{P}_{A'}$ to $\mathsf{P}_{A',A}$ and one transformation $\delta^* : \mathsf{P}_{A',A} \to \mathsf{P}_{A'}$. For these maps we have that $\delta_! \dashv \delta^* \dashv \delta_*$ and $\delta_!$ preserves finite meets. This is an easy verification from the definitions of these maps:

$$\begin{aligned}
\delta_!(V) &= V \\
\delta^*(U) &= U \cap A' \\
\delta_*(V) &= \bigcup_{U \in \mathcal{P}(A)} (U \wedge (\delta^*(U) \to V))
\end{aligned}$$

Moreover, $\delta_!$ and hence δ_* are full and faithful. That means that the geometric morphism $(\delta^*, \delta_!) : \mathsf{RT}(A', A) \to \mathsf{RT}(A')$ is *local* (definition 2.5.4), and the geometric morphism $(\delta_*, \delta^*) : \mathsf{RT}(A') \to \mathsf{RT}(A', A)$ is a section for it.

This situation is investigated in [24], and S. Awodey and L. Birkedal have analyzed these local extensions from a logical point of view (see [8]); but for my purposes, the applicability of their axioms is limited.

The relative realizability topos $\mathsf{RT}(\mathcal{K}_2^{\mathrm{rec}}, \mathcal{K}_2)$ was analyzed in [24], and $\mathsf{RT}(\mathcal{P}(\omega)^{\mathrm{re}}, \mathcal{P}(\omega))$ is studied in [11] (see also the note [154], where it is called a "topos for computable analysis").

Here I will spend a few words on $\mathsf{RT}(\mathcal{K}_2^{\mathrm{rec}}, \mathcal{K}_2)$, or the *Kleene-Vesley topos* as I will call it, because the notion of realizability it generalizes was intensively studied and described in Kleene and Vesley's famous (and notorious) book [90] (actually, an equivalent version of this realizability was already defined by Kleene in [87]). I will denote the topos by $\mathcal{KV}$. So, the logic is governed by function realizability as for $\mathsf{RT}(\mathcal{K}_2)$, with the proviso that in the end a sentence is said to be true iff it has a *recursive* realizer.

First, a few more generalities about the topos $\mathsf{RT}(A', A)$. The constant objects functor $\nabla_{A',A} : \mathsf{Set} \to \mathsf{RT}(A', A)$ sends a set X to $(X, \sim)$ where $[x \sim x'] = \{a \in A \mid x = x'\}$. As was shown in [24] and is easy to prove, $\nabla_{A',A}$ embeds Set as $\neg\neg$-sheaves in $\mathsf{RT}(A', A)$.

The subobjects of objects $\nabla_{A',A}(X)$, the $\neg\neg$-separated objects, are up to isomorphism the (A', A)-*assemblies*. The category $\mathsf{Ass}(A', A)$ of (A', A)-assemblies has the same objects as $\mathsf{Ass}(A)$, but arrows have to be tracked by an element of A'. We also have a category $\mathsf{PAss}(A', A)$ of partitioned (A', A)-assemblies, similarly defined. The partitioned (A', A)-assemblies are (up to isomorphism) the projective objects in $\mathsf{RT}(A', A)$. Every object is covered by a projective object, and $\mathsf{PAss}(A', A)$ is closed under finite limits in $\mathsf{RT}(A', A)$, so this topos is also an exact completion. Just as in $\mathsf{RT}(A)$, the notions of projective and internally projective coincide.

All this is very similar to general realizability toposes; let us see some differences.

Unlike realizability toposes, $\mathsf{RT}(A', A)$ is not 2-valued (a topos is 2-valued iff 1 has precisely two subobjects). Subobjects of 1 in $\mathsf{RT}(A', A)$ are in 1-1 correspondence with equivalence classes of subsets of A, where U is equivalent to V iff $A' \cap (U \leftrightarrow V)$ is nonempty. In the case of the Kleene-Vesley topos $\mathcal{KV}$, there is a connection with an independently studied structure.

Definition 4.5.1 The *Medvedev lattice* is the poset reflection of the preorder on $\mathcal{P}(\mathcal{K}_2)$ which is defined as: $U \leq V$ iff there is a partial recursive functional Φ such that for all $\alpha \in V$, $\Phi(\alpha)$ is defined and in U.

It is a matter of some recursion-theoretic recoding, to see that the definition of $U \leq V$ in 4.5.1 is equivalent to: $U \leq V$ iff there is an element $\beta \in \mathcal{K}_2^{\mathrm{rec}}$ such that for all $\alpha \in V$, $\beta\alpha{\downarrow}$ and $\beta\alpha \in U$.

Hence, the lattice of subobjects of 1 in $\mathcal{KV}$ is isomorphic to the *dual* of the Medvedev lattice. This gives another proof of the theorem (see, e.g.[159]), that the dual of the Medvedev lattice is a Heyting algebra.

The Medvedev lattice has been shown to be complete for embeddings of intuitionistic propositional logic by Skvortsova ([151]). Further work on the Medvedev lattice, both from the point of view of logic (study of intermediate propositional logics) and recursion theory, has been done by A. Sorbi and S. Terwijn (see e.g. [152, 159, 158]). It seems a good idea to use the higher-order structure of $\mathcal{KV}$ in order to explore also higher-order propositional logics in this lattice.

In general in $\mathsf{RT}(A', A)$, the natural numbers object is given as $(\mathbb{N}, \sim)$ with $[n \sim m] = \{\bar{n} \mid n = m\}$, $\bar{n}$ again being the Curry numeral. By the requirement of A' being an elementary sub-pca of A, these Curry numerals are in A', and also the primitive recursor from 1.3.5 is in A'.

In $\mathcal{KV}$, the function space N^N is as in $\mathsf{RT}(\mathcal{K}_2)$ and therefore projective and internally projective, so choice over N^N holds. If we have a look at the proof for Brouwer's Principle in $\mathsf{RT}(\mathcal{K}_2)$ (proposition 4.3.4), we see that a realizer can actually be found in $\mathcal{K}_2^{\mathrm{rec}}$. Therefore, BP and WCN also hold in $\mathcal{KV}$, a fact which is also in [90]. As a consequence, CT is *false* in $\mathcal{KV}$, although every arrow $N \to N$ is a recursive function!

Now if $A(x)$ is a formula of first-order arithmetic which defines a non-recursive subset of $\mathbb{N}$, then $\forall x(A(x) \vee \neg A(x))$ cannot be true in $\mathcal{KV}$ because there is no recursive function deciding $A(x)$; but since there is a logical embedding of $\mathcal{KV}$ into $\mathsf{RT}(\mathcal{K}_2)$ and the latter has classical first order arithmetic (4.3.3), we must have $\neg\neg\forall x(A(x) \vee \neg A(x))$. We see that first order arithmetic in $\mathcal{KV}$ is almost, but not entirely, classical.

The treatment of Uniformity parallels that of $\mathcal{Eff}$. An object is uniform if and only if it is covered by an object $\nabla(Y)$, and that is the case iff the object is isomorphic to an object $(X, \sim)$ for which the intersection $\bigcap_{x \in X}[x \sim x]$ contains an element of $\mathcal{K}_2^{\mathrm{rec}}$.

Let us look at $\mathcal{P}(N)$. Since every function $\phi : \mathbb{N} \to \mathcal{P}(\mathcal{K}_2)$ is automatically relational for N by the nature of the equality relation on this object, one only has to impose strictness. Define

$$E(\phi) = [\forall n(\phi(n) \to \{\bar{n}\})]$$

Then $\mathcal{P}(N)$ is $(\mathcal{P}(\mathcal{K}_2)^{\mathbb{N}}, \sim)$ with

$$[\phi \sim \psi] = E(\phi) \wedge [\forall n(\phi(n) \leftrightarrow \psi(n))]$$

Now there is certainly an element $\alpha \in \mathcal{K}_2^{\mathrm{rec}}$ such that, for each ϕ and $\beta \in E(\phi)$, $\alpha\beta{\downarrow}$ and for some ψ such that $p_1 \in E(\psi)$ we have $\alpha\beta \in [\phi \sim \psi]$.

This means that $\mathcal{P}(N)$ is a quotient of $\nabla(\mathcal{P}(\mathcal{K}_2)^{\mathbb{N}}) \simeq \mathcal{P}_{\neg\neg}(N)$; and the Uniformity Principle and Shanin's Principle hold in $\mathcal{KV}$.

It is good to observe that there are *two* functors $\Gamma_1, \Gamma_2 : \mathcal{KV} \to \mathsf{Set}$ and a natural transformation $\Gamma_1 \Rightarrow \Gamma_2$. Γ_1 is the global sections functor (and left adjoint to ∇): $\Gamma_1(X, \sim)$ is the set of equivalence classes of $\{x \in X \mid [x \sim x] \cap \mathcal{K}_2^{\mathrm{rec}} \neq \emptyset\}$ under the equivalence relation $[x \sim y] \cap \mathcal{K}_2^{\mathrm{rec}} \neq \emptyset$. The functor Γ_2 is the composition of the global sections functor from $\mathsf{RT}(\mathcal{K}_2)$ to Set with the logical embedding $\mathcal{KV} \to \mathsf{RT}(\mathcal{K}_2)$. It sends $(X, \sim)$ to the set of equivalence classes of $\{x \in X \mid [x \sim x] \neq \emptyset\}$ under the equivalence relation $[x \sim y] \neq \emptyset$. The natural transformation $\Gamma_1 \Rightarrow \Gamma_2$ is obvious.

Hence we have a functor $\mathcal{KV} \to \text{Set}^{\to}$ and this suggests we might study $\mathcal{KV}$ from the point of view of $\text{Set}^{\to}$. This is the approach taken in [25]. The axiom for an elementary sub-pca simply means that the inclusion $\mathcal{K}_2^{\text{rec}} \subset \mathcal{K}_2$ is an *internal pca* in $\text{Set}^{\to}$ (writing out the Kripke-Joyal clauses for the k- and s-axioms gives exactly the condition of being an elementary sub-pca). Then $\mathcal{KV}$ is simply the realizability topos over $\text{Set}^{\to}$, on this pca. There is a generalization in [25] of the fact that there is a local geometric morphism from $\mathcal{KV}$ to $\text{RT}(\mathcal{K}_2^{\text{rec}})$ in terms of *applicative, elementary* maps between internal pca's in a topos $\mathcal{E}$: a map $i : A \to B$ is called elementary if for every subobject R of B with global support, also $i^*(R)$ has global support. This condition is equivalent to requiring that $\mathcal{E}$ satisfies the following *rule*: if $\mathcal{E} \models \exists x{:}B\phi(x)$ then $\mathcal{E} \models \exists x{:}A\phi(ix)$ (the name 'elementary' reflects that this condition is reminiscent of the Tarski-Vaught test for elementary substructures).

An applicative map between internal pca's is like an elementary sub-pca, except the map need not be an inclusion.

There is a theorem that whenever $A \xrightarrow{i} B$ is an applicative map, there is a geometric morphism $\text{RT}_{\mathcal{E}}(B) \to \text{RT}_{\mathcal{E}}(A)$ (denoting by $\text{RT}_{\mathcal{E}}(B)$ the realizability topos over $\mathcal{E}$ on B), and moreover if i is an elementary map, this geometric morphism is local.

Then, one can consider local operators j in $\mathcal{E}$.

Definition 4.5.2 Let A be an internal pca in a topos $\mathcal{E}$ and j a local operator. The A is called *j-regular* if the following holds:

$$\mathcal{E} \models \exists c{:}A\forall ab{:}A\, j(ab\!\downarrow) \to c(pab)\!\downarrow \wedge j(c(pab) = ab)$$

For example, if $A' \subset A$ is an elementary sub-pca then the inclusion $A' \to A$ is a $\neg\neg$-regular internal pca in $\text{Set}^{\to}$.

If A is a j-regular internal pca in $\mathcal{E}$, then there is a subtripos $\mathcal{E}(-, \mathcal{P}_j(A))$ (of maps into the object of j-closed subsets of A) of the realizability tripos over $\mathcal{E}$ on A. Moreover, if j is an open local operator $(u \Rightarrow -)$ then this inclusion of triposes is also open, and we have an open subtopos $\text{RT}_{\mathcal{E}}(A, j)$ of $\text{RT}_{\mathcal{E}}(A)$. We call its closed complement the *modified realizability topos over $\mathcal{E}$ on A w.r.t. j*.

This generalizes modified realizability as given in section 4.2: in $\text{Set}^{\to}$, the local operator $\neg\neg$ is open, and for an internal pca of the form

$A = (B \xrightarrow{\text{id}} B)$, $\mathsf{RT}_{\mathrm{Set}^{\rightarrow}}(A, \neg\neg)$ is the modeified realizability topos w.r.t. B.

But one can also consider other internal pca's in $\mathrm{Set}^{\rightarrow}$; for example, an elementary inclusion $A' \subset A$. Then one obtains *modified relative realizability*.

Actually, such a construction had appeared in the literature long before the introduction of realizability toposes. In [115], J.R. Moschovakis defines modified realizability w.r.t. $\mathcal{K}_2^{\mathrm{rec}} \subset \mathcal{K}_2$. She proves that this realizability satisfies a weak form of Church's thesis (for every $f{:}N^N$, $\neg\neg(f$ is recursive)), and *Vesley's Principle*, which says:

$$\forall z \exists \alpha (\bar{\alpha}(\mathrm{lh}(z)) = z \wedge \neg A(\alpha)) \wedge \forall \alpha (\neg A(\alpha) \rightarrow \exists \beta B(\alpha, \beta))$$
$$\rightarrow \forall \alpha \exists \beta (\neg A(\alpha) \rightarrow B(\alpha, \beta))$$

which is some sort of Independence of Premiss provided the Premiss defines a dense subset of N^N. Vesley's Principle, which he called a *palatable alternative to Kripke's schema*, was introduced in [175].

4.6 Realizability toposes over other toposes than Set

We have already seen the construction of $e\mathcal{E}$, the effective topos over a topos $\mathcal{E}$, in section 3.8.3, and the general realizability topos $\mathsf{RT}_{\mathcal{E}}(A)$ over $\mathcal{E}$ on an internal pca in $\mathcal{E}$; but apart from $\mathcal{E} = \mathcal{E}\!f\!f$ and $\mathcal{E} = \mathrm{Set}^{\rightarrow}$, no concrete examples. In this section I give two such examples: the *free topos* $\mathcal{F}$ and a *sheaf model of realizability*.

4.6.1 The free topos with NNO

In the book [95], an adjunction is defined between a category Lang of type theories (which, for them, are internal languages of toposes) and interpretations between them, and the category Top of toposes with natural numbers object and logical functors. Actually these are both 2-categories, with provable equivalences and natural isomorphisms as respective 2-cells, but I ignore this. The left adjoint, the functor from Lang to Top, constructs the topos freely generated by a type theory. It is a construction that is paramount in category theory, and has a number of applications:

1)   The free topos with NNO. Lang has an initial object, the pure type theory, and the topos freely generated by it, is initial in Top (for another syntactic construction, see [19]);

2)   similarly, we have the free Boolean topos;

3)   constructions on toposes like "freely adding an arrow", "inverting an arrow", are available.

The free topos with NNO, denoted $\mathcal{F}$ is (up to equivalence of categories) determined by the fact that for every topos with NNO there is a unique (up to isomorphism) logical functor from $\mathcal{F}$ to it (note that a logical functor always preserves the NNO).

The free topos harbors an interpretation of higher order intuitionistic arithmetic HAH, such that for any statement ϕ in its language, $\mathcal{F} \models \phi$ precisely if HAH $\vdash \phi$.

We can now apply some simple topos theory to $\mathcal{F}$ in order to derive proof theoretic properties of HAH, which are similar to a number of so-called *derived rules* for HA, proved by various techniques. Here are some examples of such derived rules for HA:

If HA $\vdash \forall x (A(x) \vee \neg A(x)) \wedge \neg\neg \exists x A(x)$, then HA $\vdash \exists x A(x)$
(Markov's Rule)

If HA $\vdash \exists n \varphi(n)$ then there exists a number $n \in \mathbb{N}$ such that HA $\vdash \varphi(n)$
(Numerical existence property)

If HA $\vdash \forall x (\neg A(x) \rightarrow \exists y B(x,y))$ then HA $\vdash \forall x \exists y (\neg A(x) \rightarrow B(x,y))$
(Independence of Premiss Rule)

If HA $\vdash \forall x (A(x) \rightarrow \exists y B(x,y))$ and $A(x)$ is almost negative, then

$$HA \vdash \exists e \forall x (A(x) \rightarrow ex\!\downarrow \wedge B(x,ex))$$

(Extended Church's Rule)

For HAH, we can consider the extensions of these rules, and moreover other rules:

If $\text{HAH} \vdash \forall\alpha{:}\mathcal{P}(N)\exists n{:}N\phi(\alpha,n)$ then $\text{HAH} \vdash \exists n{:}N\forall\alpha{:}\mathcal{P}(N)\phi(\alpha,n)$
(Uniformity Rule)

If $\text{HAH} \vdash \forall\alpha{:}N^N\exists n{:}N\phi(\alpha,n)$ then

$$\text{HAH} \vdash \forall\alpha{:}N^N\exists nm{:}N\forall\beta{:}N^N(\bar\beta m = \bar\alpha m \to \phi(\beta,n))$$

(Weak Continuity Rule)

This list is by no means exhaustive.

The main method of proving these rules for HAH is *glueing*. Lambek and Scott used glueing of the free topos $\mathcal{F}$ to Set along the global sections functor $\Gamma = \mathcal{F}(1,-) : \mathcal{F} \to \text{Set}$. This method is the topos theoretic analogue and generalization of what in the context of HA was known as the *Kleene slash* (see [163]).

I shall look briefly at a realizability variant of glueing, namely glueing of the subobject tripos $P(X) = \text{Sub}_{\mathcal{F}}(X)$ on $\mathcal{F}$, and the effective tripos P_e on $\mathcal{F}$. Of course, $\mathcal{F}[P]$ is equivalent to $\mathcal{F}$ and this is very similar to glueing $\mathcal{F}$ to $e\mathcal{F}$ along ∇.

We have a transformation of triposes $P \overset{\Phi}{\to} P_e$, such that Φ_X sends a subobject U of X to the map

$$x \mapsto \{n \in N \mid x \in U\}$$

This gives (by the theory in section 2.8) the glued tripos $P_{qe} = (P{\downarrow}\Phi)$, defined by

$$P_{qe}(X) = \{(U,\psi) \mid U \subseteq X, \psi \in \mathcal{P}(N)^X, \forall xn(n \in \psi(x) \to x \in U)\}$$

and the order is given by: $(U,\psi) \leq (U',\psi')$ iff $U \subseteq U'$ and for some number $n \in \mathbb{N}$,

$$\mathcal{F} \models \forall x\forall a \in \psi(x)(na{\downarrow} \wedge na \in \psi'(x))$$

Heyting implication in $P_{qe}(X)$ is given by $[(U,\psi) \Rightarrow (U',\psi')] = (V,\chi)$, where $V = \{x \in X \mid x \in U \to x \in U'\}$ and

$$\chi(x) = \{n \in N \mid x \in V \wedge \forall a \in \psi(x)(na{\downarrow} \wedge na \in \psi'(x))\}$$

This tripos generalizes a construction which is essentially already in Kleene's 1945 paper [88] and was later called *q-realizability* by Troelstra ([161]). The tripos analogue was first formulated by R. Grayson ([61]).

In $\mathcal{F}[\mathsf{P}_{qe}]$ we have objects $(X, \equiv, \sim)$ such that $\equiv$ is a partial equivalence relation on X in $\mathcal{F}$, and $(X, \sim)$ is an object of $e\mathcal{F}$ (that is, $\sim$ is a map $X \times X \to \mathcal{P}(N)$ in $\mathcal{F}$ which is symmetric and transitive in the realizability sense), and moreover the sentence

$$\forall xyn(n \in [x \sim y] \to x \equiv y)$$

holds in $\mathcal{F}$.

In section 2.8 we have seen that the projection $(X, \equiv, \sim) \to (X, \equiv)$ is a logical functor from $\mathcal{F}[\mathsf{P}_{qe}]$ to $\mathcal{F}[\mathsf{P}]$. The equivalence $\mathcal{F}[\mathsf{P}] \to \mathcal{F}$ is given by $(X, \equiv) \mapsto U/\equiv$, where U is the field of $\equiv$. Since $\mathcal{F}$ is the free topos, we also have a logical functor $\mathcal{F} \to \mathcal{F}[\mathsf{P}_{qe}]$ and the composition of the two is isomorphic to the identity on $\mathcal{F}$.

It is readily calculated that the NNO in $\mathcal{F}[\mathsf{P}_{qe}]$ is given by $(N, =, \sim)$ where $[n \sim m] = \{n | n = m\}$.

As an example I shall use $\mathcal{F}[\mathsf{P}_{qe}]$ to derive Church's Rule for HAH: if ϕ is a definable subobject of $N \times N$ and $\mathrm{HAH} \vdash \forall n \exists m \phi(n, m)$, then there is a number e such that $\mathrm{HAH} \vdash \forall n(en{\downarrow} \wedge \phi(n, en))$.

So assume $\mathrm{HAH} \vdash \forall n \exists m \phi(n, m)$. Since $\mathcal{F} \to \mathcal{F}[\mathsf{P}_{qe}] \to \mathcal{F}$ is isomorphic to the identity, we may assume that the interpretation of ϕ as subobject of $N \times N$ in $\mathcal{F}[\mathsf{P}_{qe}]$ is given by a strict relation on $N \times N$ of the form

$$(\phi_{\mathcal{F}}, \chi)$$

with $\phi_{\mathcal{F}} \subseteq N \times N$ the interpretation of ϕ in $\mathcal{F}$ and $\chi : N \times N \to \mathcal{P}(N)$ satisfies

$(*)$ $\mathcal{F} \models \forall nmk(k \in \chi(n, m) \to \phi(n, m))$

Because $\mathrm{HAH} \vdash \forall n \exists m \phi(n, m)$, this sentence is true in $\mathcal{F}[\mathsf{P}_{qe}]$. By definition of truth in this topos, there is therefore a number a such that

$$\mathcal{F} \models \forall n(an{\downarrow} \wedge p_1(an) \in \chi(n, p_0(an)))$$

By $(*)$ then, if $e = \langle n \rangle p_0(an)$,

$$\mathcal{F} \models \forall n(en{\downarrow} \wedge \phi(n, en))$$

so HAH proves this sentence, and we are done.

With a little further analysis of the tripos P_{qe} this could have been strengthened to yield Extended Church's Thesis too.

The method is quite versatile. There is a similar glueing of P to the modified realizability tripos on $\mathcal{F}$, which enables one to derive the Independence of Premiss Rule for HAH. In [171], a syntactical form of glueing with extensional realizabiity is used to obtain an 'Extensional Church's Rule' for HA:

> Suppose HA $\vdash \forall e(\forall x \exists y B(e, x, y) \rightarrow \exists z C(e, z))$, where B is an almost negative formula.
>
> Then there is a number n such that

$$\text{HA} \vdash \forall e(ne{\downarrow} \wedge \forall f f'(\forall x(fx{\downarrow} \wedge f'x{\downarrow} \wedge fx = f'x \wedge B(e, x, fx)) \rightarrow$$
$$nef{\downarrow} \wedge nef'{\downarrow} \wedge nef = nef' \wedge C(e, nef)))$$

(note, that this rule contains Extended Church's Rule)

4.6.2   A sheaf model of realizability

D. de Jongh was, to my knowledge, the first who had the idea of combining realizability with Kripke forcing, in the unpublished manuscript [35]. He built an internal pca in the topos of the form Set^P, with P a poset. Concretely, this is a P-indexed system of pas's $(A_p \,|\, p \in P)$ and transition maps $i_{pq} : A_p \rightarrow A_q$ for $p \leq q$, such that the Kripke interpretation of the pca-axiom holds. For example, for each $p \in P$ there is an element k_p such that for all $q \geq p$ and all $a, b \in A_q$, $i_{pq}(k_p)ab{\downarrow}$ in A_q, and equal to a.

De Jongh's aim was to use such a realizability interpretation to prove what is now known as De Jongh's Theorem (see the remark following theorem 3.1.5 for a statement of it). He only succeeded for a restricted class of predicate formulas.

A very similar construction, by N. Goodman, appeared 9 years later, in [58]. Here the application was different, but what matters for us is the construction.

Consider a Gödel numbering of partial recursive functions which consult an *oracle* U. We think of U as a partial function on $\mathbb{N}$; the computer may ask questions like $U(n) = ?$, and receives the right answer if $n \in \text{dom}(U)$; if $n \notin \text{dom}(U)$ the computation diverges at this point. It is important to realize that there is a Gödel numbering of such partial recursive functions consulting an oracle, which does not depend on the oracle; and also, for this numbering, the *Smn*-theorem holds and the *Smn*-functions are primitive recursive (and don't use the oracle). That is, if we denote partial recursive application using oracle U by $a^U b$, then $(\mathbb{N}, (\cdot)^U(\cdot))$ is a pca, and k and s can be chosen independent of U.

If V is a partial function which extends U, then clearly whenever $a^U b = c$, also $a^V b = c$.

So if P is a poset, and $p \mapsto U_p$ is an order-preserving map which assigns to each $p \in P$ a partial function on $\mathbb{N}$, we have an internal pca A in Set^P, with $A_p = (\mathbb{N}, (\cdot)^{U_p}(\cdot))$, and the identity function as transition map. Let us denote the realizability tripos on Set^P w.r.t. A by P_A.

Of course, by iteration the topos $\text{Set}^P[\mathsf{P}_A]$ is equivalent to $\text{Set}[\mathsf{P}_A \circ \Delta^{\text{op}}]$ where $\Delta : \text{Set} \to \text{Set}^P$ is the constant presheaf functor. One can now easily write out a truth definition for first order arithmetic in this topos, in clauses which combine Kleene realizability with Kripke forcing. The basic notion is the relation '$p \Vdash n \; \mathbf{r} \; \phi$', for $p \in P$, $n \in \mathbb{N}$ and ϕ a sentence of arithmetic. For example, the implication clause reads

$p \Vdash n \; \mathbf{r} \; (\phi \to \psi)$ iff for every $q \geq p$ and every m such that $q \Vdash m \; \mathbf{r} \; \phi$, $n^{U_q}m\downarrow$ and $q \Vdash n^{U_q}m \; \mathbf{r} \; \psi$.

This is not exactly what Goodman did; he combined this with the $\neg\neg$-operator in Set^P, and his definition therefore went

$p \Vdash n \; \mathbf{r} \; (\phi \to \psi)$ iff for every $q \geq p$ and every m such that $q \Vdash m \; \mathbf{r} \; \phi$, there is an $r \geq q$ such that $n^{U_r}m\downarrow$ and $r \Vdash n^{U_r}m \; \mathbf{r} \; \psi$.

In [168], another version of the idea is developed. The application here is a proof of de Jongh's Theorem. Instead of the $\neg\neg$-operator, another local operator was used, which corresponds to a so-called *fallible Beth model*.

We consider the full binary tree T of finite 01-sequences, ordered $\sigma \sqsubseteq \tau$ if σ is an initial segment of τ. A subset U of T is specified, which is upwards closed and has the property that if σ is such that every path through σ meets U somewhere, then already $\sigma \in U$.

We consider the topos Set^T and the following local operator on it: for an upwards closed subset R of T, let $j_U(R)$ be the set of those $\sigma \in T$ such that every path through σ meets $R \cup U$. So j_U is the closed local operator corresponding to the subobject of 1 determined by U.

Now suppose $\mathcal{L}$ is a language in predicate logic with only relation symbols. A *Beth structure* for $\mathcal{L}$ w.r.t. U assigns to every n-place relation symbol R a subfunctor of the constant functor $\Delta(\mathbb{N}^n)$ in Set^T, which is closed for j_U. That is, we have subsets $R_\sigma \subseteq \mathbb{N}^n$ such that for every n-tuple $x_1, \ldots, x_n$ the set

$$\{\sigma \in T \mid (x_1, \ldots, x_n) \in R_\sigma\}$$

is an upwards closed, j_U-closed set.

Given such a Beth structure, we have an obvious interpretation of intuitionistic logic, formulated in Kripke-style clauses, the only differences being:

$$\sigma \Vdash (\phi \vee \psi)(\vec{x}) \text{ iff } \sigma \in j_U(\{\tau \mid \tau \Vdash \phi(\vec{x}) \text{ or } \tau \Vdash \psi(\vec{x})\})$$

$$\sigma \Vdash (\exists y \phi)(\vec{x}) \text{ iff } \sigma \in j_U(\{\tau \mid \text{for some } y, \tau \Vdash \phi(\vec{x}, y)\})$$

Note that if $\sigma \in U$, then $\sigma \Vdash \phi$ for any ϕ.

The theorem (to be found in [163], chapter 13) is that for every r.e. theory $\mathcal{T}$ in a language $\mathcal{L}$ with only relation symbols, there is a subset U of T as above, and a Beth structure for $\mathcal{L}$ w.r.t. U, such that for the empty sequence $\langle \rangle$ it holds that for every ϕ:

$$\langle \rangle \Vdash \phi \Leftrightarrow \mathcal{T} \vdash \phi$$

Moreover, there is an enumeration ϕ_i of te $\mathcal{L}$-formulas such that the relation $\sigma \Vdash \phi_i(x_1, \ldots, x_n)$ is r.e. in $\sigma, i, \vec{x}$.

The next step is to build a realizability model on this Beth structure, and take care that the pca is a sheaf for the operator j_U. So we need to pick partial functions U_σ for each σ which will be oracles.

It is possible, using a trick from Recursion theory, to pick the oracle functions sufficiently independent from each other (in a recursion-theoretic sense), so that to each relation symbol R_i an arithmetical formula of the form

$$C_i(\vec{x}) \; \equiv \; \forall y(D_i(\vec{x}, y) \lor \neg D_i(\vec{x}, y))$$

can be associated, in such a way that no predicate logical relations between the C_i are realizable, than already provable (for the R_i) in $\mathcal{T}$. That means, we have an interpretation of $\mathcal{T}$ into HA which reflects provability.

Bibliography

[1] M. Abadi and G.D. Plotkin. A per model of polymorphism and recursive types. In J. Mitchell, editor, *5th Annual IEEE Symposium on Logic in Computer Science*, pages 355–365, Philadelphia, 1990. IEEE Computer Society Press.

[2] P Aczel. The type-theoretic interpretation of constructive set theory. In *Logic Colloquium '77*, number 96 in Studies in Logic, pages 55–66. North-Holland, 1978.

[3] P Aczel. The type-theoretic interpretation of constructive set theory:choice principles. In *Te L.E.J.Brouwer Centenary Symposium*, number 110 in Studies in Logic, pages 1–40. North-Holland, 1982.

[4] P Aczel. The type-theoretic interpretation of constructive set theory:inductive definitions. In *Logic, Methodology and Philosophy of Science VII*, number 114 in Studies in Logic, pages 17–49. North-Holland, 1986.

[5] P. Aczel and M. Rathjen. Notes on Constructive Set Theory. Technical Report 40, Institut Mittag-Leffler, 2000. ISSN 1103-467X.

[6] R. Amadio. On the adequacy of per models. In *Mathematical Foundations of Computer Science*, pages 222–231. Springer, LNCS 711, 1993.

[7] R.M. Amadio and P.-L. Curien. *Domains and Lambda Calculi*. Cambridge University Press, 1998.

[8] S. Awodey and L. Birkedal. Elementary axioms for local maps of toposes. *Journ.Pure Appl.Alg.*, 177(3):215–230, 2003.

[9] S. Awodey, L. Birkedal, and D.S. Scott. Local realizability toposes and a modal logic for computability. *Mathematical Structures in Computer Science*, 12(3):319–334, 2002.

[10] S. Bainbridge, P.J. Freyd, A. Scedrov, and P. Scott. Functorial polymorphism. *Theoretical Computer Science*, 70:35–64, 1990.

[11] A. Bauer. *The Realizability Approach to Computable Analysis and Topology*. PhD thesis, Carnegie Mellon University, Pittsburgh, 2000.

[12] A. Bauer. A relationship between equilogical spaces and type two effectivity. *Electr. Notes in Theor. Comp. Science*, 45, 2001.

[13] A. Bauer. First steps in synthetic computability theory. *Electr. Notes in Theor. Comp. Science*, 155, 2006.

[14] A. Bauer, L. Birkedal, and D. Scott. Equilogical spaces. *Theor. Comp. Science*, 315(1):35–59, 2004.

[15] A. Bauer and A. Simpson. Two constructive embedding-extension theorems with applications to continuity principles and to banach-mazur computability. *Math.Logic Quarterly*, 50:351–369, 2004.

[16] M.J. Beeson. Recursive models for constructive set theories. *Annals of Pure and Applied Logic*, 23:127–178, 1982.

[17] M.J. Beeson. *Foundations of constructive mathematics*. Springer-Verlag, 1985.

[18] J.L. Bell. *Boolean-valued Models and Independence Proofs in Set Theory*. Clarendon Press, Oxford, 1977.

[19] J.L. Bell. *Toposes and Local Set Theories*. Number 14 in Oxford Logic Guides. Clarendon Press, Oxford, 1988.

[20] S. Berardi. An application of per models to program extraction. *Math.Struct. Comp.Science*, 3(3):309–331, 1993.

[21] I. Bethke. On the existence of extensional partial combinatory algebras. *Journal of Symbolic Logic*, 52:819–833, 1987.

[22] I. Bethke. *Notes on Partial Combinatory Algebras*. PhD thesis, Universiteit van Amsterdam, 1988.

[23] M. Bezem. Isomorphisms between heo and hro^e, ecf and icf^e. *Journal of Symbolic Logic*, 50(2):359–371, 1985.

[24] L. Birkedal. Developing theories of types and computability via realizability. *Electronic Notes in Theoretical Computer Science*, 34:viii+282, 2000. Book version of PhD-thesis.

[25] L. Birkedal and J. van Oosten. Relative and modified relative realizability. *Ann.Pure Appl.Logic*, 118:115–132, 2002.

[26] A. Blass. Words, free algebras, and coequalizers. *Fundamenta Mathematicae*, 117:117–160, 1983.

[27] A. Blass and A. Scedrov. Small decidable sheaves. *Journal of Symbolic Logic*, 51(3):726–731, 1986.

[28] F. Borceux. *Handbook of Categorical Algebra*, volume 50 of *Encyclopedia of Mathematics and its Applications*. Cambridge University Press, 1994. 3 vols.

[29] A. Bucciarelli and T. Ehrhard. Sequentiality and strong stability. In *Proc. Logic in Computer Science*, 1991.

[30] A. Carboni. Some free constructions in realizability and proof theory. *Journal of Pure and Applied Algebra*, 103:117–148, 1995.

[31] A. Carboni, P.J. Freyd, and A. Scedrov. A categorical approach to realizability and polymorphic types. In M. Main, A. Melton, M. Mislove, and D.Schmidt, editors, *Mathematical Foundations of Programming Language Semantics*, volume 298 of *Lectures Notes in Computer Science*, pages 23–42, New Orleans, 1988. Springer-Verlag.

[32] A. Carboni and R. Celia Magno. The free exact category on a left exact one. *Journal of Australian Mathematical Society*, 33(A):295–301, 1982.

[33] A. Carboni and E.M. Vitale. Regular and exact completions. *Journal of Pure and Àpplied Algebra*, 125:79–117, 1998.

[34] L. Cardelli and G. Longo. A semantic basis for Quest. Technical Report 55, Digital Equipment Corporation, 1989.

[35] D.H.J. de Jongh. The maximality of the intuitionistic predicate calculus with respect to Heyting's Arithmetic, 1969. Typed manuscript from University of Wisconsin, Madison.

[36] J. Diller and A.S.Troelstra. Realizability and intuitionistic logic. *Synthese*, 60:253–282, 1984.

[37] A.G. Dragalin. Transfinite completions of constructive arithmetical calculus (Russian). *Doklady*, 189:458–460, 1969. Translation *SM* 10, pp. 1417–1420.

[38] M. Droste. Concurrent automata and domains. *Internat.Journ.Found.Comp.Science*, 3(4):389–418, 1992.

[39] S. Eielenberg and S. MacLane. General theory of natural equivalences. *Trans.Amer.Math.Soc.*, 58:231–294, 1945.

[40] E. Engeler. Algebras and combinators. *Algebra Universalis*, 13:389–392, 1981.

[41] M. Escardó and T. Streicher. In domain realizability, not all functionals on $\mathcal{C}[-1,1]$ are continuous. *Math. Log. Quarterly*, 48(1):41–44, 2002.

[42] S. Feferman. A language and axioms for explicit mathematics. In J.N. Crossley, editor, *Algebra and Logic*, pages 87–139. Springer-Verlag, 1975.

[43] M. Fiore. *Axiomatic Domain Theory in Categories of Partial Maps*. Distinguished Dissertations in Computer Science. Cambridge Univerity Press, 1996.

[44] M.P. Fourman and D.S. Scott. Sheaves and logic. In M.P. Fourman, C.J. Mulvey, and D.S. Scott, editors, *Applications of Sheaves*, pages 302–401. Springer-Verlag, 1979.

[45] P.J. Freyd. POLYNAT in PER. In J.W. Gray and A. Scedrov, editors, *Categories in Computer Science and Logic*, volume 92 of *Contemporary Mathematics*, pages 67–68, Boulder, June 1987, 1989. American Mathematical Society.

[46] P.J. Freyd. Algebraically complete categories. In A. Carboni, M.C. Pedicchio, and G. Rosolini, editors, *Category Theory - Proceedings Como 1990*, pages 95–104. Springer, LNM 1488, 1991.

[47] P.J. Freyd, P. Mulry, G. Rosolini, and D.S. Scott. Extensional PERs. *Information and Computation*, 98:211–227, 1992.

[48] P.J. Freyd and A. Scedrov. *Categories, Allegories*. North Holland Publishing Company, 1991.

[49] H. M. Friedman and A. Scedrov. Set existence property for intuitionistic theories with dependent choice. *Annals of Pure and Applied Logic*, 25:129–140, 1983. Corrigendum in *APAL* **26** (1984), p.101.

[50] H. M. Friedman and A. Scedrov. The lack of definable witnesses and provably recursive functions in intuitionistic set theories. *Advances in Mathematics*, 57:1–13, 1985.

[51] H.M. Friedman. Some applications of Kleene's methods for intuitionistic systems. In A. R. D. Mathias and H. Rogers, editors, *Cambridge Summer School in Mathematical Logic*, pages 113–170. Springer-Verlag, 1973.

[52] H.M. Friedman. Set theoretic foundations of constructive analysis. *Annals of Mathematics, Series 2*, 105:1–28, 1977.

[53] H.M. Friedman. Classically and Intuitionistically Provably Recursive Functions. In G.H. Müller and D.S. Scott, editors, *Higher Set Theory*, pages 21–27. Springer (Lecture Notes in Mathematics 669), 1978.

[54] H.M. Friedman and A. Scedrov. Large sets in intuitionistic set theory. *Annals of Pure and Applied Logic*, 27:1–24, 1984.

[55] H.M. Friedman and A. Scedrov. Intuitionistically provable recursive well-orderings. *Annals of Pure and Applied Logic*, 30:165–171, 1986.

[56] J.-Y. Girard. Une extension de l' interpretation fonctionelle de gödel à l'analyse et son application à l'élimination des coupures dans l'analyse et la théorie des types. In J.F. Fenstad, editor, *Proc. 2nd Scand. Logic Symp.*, pages 63–92. North-Holland, Amsterdam, 1971.

[57] J.-Y. Girard. The system F of variable types, fifteen years later. *Theoretical Computer Science*, 45 (2):159–192, 1986.

[58] N.D. Goodman. Relativized realizability in intuitionistic arithmetic of all finite types. *Journal of Symbolic Logic*, 43:23–44, 1978.

[59] L. Gordeev. Constructive models for set theory with extensionality. In A.S. Troelstra and D. van Dalen, editors, *The L.E.J. Brouwer Centenary Symposium*, pages 123–148, Amsterdam, 1982. North Holland.

[60] R.J. Grayson. Heyting-valued models for intuitionistic set theory. In M. Fourman, C. Mulvey, and D.S. Scott, editors, *Application of Sheaves*, volume 743 of *Lecture Notes in Mathematics*, pages 402–414, Berlin, 1979. Springer.

[61] R.J. Grayson. Derived rules obtained by a model-theoretic approach to realisability, 1981. Handwritten notes from Münster University.

[62] R.J. Grayson. Modified realisability toposes, 1981. Handwritten notes from Münster University.

[63] A. Heyting, editor. *Constructivity in Mathematics*. North-Holland Publishing Company, 1959.

[64] D. Higgs. A category approach to boolean-valued set theory. Technical report, University of Waterloo, 1973.

[65] D. Higgs. Injectivity in the topos of complete heyting algebra valued sets. *Canadian Journal of Mathematics*, 36:550–568, 1984.

[66] M. Hofmann, J. van Oosten, and T. Streicher. Well-foundedness in realizability. *Arch.Math.Log.*, 45:795–805, 2006.

[67] P. Hofstra. Relative completions. *Journ.Pure Appl.Alg.*, 192:129–148, 2004.

[68] P. Hofstra. All realizability is relative. *Math. Proc. Camb. Phil. Soc.*, 141:239–264, 2006.

[69] P. Hofstra and J. van Oosten. Ordered partial combinatory algebras. *Math. Proc. Camb. Phil. Soc.*, 134:445–463, 2003.

[70] J.M.E. Hyland. The effective topos. In A.S. Troelstra and D. Van Dalen, editors, *The L.E.J. Brouwer Centenary Symposium*, pages 165–216. North Holland Publishing Company, 1982.

[71] J.M.E. Hyland. A small complete category. *Journal of Pure and Applied Logic*, 40:135–165, 1988.

[72] J.M.E. Hyland. First steps in synthetic domain theory. In A. Carboni, M.C. Pedicchio, and G. Rosolini, editors, *Category Theory '90*, volume 1144 of *Lectures Notes in Mathematics*, pages 131–156, Como, 1992. Springer-Verlag.

[73] J.M.E. Hyland. Variations on realizability: realizing the propositional axiom of choice. *Math.Structures Comput.Sci.*, 12:295–317, 2002.

[74] J.M.E. Hyland, P.T. Johnstone, and A.M. Pitts. Tripos theory. *Math. Proc. Camb. Phil. Soc.*, 88:205–232, 1980.

[75] J.M.E. Hyland and C.-H. L. Ong. Modified realizability toposes and strong normalization proofs. In J.F. Groote and M. Bezem, editors, *Typed Lambda Calculi and Applications*, volume 664 of *Lecture Notes in Computer Science*, pages 179–194. Springer-Verlag, 1993.

[76] J.M.E. Hyland, E.P. Robinson, and G. Rosolini. Algebraic types in PER models. In M. Main, A. Melton, M. Mislove, and D.Schmidt, editors, *Mathematical Foundations of Programming Language Semantics*, volume 442 of *Lecture Notes in Computer Science*, pages 333–350, New Orleans, 1990. Springer-Verlag.

[77] J.M.E. Hyland, E.P. Robinson, and G. Rosolini. The discrete objects in the effective topos. *Proceedings of the London Mathematical Society*, 60:1–60, 1990.

[78] B. Jacobs. *Categorical Logic and Type Theory*. Number 141 in Studies in Logic. North-Holland, 1999.

[79] M. Jibladze. A presentation of the initial lift algebra. *Journal of Pure and Applied Algebra*, 116:185–198, 1997.

[80] P.T. Johnstone. *Topos Theory*. Number 10 in LMS Mathematical Monographs. Academic Press, London, 1977.

[81] P.T. Johnstone. *Stone Spaces*, volume 3 of *Cambridge Studies in Advanced Mathematics*. Cambridge University Press, 1982.

[82] P.T. Johnstone. Quotients of decidable objects in a topos. *Mathematical Proceedings of Cambridge Philosophical Society*, 93:409–419, 1983.

[83] P.T. Johnstone. *Sketches of an Elephant (2 vols.)*, volume 43 of *Oxford Logic Guides*. Clarendon Press, Oxford, 2002.

[84] P.T. Johnstone and E.P. Robinson. A note on inequivalence of realizability toposes. *Mathematical Proceedings of Cambridge Philosophical Society*, 105:1–3, 1989.

[85] A. Joyal and I. Moerdijk. *Algebraic Set Theory*, volume 220 of *London Mathematical Society Lecture Note Series*. Cambridge University Press, Cambridge, 1995.

[86] A. Joyal and M. Tierney. *An extension of the Galois theory of Grothendieck*, volume 309 of *Memoirs of the American Mathematical Society*. American Mathematical Society, Providence, R.I., 1984.

[87] S. C. Kleene. Realizability. In *Summaries of Talks presented at the Summer Institute for Symbolic Logic*, pages 100–104. Institute for Defense Analyses, Communications Research Division, Princeton, 1957. Also in *[63]*, pp. 285–289. Errata in *[90]*, page 192.

[88] S.C. Kleene. On the interpretation of intuitionistic number theory. *Journal of Symbolic Logic*, 10:109–124, 1945.

[89] S.C. Kleene. Logical calculus and realizability. *Acta Philosophica Fennica*, 18:71–80, 1965.

[90] S.C. Kleene and R.E. Vesley. *The Foundations of Intuitionistic Mathematics, especially in relation to recursive functions*. North-Holland Publishing Company, 1965.

[91] A. Kock. *Synthetic Differential Geometry*. Number 333 in London Math.Soc.Lecture Note Series. Cambridge University Press, 2006. second edition.

[92] C. Kouwenhoven-Gentil and J. van Oosten. Algebraic set theory and the effective topos. *Journal of Symbolic Logic*, 70 (3):879–890, 2005.

[93] G. Kreisel. Interpretation of analysis by means of functionals of finite type. In A. Heyting, editor, *Constructivity in Mathematics*, pages 101–128. North-Holland, 1959.

[94] K. Kunen. *Set Theory*, volume 102 of *Studies in Logic*. North-Holland, Amsterdam, 1980.

[95] J. Lambek and P. J. Scott. *Introduction to Higher Order Categorical Logic*. Cambridge University Press, Cambridge, 1986.

[96] D. Leivant. *Absoluteness of Intuitionistic Logic*. PhD thesis, University of Amsterdam, 1975.

[97] P. Lietz. *From Constructive Mathematics to Computable Analysis via the Realizability interpretation*. PhD thesis, TU Darmstadt, 2004. available at http://deposit.d-nb.de/cgi-bin/dokserv?idn=974032735.

[98] V. Lifschitz. CT_0 is stronger than CT_0! *Proceedings of the American Mathematical Society*, 73:101–106, 1979.

[99] J. Longley. *Realizability Toposes and Language Semantics*. PhD thesis, Edinburgh University, 1995.

[100] J.R. Longley and A.K. Simpson. A uniform approach to domain theory in realizability models. *Mathematical Structures in Computer Science*, 7:469–505, 1997.

[101] R.S. Lubarsky. CZF and Second Order Arithmetic. *Annals of Pure and Appl. Logic*, 141(1-2):29–34, 2006.

[102] S. Mac Lane and I. Moerdijk. *Sheaves in Geometry and Logic*. Springer Verlag, 1992.

[103] D.C. McCarty. Realizability and recursive mathematics. Technical Report CMU–CS–84–131, Department of Computer Science, Carnegie-Mellon University, 1984. Report version of the author's PhD thesis, Oxford University 1983.

[104] D.C. McCarty. Realizability and recursive set theory. *Annals Pure Appl. Logic*, 32:153–183, 1986.

[105] D.C. McCarty. Subcountability under realizability. *The Notre Dame Journal of Formal Logic*, 27:210–220, 1986.

[106] D.C. McCarty. Markov's principle, isols and Dedekind finite sets. *Journal of Symbolic Logic*, 53:1042–1069, 1988.

[107] Yu.T. Medvedev. Degrees of difficulty of the mass problems. *Doklady Akad.Nauk.SSSR*, 140(4):501–504, 1955.

[108] M. Menni. *Exact Completions and Toposes*. PhD thesis, University of Edinburgh, 2000.

[109] M. Menni. More exact completions that are toposes. *Annals of Pure and Applied Logic*, 116:187–203, 2002.

[110] R. Milner. Fully abstract models of typed lambda calculi. *Theor. Comp. Science*, 4, 1977.

[111] J.C. Mitchell. *Foundations of Programming Languages*. MIT Press, 1996.

[112] I. Moerdijk and E. Palmgren. Wellfounded trees in categories. *Annals of Pure and Applied Logic*, 104:189–218, 2000.

[113] I. Moerdijk and E. Palmgren. Type theories, toposes and constructive set theory: predicative aspects of AST. *Annals of Pure and Applied Logic*, 114:155–201, 2002.

[114] I. Moerdijk and G. Reyes. *Models for Smooth Infinitesimal Analysis*. Springer, 1991.

[115] J.R. Moschovakis. Can there be no nonrecursive functions? *Journal of Symbolic Logic*, 36:309–315, 1971.

[116] P. Mulry. Generalized Banach-Mazur functionals in the topos of recursive sets. *Journal of Pure and Applied Algebra*, 26:71–83, 1982.

[117] J.R. Myhill. Some properties of intuitionistic Zermelo-Fraenkel set theory. In A.R.D. Mathias and H. Rogers, editors, *Cambridge Summer School in Mathematical Logic*, pages 206–231. Springer, 1973.

[118] J.R. Myhill. Constructive set theory. *Journal of Symbolic Logic*, 40:347–382, 1975.

[119] D. Nelson. Recursive functions and intuitionistic number theory. *Transactions of the American Mathematical Society*, 61:307–368,556, 1947.

[120] C.-H.L. Ong and E. Ritter. A generic strong normalization proof: application to the calculus of constructions. In *Computer Science Logic: 7th workshop, Swansea '93*, volume 832 of *LNCS*, pages 261–279. Springer, 1994.

[121] W. Phoa. Relative computability in the effective topos. *Mathematical Proceedings of the Cambridge Philosophical Society*, 106:419–422, 1989.

[122] W. Phoa. *Domain Theory in Realizability Toposes*. PhD thesis, Cambridge University, 1990.

[123] A.M. Pitts. *The Theory of Triposes*. PhD thesis, Cambridge University, 1981.

[124] A.M. Pitts. Comprehension without extensionality. Handwritten note, November 1983.

[125] A.M. Pitts. Tripos theory in retrospect. *Math. Struct. Comp. Science*, 12:265–279, 2002.

[126] G. Plotkin. LCF considered as a programming language. *Theor. Computer Science*, 5:223–255, 1977.

[127] M.B. Pour-El and J.Ian Richards. *Computability in Analysis and Physics*. Springer-Verlag, 1989.

[128] W. Powell. Extending Gödel's Negative Interpretation to ZF. *Journ.Symb.Logic*, 40(2):221–229, 1975.

[129] G.R. Renardel de Lavalette. Extended bar induction in applicative theories. *Annals of Pure and Applied Logic*, 50:139–189, 1990.

[130] B. Reus. Realizability Models for Type Theories. *Electronic Notes in Theoretical Computer Science*, 23(1):1–31, 1999.

[131] J. Reynolds. Polymorphism is not set-theoretic. In G. Kahn, D.B. MacQueen, and G.D. Plotkin, editors, *Semantics of Data Types*, volume 173 of *Lecture Notes in Computer Science*, pages 145–156. Springer, 1984.

[132] E.P. Robinson. How complete is PER? In A.R. Meyer, editor, *Proceedings of the 4th Annual IEEE Symposium on Logic in Computer Science*, pages 106–111, Asilomar, 1989. IEEE Computer Society Press.

[133] E.P. Robinson and G. Roslini. An abstract look at realizability. In *Proc. CSL 15*, volume 2142 of *LNCS*, pages 173–187. Springer, 2001.

[134] E.P. Robinson and G. Rosolini. Colimit completions and the effective topos. *Journal of Symbolic Logic*, 55:678–699, 1990.

[135] H. Rogers. *Theory of Recursive Functions and Effective Computability*. McGraw-Hill, 1967. (reprinted by MIT Press, Cambridge MA, 1987).

[136] G. Rosolini. *Continuity and Effectiveness in Topoi.* PhD thesis, University of Oxford, 1986.

[137] G. Rosolini. Categories and effective computations. In D.H. Pitt, A. Poigné, and D.E. Rydeheard, editors, *Category Theory and Computer Science*, volume 283 of *Lectures Notes in Computer Science*, pages 1–11, Edinburgh, 1987. Springer-Verlag.

[138] G. Rosolini. About modest sets. *International Journal of Foundations of Computer Science*, 1:341–353, 1990.

[139] G. Rosolini. An ExPer model for Quest. In S. Brookes, M. Main, A. Melton, M. Mislove, and D. Schmidt, editors, *MFPS'91*, volume 598 of *Lecture Notes in Computer Science*, pages 436–445. Springer, 1991.

[140] I. Rummelhoff. Polynat in PER models. *Theor. Comp. Sci.*, 316:215–224, 2004.

[141] A. Scedrov. Differential equations in constructive analysis and in the recursive realizability topos. *Journal of Pure and Applied Algebra*, 33:69–80, 1984.

[142] A. Scedrov. Intuitionistic set theory. In *Harvey Friedman's research on the foundations of mathematics*, number 117 in Studies in Logic, pages 257–284. North-Holland, 1985.

[143] M. Schönfinkel. Über die Bausteine der Mathematischen Logik. *Mathematische Annalen*, 92:305–316, 1924.

[144] D.S. Scott. Continuous lattices. In W. Lawvere, editor, *Toposes, Alebraic Geometry and Logic*, pages 97–136, Berlin, 1972. Springer (LNM 274).

[145] D.S. Scott. Lambda calculus and recursion theory. In S. Kanger, editor, *Proc. Third Scand. Log. Symp*, pages 154–193. North Holland, 1975.

[146] D.S. Scott. Data types as lattices. *SIAM Journal of Computing*, 5(3):522–587, 1976.

[147] D.S. Scott. Identity and existence in intuitionistic logic. In M. Fourman, C.J. Mulvey, and D.S. Scott, editors, *Applications of Sheaves*, pages 660–696, Berlin, 1979. Springer (LNM 753).

[148] D.S. Scott. A new category? Domains, spaces and equivalence relations. Manuscript, available at
`http://www.cs.cmu.edu/Groups/LTC/`, 1996.

[149] A. Simpson. Computational adequacy in an elementary topos. In *Computer Science Logic - Proceedings CSL '98*, pages 323–342, 1999.

[150] A. Simpson. Computational adequacy for recursive types in models of intuitionistic set theory. *Ann.Pure Appl. Logic*, 130:207–275, 2004.

[151] E.Z. Skvortsova. A faithful interpretation of the intuitonistic propositional calculus by means of an initial segment of the Medvedev lattice. *Sibirsk.Math.Zh.*, 29(1):171–178, 1988. (Russian).

[152] A. Sorbi. Some remarks on the structure of the Medvedev lattice. *Journal of Symbolic Logic*, 55(2):831–853, 1990.

[153] T. Streicher. Investigations into intensional type theory. Habilitationsschrift, Universität München, 1994.

[154] T. Streicher. A topos for computable analysis, 1997. Note of a talk presented at PSSL, May 1997 in Utrecht, Holland. Available electronially at www.mathematik.uni-darmstadt.de/ streicher.

[155] T. Streicher. Realizability models for czf+¬pow, 2005. Note of a talk presented at workshop, May 2006 in Utrecht, Holland. Available electronially at www.mathematik.uni-darmstadt.de/ streicher.

[156] P. Taylor. The fixed point property in synthetic domain theory. In *6th Symp. on Logic in Computer Science*, pages 152–160. IEEE Computer Society Press, 1991.

[157] P. Taylor. *Practical Foundations of Mathematics*, volume 59 of *Cambridge Studies in Advanced Mathematics*. Cambridge University Press, 1999.

[158] S. Terwijn. Constructive logic and the Medvedev lattice. *Notre Dame Journ. formal Logic*, 47(1):73–82, 2006.

[159] S. Terwijn. The Medvedev lattice of computably closed sets. *Arch. Math. Logic*, 45(2):179–190, 2006.

[160] A.S. Troelstra. Notions of realizability for intuitionistic arithmetic and intuitionistic arithmetic in all finite types. In J.E. Fenstad, editor, *The Second Scandinavian Logic Symposium*, pages 369–405. North-Holland, 1971.

[161] A.S. Troelstra, editor. *Metamathematical Investigation of Intuitionistic Arithmetic and Analysis*. Springer (Lecture Notes in Mathematics 344), 1973. With contributions by A.S. Troelstra, C.A. Smoryński, J.I. Zucker and W.A. Howard.

[162] A.S. Troelstra. A note on non–extensional operations in connection with continuity and recursiveness. *Indagationes Mathematicae*, 39:455–462, 1977.

[163] A.S. Troelstra and D. van Dalen. *Constructivism in Mathematics*. North-Holland, 1988. 2 volumes.

[164] B. van den Berg. *Predicative topos theory and models for constructive set theory*. PhD thesis, Utrecht University, 2006.

[165] J. van Oosten. Lifschitz' realizability. *Journal of Symbolic Logic*, 55:805–821, 1990.

[166] J. van Oosten. *Exercises in Realizability*. PhD thesis, Universiteit van Amsterdam, 1991.

[167] J. van Oosten. Extension of Lifschitz' realizability to higher order arithmetic, and a solution to a problem of F. Richman. *Journal of Symbolic Logic*, 56:964–973, 1991.

[168] J. van Oosten. A semantical proof of De Jongh's theorem. *Archive for Mathematical Logic*, pages 105–114, 1991.

[169] J. van Oosten. Axiomatizing higher-order Kleene realizability. *Annals of Pure and Applied Logic*, 70:87–111, 1994.

[170] J. van Oosten. Two remarks on the Lifschitz realizability topos. *Journal of Symbolic Logic*, 61:70–79, 1996.

[171] J. van Oosten. Extensional realizability. *Annals of Pure and Applied Logic*, 84:317–349, 1997.

[172] J. van Oosten. The modified realizability topos. *Journal of Pure and Applied Algebra*, 116:273–289, 1997.

[173] J. van Oosten. A combinatory algebra for sequential functionals of finite type. In S.B. Cooper and J.K. Truss, editors, *Models and Computability*, pages 389–406. Cambridge University Press, 1999.

[174] J. van Oosten and A.K. Simpson. Axioms and (counter)examples in synthetic domain theory. *Annals of Pure and Applied Logic*, 104:233–278, 2000.

[175] R.E. Vesley. A palatable substitute for Kripke's schema. In A. Kino, J.R. Myhill, and R.E. Vesley, editors, *Intuitionism and Proof Theory*, pages 197–207. North-Holland, 1970.

[176] S. Vickers. Locales and toposes as spaces. In M. Aiello, E. Pratt-Hartmann, and J. Van Benthem, editors, *Handbook of spatial logics*, 2007.

[177] K. Weihrauch. *Computable Analysis - an Introduction*. Springer Verlag, 2000. 285 pp.

[178] G. Wraith. Artin glueing. *Journal of Pure and Applied Algebra*, 4:345–348, 1974.

Index